Changing Welfare Services
Case Studies of Local Welfare Reform Programs

Changing Welfare Services
Case Studies of Local Welfare Reform Programs

Michael J. Austin, PhD
Editor

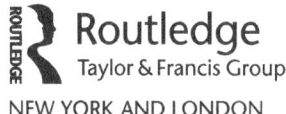
Routledge
Taylor & Francis Group
NEW YORK AND LONDON

First published 2004 by The Haworth Press, Inc.

This edition published 2012 by Routledge
605 Third Avenue, New York, NY 10017
2 Park Square, Milton Park, Abingdon, Oxon OX14 4RN

Routledge is an imprint of the Taylor & Francis Group, an informa business

Copyright © 2004 by Taylor & Francis.

All rights reserved. No part of this book may be reprinted or reproduced or utilised in any form or by any electronic, mechanical, or other means, now known or hereafter invented, including photocopying and recording, or in any information storage or retrieval system, without permission in writing from the publishers.

Notice:
Product or corporate names may be trademarks or registered trademarks and are used only for identification and explanation without intent to infringe.

ISBN 13: 978-0-7890-2314-8 (pbk)

PUBLISHER'S NOTE
Identities and circumstances of individuals discussed in this book have been changed to protect confidentiality.

Cover design by Lora Wiggins.

Library of Congress Cataloging-in-Publication Data

Changing welfare services : case studies of local welfare reform programs / Michael J. Austin, editor.
    p. cm.
  Includes bibliographical references and index.
  ISBN 0-7890-2313-X (case : alk. paper)—ISBN 0-7890-2314-8 (pbk. : alk. paper)
    1. Public welfare—United States—Case studies. 2. Welfare recipients—Employment—United States—Case studies. 3. Public welfare administration—United States—Case studies. I. Austin, Michael J.

HV95.C415 2004
361.6'8'0973—dc22
                                                    2003021004

CONTENTS

Foreword   xi
    Maureen Borland

Acknowledgments   xv

Introduction   xvii
    Michael J. Austin

SECTION I:
AN OVERVIEW OF WELFARE REFORM IMPLEMENTATION AND PRACTICE

Chapter 1. Implementing Welfare Reform and Guiding Organizational Change   3
    Sarah Carnochan
    Michael J. Austin

Chapter 2. Overview of Innovative Programs and Practices   27
    Jonathan Prince
    Michael J. Austin

SECTION II:
REDEFINING SERVICE DELIVERY

REMOVING BARRIERS TO WORKFORCE PARTICIPATION

Chapter 3. Connections Shuttle: Transportation for CalWORKs Participants   53
    Debbie Downes
    Michael J. Austin

Chapter 4. The Guaranteed Ride Home Program: Transportation Services for Welfare-to-Work Participants   65
    Christine M. Schmidt
    Michael J. Austin

Chapter 5. Training Exempt Providers to Deliver High-Quality
   Child Care Programs   77
      Jonathan Prince
      Michael J. Austin

Chapter 6. Integrating Mental Health and Substance Abuse
   Services into a County Welfare-to-Work Program   91
      Christine M. Schmidt
      Michael J. Austin

SELF-SUFFICIENCY SUPPORT SERVICES

Chapter 7. Combining Business with Rehabilitation
   in a Public Work Center for Disabled
   and Low-Income Participants   103
      Jonathan Prince
      Michael J. Austin

Chapter 8. The Family Loan Program
   As a Public-Private Partnership   117
      Susan E. Doyle
      Michael J. Austin

Chapter 9. The Adopt-A-Family Program: Building
   Networks of Support   131
      Susan E. Doyle
      Michael J. Austin

Chapter 10. Utilizing Hotline Services to Sustain
   Employment   143
      Christine M. Schmidt
      Michael J. Austin

Chapter 11. Hiring TANF Participants to Work
   in a County Human Services Agency   153
      Kirsten A. Deichert
      Michael J. Austin

Chapter 12. Promoting Self-Sufficiency Through
Individual Development Accounts (IDAs)   165
    Judie Svihula
    Michael J. Austin

SECTION III:
ENHANCING COMMUNITY PARTNERSHIPS

NEIGHBORHOOD PARTNERSHIPS

Chapter 13. Fostering Neighborhood Involvement
in Workforce Development: The Alameda County
Neighborhood Jobs Pilot Initiative   189
    Judie Svihula
    Michael J. Austin

Chapter 14. Neighborhood Self-Sufficiency Centers   217
    Christine M. Schmidt
    Michael J. Austin

COMMUNITY-WIDE PARTNERSHIPS

Chapter 15. A Community Partnership Approach
to Serving the Homeless   231
    Margaret K. Libby
    Michael J. Austin

Chapter 16. Wraparound Services for Homeless TANF
Families Recovering from Substance Abuse   251
    Debbie Downes
    Michael J. Austin

Chapter 17. Building a Coalition of Nonprofit Agencies
to Collaborate with a County Health and Human
Services Agency   267
    Margaret K. Libby
    Michael J. Austin

Chapter 18. Collaborative Partnerships Between a Human
  Services Agency and Local Community Colleges   285
  Kirsten A. Deichert
  Michael J. Austin

SECTION IV:
PROMOTING AGENCY RESTRUCTURING

Chapter 19. Introducing Organizational Development
  (OD) Practices into a County Human Service Agency   297
  Andrea DuBrow
  Donna Wocher
  Michael J. Austin

Chapter 20. Preparing Human Service Workers
  to Implement Welfare Reform: Establishing the Family
  Development Credential in a Human Services Agency   317
  Judie Svihula
  Michael J. Austin

Chapter 21. Merging a Workforce Investment Board
  and a Department of Social Services into a County
  Department of Employment and Human Services   339
  Jonathan Prince
  Michael J. Austin

Chapter 22. Blending Multiple Funding Streams
  into County Welfare-to-Work Programs   353
  Christine M. Schmidt
  Michael J. Austin

Chapter 23. Crossover Services Between Child Welfare
  and Welfare-to-Work Programs   363
  Jonathan Prince
  Michael J. Austin

SECTION V:
CONCLUSION AND FUTURE CONSIDERATIONS

Chapter 24. Managing Out: The Community Practice
   Dimensions of Effective Agency Management   379
      Michael J. Austin

Index   395

ABOUT THE EDITOR

Michael J. Austin, PhD, is Professor of Management and Planning at the School of Social Welfare at the University of California in Berkeley and former Dean of the School of Social Work at the University of Pennsylvania in Philadelphia. His teaching and research are in the areas of client-centered agency management, strategic planning, community organizing, and policy implementation in both the public social services and nonprofit Jewish communal organizations. Since 1992, Dr. Austin has served as Staff Director of the Bay Area Social Services Consortium (BASSC), a university-agency-foundation collaborative whose activities include an applied research program, an executive development program, and a policy analysis/implementation program.

Dr. Austin has authored and edited numerous books, articles, and reports in the area of human service administration, including *Management Simulations for Mental Health and Human Services Administration* and *Human Services Integration*. He serves on the editorial boards of seven journals and is Associate Editor of *Administration in Social Work*. For over thirty years he has served as a consultant to a variety of nonprofit communal organizations related to strategic planning, program evaluation, and organizational development and restructuring. Over the past decade he has facilitated the development of strategic plans for ten nonprofit organizations in California, New York, and New Jersey.

Foreword

This volume of promising practices that emerged out of the implementation of welfare reform arrives at an opportune time. We have just completed the first seven years of implementation and continue to await the federal reauthorization of the 1996 Personal Responsibility and Work Opportunity Reconciliation Act. Our efforts in California to promote welfare reform are embedded in the state legislation known as CalWORKs. The challenges that we all faced as county social service directors in 1996 were staggering. For the first time in the sixty-one years of federal legislation authorizing public social services (dating back to the 1935 Social Security Act), we had the freedom and financial capacities to develop local strategies to address the varying needs of our local welfare populations.

Although many of the case studies described in this book took place in my county, they reflect a broad spectrum of experience throughout the counties that make up the Bay Area in northern California. The cases grew out of an interest among county social service directors to describe some of the innovative aspects of our work to share with other counties. Given the rapid pace of change experienced by those hardworking staff members implementing welfare reform, it was clear that they would not have the time or perspective to describe their own innovative work. As a result, the directors who compose the Bay Area Social Services Consortium, along with university and foundation representatives, decided that they should invest in the development of case studies to share with others. This book details the first round of promising practices that were supported, in large part, by the federal incentive funds used to encourage caseload reductions as part of the welfare reform legislation. Many of the cases reflect the early experiences of staff seeking to provide specialized services to those moving from welfare to work, and it will take many more years to adequately document the specific outcomes for TANF (Temporary Assistance to Needy Families) participants. In the meantime, it is clear that the practices described in this book are truly promising, even if they are not yet ready to serve as evidence-based benchmarks for best practices.

It is difficult to capture the full range of experiences and emotions that surrounded the early years of welfare reform implementation. For some of us, the new legislation represented an unusual opportunity to shift from a very bureaucratic system of eligibility determination to a more community-focused system of employability. We recognized early on that the process of reducing the welfare rolls would not necessarily result in reducing poverty in the United States. Many of us worried that we might only be changing the labels from "welfare recipient" to "working poor." Others of us worried about the authorizing legislation itself, as it represented the first time in our country's history that we had passed legislation which required poor women to work but did not establish an entitlement to the child care necessary for many of them to do so. We also worried about the impact of welfare reform on the well-being of children. Would children be helped or hindered when their mothers were working outside the home?

Despite all these reservations, we proceeded to open up our organizations to new ways of thinking and doing, sought broad-based community involvement, and began experimenting with new approaches to support services. Many of the examples of this innovative process are found in this book.

Since the passage of the welfare reform legislation, we have all been in a learning mode. The following are some of the lessons we learned as county social services directors:

- Partnerships with community service providers are essential for the rapid deployment of new services requiring local expertise and cultural competence.
- Despite our service innovations related to fostering employment, we are still in the eligibility business, with increasing roles related to Medicaid and Food Stamp outreach and eligibility, often as unfunded workloads.
- Integrating welfare, employment services, and child welfare services is a classic service-integration challenge, whether done inside the agency at the line-worker level, outside the agency at the neighborhood level, or departmentally at the county level.
- The challenges facing the "hard-to-employ" TANF participants are testing all of us with respect to finding the appropriate array of supports needed to help participants move from welfare to work and sustain their self-sufficiency.
- The focus on service delivery has now expanded to include service outcomes. The lack of capacities of our information systems to meet the challenge of providing accurate and useful data for decision making is evident.
- Although a high level of media coverage and policy interest surrounded the launch of welfare reform, it is not clear that this interest

- can be sustained during the difficult years of economic instability and program maturity.
- Although much has been accomplished, relationships inside and outside the social service agency continue to be unstable due to limited resources (many states are operating in 2004 with significant deficits), the financial precariousness of some nonprofit service providers in the community, and the overwhelming challenges facing the hard to employ.

It is not yet clear how the reauthorization of welfare reform will play itself out at the local level. What is clear is that the traditional role of public social services will continue to change, especially when TANF participants who have either been sanctioned or timed out face the prospect of devastating poverty. Recognition is growing that the future of public social services will increasingly involve specialized services to low-income working families regardless of prior involvement with TANF programs. These services may include the promotion of safety net measures such as EITC (Earned Income Tax Credit), Child Care Tax Credit, Medicaid eligibility, Food Stamps eligibility, and the promotion of neighborhood supports in the form of housing, child care, and transportation assistance.

Although the future is uncertain, the recent past is clear. Local social service agencies can demonstrate the necessary creativity, responsiveness, and collaborative spirit needed to find new ways to serve the needs of low-income residents. This volume documents this creativity and provides a welcome addition to all the national quantitative studies of the welfare population. The rich qualitative descriptions of the case studies in this book are needed to capture the totality of the welfare reform implementation experience. Without a doubt, more promising practices are being developed and hopefully will be reported on in subsequent volumes like this one.

On behalf of the members of the Bay Area Social Services Consortium, we applaud the work of our staff director, Mike Austin (who is also Professor of Management and Planning at the School of Social Welfare, University of California, Berkeley), and his very able group of graduate students who helped develop the chapters in this book. Rarely do we as practicing administrators see the work of our staff members so closely and thoroughly documented and reported. I appreciate the opportunity to contribute to this volume.

Maureen Borland, Director
Human Services Agency
San Mateo County, California

Acknowledgments

Many individuals deserve credit for this publication. First, the dedicated and hardworking staff members in county social service agencies and nonprofit community-based organizations deserve much of the credit for the promising programs and practices described in the case studies. They are so busy being creative and innovative that they rarely have the time to reflect in writing on their practice. Second, the dynamic and visionary directors of county social service agencies in the San Francisco Bay Area deserve considerable credit for designing and/or facilitating the implementation of these promising practices and programs. Third, these case studies would not have seen the light of day without the dedication and curiosity of the graduate research assistants at the University of California School of Social Welfare. They included a very talented group of doctoral students (Sarah Carnochan, Jonathan Prince, and Judie Svihula) and master's students (Kirsten Deichert, Debbie Downes, Susan E. Doyle, Andrea DuBrow, Margaret K. Libby, and Christine M. Schmidt). Fourth, the financial support of the Bay Area Social Services Consortium, The Zellerbach Family Foundation, and the VanLobenSels/RembeRock Foundation made it possible for me to pull all this creativity together into one publication. Finally, without the patience and good cheer of my loyal and able administrative assistant, Sharon Ikami, I could have never completed this complex project.

I assume full responsibility for any errors that may be found in this effort to capture the dynamic and ever-changing environment of welfare reform implementation.

Introduction

Michael J. Austin

While most of the attention during the first eight years of welfare reform (1996-2003) in the United States has focused on reduced caseloads and a growing economy, little attention has been given to the organizational changes in local social service delivery (Hagen and Owens-Manley, 2002; Lurie, 2001; Meyers, Glasser, and MacDonald, 1998). As Gais and colleagues (2001) have noted in their assessment of early years of welfare reform implementation, "we see a broader movement toward complex combinations of diverse institutions drawn from both the public and private sector" (p. 43). This diversity is reflected in this collection of case studies on promising practices and programs emerging at the local level from the implementation of welfare reform.

THE IMPACT OF WELFARE REFORM

Welfare reform in the United States (the Personal Responsibility and Work Opportunity Reconciliation Act [PRWORA] of 1996) and the various state legislative acts passed in the wake of the federal legislation have had a profound impact on the mission and structure of social service agencies at the state and local levels. The legislation focuses on moving former recipients from welfare to work with policies to address barriers to work as well as opportunities to sustain employability. Former *recipients* of the income maintenance program (Aid to Families with Dependent Children [AFDC]) became *participants* in the program of Temporary Assistance to Needy Families (TANF) which promoted publicly funded workforce development services, often in collaboration with community-based nonprofit organizations. All of this change was implemented in a policy environment of time-limited benefits and sanctions for noncompliance.

As Glazer (2002) noted, the major federal 1996 TANF provisions included the following:

- The individual entitlement to cash benefits provided by AFDC was repealed and replaced by a system of mutual responsibilities in which cash benefits are conditioned on attempts to prepare for self-support.
- The funding mechanism of open-ended federal payments for every person added to the welfare rolls by states was replaced by a block grant with a fixed amount of funding for each state for six years and more discretion than under AFDC to spend funds for purposes other than cash assistance (transportation, wage subsidies, pregnancy prevention, and family formation).
- States were required to place an escalating percentage of their caseload in work programs.
- Financial sanctions were placed both on states and individuals who fail to meet the work standards. In the case of individuals, states must reduce the cash benefit and sometimes the Food Stamp benefit of adults who fail to meet the work requirements designed by the states. Similarly, the federal government will reduce the block grant of states that fail to meet the percentage work requirement. This requirement stipulates that states must have 50 percent of their caseload involved in work programs for a minimum of thirty hours per week by 2002.
- States are generally not allowed to use federal dollars to pay the benefits of families who have been on welfare for more than five years.

Based on these federal policy mandates and the policy guidelines noted in Box I.1 (Weil and Finegold, 2002), state and local governments began to transform their delivery of welfare services. For state-administered welfare services, state human service agencies took the lead, while for county-administered services, county social service agencies took the lead.

The welfare services can be viewed in three different but overlapping ways (Seefeldt, 2002). First, many state and local governments adopted the *work-first* service philosophy that encourages TANF program participants to find employment quickly and, if needed, to acquire job-readiness skills (interviewing, résumé writing, money management, parenting, time management, job searching, etc.). With a job, participants are then encouraged to advance themselves by assuming increased job responsibilities as well as seeking additional training and education. The second change in service delivery involved the staff and changing the culture of the welfare agency from a preoccupation with work activities related to eligibility and benefits to the increasing importance of support services related to employability. In some agencies, this transition to *case management* involved working intensively with TANF participants (counseling) to assist them in finding work or de-

BOX I.1. Key Provisions of the Personal Responsibility and Work Opportunity Reconciliation Act of 1996 (PRWORA)

Temporary Assistance for Needy Families (TANF)

Purposes: Increase state flexibility; keep children in own homes or homes of other relatives; end parental dependence on government benefits by promoting job preparation, work, and marriage; discourage pregnancies outside of marriage; encourage formation and maintenance of two-parent families.

Block grant: Replaced Aid to Families with Dependent Children entitlement with TANF block grant. Allocation to states based primarily on historic spending levels.

Time limits: Federal lifetime limit of sixty months on cash assistance. Period of time may be shorter at state option. States may exempt up to 20 percent of recipients and may continue benefits beyond federal time limits with own funds.

Work requirements: Recipients required to work after two years of case assistance. States must meet targets for percentage of cases in work activities or face financial penalties.

Family cap: States may deny additional benefits when children are born to families already receiving cash assistance.

Immigrants

Restricted eligibility of noncitizen immigrants for Supplemental Security Income (SSI) and Food Stamps.
States may restrict eligibility of noncitizen immigrants for TANF and Medicaid.

Child Care

Consolidated four existing programs into Child Care and Development Fund (CCDF) block grants.
Eliminated entitlements for child care for current/former welfare recipients.
Allowed states to transfer TANF funds into CCDF or spend directly for child care.
Increased CCDF funding levels.

Medicaid

Delinked Medicaid eligibility from welfare.
Froze state eligibility standards as of the date the law was enacted.
States may cover all members of a family using a single, higher income eligibility standard.

(continued)

> *(continued)*
>
> **Child Support**
>
> States required to strengthen child support enforcement.
> Eliminated requirements that states disregard first fifty dollars of monthly child support in calculating TANF eligibility and benefits.
>
> **Food Stamps**
>
> Reduced maximum benefit and limited deductions.
> Able-bodied adults without dependents are limited to three months of benefits if not working at least twenty hours per week.
>
> **Supplemental Security Income**
>
> Narrowed standards for disability for children.
> Increased frequency of review of disability status for children and adults.

veloping a plan to prepare for work (including the identification of services related to domestic violence, substance abuse, mental health, health and nutrition, etc.). The third change in service delivery involved the increased involvement of *nonprofit, community-based organizations* to provide support services (education and training, child care, transportation, mental health and substance abuse, etc.). In only a few locales around the country nonprofits also assumed responsibility for eligibility determination and benefits administration. In addition, in some locales, for-profit organizations have also been involved in delivery services to TANF participants.

From the perspective of the public social service agency, the changes have been most apparent in the mission of the agency as it transformed its income maintenance programs from client eligibility determination to client employability enhancement. This change required extensive organizational restructuring, cultural change, and staff training (Hagen, 1999). At the same time, county social service agencies began to actively promote more community outreach and collaboration. These efforts led to promising programs and practices in the areas of service delivery, community partnerships, and organizational change.

Social service agencies are in transition from operating as public bureaucracies preoccupied with accounting for taxpayer funds to functioning as community-building institutions which provide leadership in partnership with others (see Chapter 1 Appendix; Carnochan and Austin, 2002). The organizational changes involve the agency's mission, location of services, and the role of staff as highlighted in the following list.

1. Welfare reform required a new operating philosophy and mission. The philosophy includes a social development approach to investing in community resource development in order to develop a career-resilient workforce able to move permanently from welfare to work and self-sufficiency. For example, new ways for social service agencies to invest in human capital development include helping the low-wage working poor learn new skills through specially developed community college programs or learning how to save by using individual development accounts. Modifying the mission statement also required confronting the tensions built into the welfare reform legislation where county social service agencies, as well as community nonprofits, struggled to deal with the short-term goals of reducing welfare caseloads and the long-term goals of preparing low-income program participants for self-sufficiency. Many feared that the legislation would simply relabel low-income welfare recipients with the term *working poor* and not substantially add to the resources or capabilities of the least advantaged in our society.
2. Welfare reform required an expanded agency mission that creates a public forum and consciousness about promoting a civil society and open dialogue about future public policy directions. This change requires the social service agency to serve as a catalyst for private action to ensure that communities address the needs of their most disadvantaged members; for example, welfare reform in California (the federal TANF program is known as CalWORKs) called for community-wide meetings and needs assessment strategies to document and address local needs, where much debate took place.
3. There needed to be a shift from a preoccupation with the individual to a focus on the family and neighborhood in the form of neighborhood-based family support services. For example, efforts were renewed to explore ways to decentralize governmental services into neighborhood offices, often colocated with other nonprofit service providers, with renewed attention to such family support services as child care, transportation, and the promotion of affordable housing.
4. The transformation of the social service agency included changing roles for agency staff in order to acquire more community-building knowledge and skills (outreach, interagency collaboration, local economic development) as well as to transform public social service agencies into learning organizations (new information systems, teamwork, intra-agency coordination). For example, the increased flexibility in the use of federal and state funding has allowed local county social service agencies to develop new services, including those with

nonprofit organizations, that more effectively meet the needs of the working poor and help to build community.

As these changes in agency vision and mission were unfolding, large-scale national research projects were launched, generating new and important findings.

RESEARCH ON WELFARE REFORM

Although there is no attempt here to capture the volumes of research on welfare reform that have been flowing out of national research centers since the passage of the 1996 legislation, it is important to provide an overview of the major questions and selected findings. The major questions can be categorized into the following three areas: (1) population, (2) public policies, and (3) service programs. Of course, research takes place within society's political, social, and economic environment. As a result, many argue that the preliminary results of welfare reform studies are greatly influenced by the booming American economy of the 1990s. It is too early to tell whether the economic slowdown of 2000-2003 will return the *working poor* to the age-old prophecy of "last hired, first fired."

Population

With respect to the welfare population, the vast majority of TANF recipients are single-parent families composed of women and children. For this population, the major questions seem to focus on those who (1) left welfare and never returned, (2) left and returned, and (3) never left and are exhausting their five-year time limit. A sampling of the findings of the Urban Institute's National Survey of America's Families (Loprest, 2002) provides the following preliminary picture of the impact of welfare reform on poor families:

- Many TANF participants have found work; about 50 percent of those who left welfare between 1997 and 1999 were employed in 1999, predominantly in low-wage, service-sector jobs, with only one-third receiving health benefits or paid sick leave.
- Food Stamps and Medicaid benefits are greatly underutilized by former TANF recipients.
- About 25 percent of former TANF participants who lost their jobs between 1997 and 1999 returned to TANF in 1999.

- Among 40 percent of the long-term TANF participants in 1999, the barriers to work included two or more of the following factors:
  1. poor physical or mental health,
  2. less than high school education,
  3. child under the age of one,
  4. disabled child on SSI,
  5. low English proficiency, or
  6. lack of work experience.
- Some TANF participants (12 percent in 1999) were off welfare but not working (living with others or homeless).

One of the most significant findings from research on poor families over the past decade has been their capacities to survive through involvement in the informal economy of intermittent work (baby-sitting, laundry work, waitress work, piecework, etc.) as a supplement to public assistance (Edin and Lein, 1997). In addition, the Urban Institute study (Zedlewski, 2002) found that half the families in the bottom quintile continued to receive Food Stamps and health care coverage under Medicaid. The study noted that although the official measures of poverty based on pretax cash income declined between 1996 and 1998, measures of disposable income showed that the percentage of people living in extreme poverty did not change and the number of independent single families living in extreme poverty slightly increased.

Other questions also exist about the population on welfare. Are immigrants and other racial/ethnic groups affected differently, and if so, how? How has welfare reform fostered marriage and/or two-parent families? How has childbearing been affected? What has been the impact on children in TANF households with respect to child care, child support, school success, and delinquency rates? These questions simply demonstrate the complexity of evaluating such a comprehensive piece of federal legislation that is being implemented through a diversity of state and local programs.

Public Policy

The second area of research relates to evaluating the impact of public policy (the Personal Responsibility and Work Opportunity Reconciliation Act of 1996). The two most controversial aspects of the welfare reform legislation are sanctions for not complying and time limits to receiving benefits. The sanctioning process varies by state, as each decided on its own approach to sanctioning and ways of determining compliance. Similarly, states are only now beginning to determine who has exhausted the five-year time limit for the receipt of TANF benefits. So the obvious research questions relate to who has been sanctioned, for what reasons, and what has been the impact of the sanctions? With respect to time limits, more time will need to pass in order to get answers to such questions as who exhausted their time limits, what were the reasons, and how did they cope without their TANF benefits? According to Pavetti and Bloom (2001), sanctions are influencing the behavior of many TANF participants, but many have not responded to the loss of all their cash assistance (full-family sanction). Although the evidence is mixed with regard to the ways in which time limits affect the behaviors of recipients, Pavetti and Bloom (2001) note that implementation studies have found that the presence of a time limit can (1) create a sense of urgency for staff and managers, (2) push programs to work harder to identify long-hidden barriers facing their clients, and (3) stimulate creative strategies for helping recipients address such issues.

Other policy research areas include the impact of the *work-first* policy, the nature and extent of the maintenance of financial effort by the states (contributing 75 percent or more to their TANF program of what they were contributing to AFDC in 1994), and the impact of the 2002 federal reauthorization legislation. As with the population research, the policy implementation research takes years to allow enough time for the impact to unfold and the data to be collected.

Service Programs

The third area of welfare reform research relates to program implementation. The research issues in this area include (1) the depth and breadth of welfare-to-work services offered by state or local governments, (2) the nature of barriers to employing TANF participants and how these barriers are addressed, (3) the breadth and depth of work supports (transportation, child care, health care, affordable housing, etc.), (4) the role of staff in acquiring the skills and experience in delivering effective services related to welfare reform, and (5) the extent to which TANF participants understand the new system of welfare reform and fully utilize available services. For example, Cherlin (2000) found that although TANF participants understood the concept of time limits, there was considerable uncertainty about the details of time limits and related policies. Similarly, Gais and colleagues (2001) found states expanded the array of services as a result of the welfare reform legislation to include pregnancy prevention, mental health services, substance abuse services, and child care services.

Research on service implementation is further compounded by the complexity of administrative structures and processes. As Gais and colleagues (2001) point out, the complexity is related to (1) the need for sophisticated information systems to account for the multiple contacts with TANF participants over time; (2) blending the TANF work-first service philosophy with the old AFDC eligibility systems; (3) new multiservice system approaches involving many more service providers, increased attention to service coordination, and expanded contract monitoring activities; and (4) significant transfers of administrative control from states to intricate local coalitions of public and private institutions.

However, when it comes to the staff members who have carried the burden of welfare reform implementation, very little research has been done. As Hagen (1999) accurately predicted,

> The flexibility allowed under TANF combined with the federal work requirements and time-limited benefits may serve as an impetus for major organizational and service delivery changes in public welfare agencies at both the state and local levels. However, changing the organizational culture of welfare agencies is extremely difficult and intra-organizational leadership and management may well be key variables in bringing it about. (p. 85)

In summary, it is important to note that the three sets of research questions related to population, public policy, and service programs focus primarily on the reduction of the welfare rolls and not necessarily on the reduction of poverty. In most of the preliminary findings, the rolls have been reduced but not the incidence of poverty. Some have argued that we have simply changed the labels from welfare recipient to working poor; yet there appears to be more emerging public and political support for supporting the needs of the working poor to get out of poverty than there ever was for the long-term support of welfare recipients. It will take generations of research to determine whether the costs of keeping mothers of young children at home are less than promoting work first with child care and other supports to keep mothers working. Numerous child development and parenting issues are buried under the surface, and the impact of welfare reform on children is only beginning to receive research attention (Duncan and Chase-Landsale, 2001).

FROM POLICY DEVOLUTION TO COMMUNITY BUILDING

In the context of devolving the implementation of welfare reform policy from the federal level down to state and local governments, the previous research questions place more attention on the impact of public policy than on the service delivery dimensions of community building and networking. The emphasis is more on reducing dependency and costs than on expanding the social capital (safety net) and human capital (education and training) of those trapped in the low-income sector of our American communities.

With the growing shift to multiyear contracting with community-based organizations, public social service agencies are viewing themselves increasingly as one agency among many in a community (i.e., not the old dominating public bureaucracy). The contracting process appears to be increasingly directed toward providing needed services through nonprofits as well as strengthening the infrastructure of community-based organizations. The goal of the contracting relationship then becomes service provision *and* community building (Austin, 2003).

Weil (1996) defines community building as activities, practices, and policies that support and foster positive connections among individuals, groups, organizations, neighborhoods, and geographic and functional communities. This process definition suggests, for example, that county social service agencies need to orient their programs and operating style to make community partnerships central to their service-delivery agenda. Kingsley, McNeely, and Gibson (1997) use community-building concepts of shared values, planning, and networking. For example, strengthening the public-private partnership involves the reinforcement of shared values whereby trust building and interagency networking (building social capital) are complemented by staff learning new ways to communicate and collaborate over time (building human capital). In addition, the partnership needs to reflect sufficiently broad participation by staff in both agencies (public and nonprofit) to foster a high level of ownership and self-reliance.

Multiple examples of community building are reflected in this collection of case studies. For example, when it comes to removing barriers to workforce participation, county social service agencies have contracted with nonprofits to provide transportation services for TANF participants as well as to train them as drivers for future jobs in transit systems. In other situations, contracted services with nonprofits were based on colocating nonprofit mental health services with the public TANF services to create one-stop neighborhood-based service centers. In another example, community building involved the collaboration of three public agencies (social services, mental health, and public housing) with a community nonprofit to create wraparound family services for formerly addicted TANF mothers and their children in housing on a former army base. Community building can also be found in the establishment of new organizational partnerships, such as those between public social service agencies and local community colleges for TANF job training, as well as coalitions of nonprofit service providers supported by public social service agencies.

OVERVIEW OF BOOK

The cases in this book grew out of the interests and leadership of local county public welfare directors who have been working collaboratively since 1987 as part of the twelve-county Bay Area Social Services Consortium (BASSC) in northern California (Austin et al., 1999). This innovative partnership between universities, county social service agencies, and local foundations has developed an extensive research program, an executive development program, and a policy development and implementation program. The consortium is guided by a multicounty vision statement that is highlighted in Box I.2 and described in the Appendix of Chapter 1.

Preceding the cases are two chapters that set the stage. Chapter 1 captures the early experiences of county social service directors as they launched the welfare reform implementation process. It features the lessons learned and provides insights into the leadership challenges. Chapter 2 provides an overview of the cases as well as a cross-case comparison. The comparison demonstrates how welfare reform policy and funding helped to increase the social capital needed to provide a new safety net for the poor. It also reflects a decrease in the traditional emphasis on job training or human capital development in favor of work first. Chapter 3 begins the series of case studies that feature services, partnerships, and agency restructuring.

The topics for the cases were identified by the agency directors as reflecting the most promising programs and practices emerging out of welfare reform implementation in the San Francisco Bay Area. The cases are separated into the following three sections:

1. *Redefining service delivery:* This set of cases captures two dimensions of service delivery redesign. The first focuses on the removal of barriers to workforce participation and features cases in the area of transportation (relating to work and child care), child care services (preparing TANF recipients and other low-income women for jobs in child care), and colocated services (increasing access to multiple services). The second dimension illustrates the nature of self-sufficiency support services. This set of cases features sheltered workshops for skill enhancement, loan programs for work-related expenses, support networks between families, hotlines to promote job retention, employment of TANF participants in social service agencies, and a savings account program for the working poor.
2. *Enhancing community partnerships:* This set of cases includes two approaches to partnerships between and among community-based nonprofit organizations and county social service agencies. The neigh-

borhood partnerships reflect the initiatives of urban counties as they decentralize job readiness and support services into local neighborhoods. One case focuses on outreach and job readiness while the other emphasizes assistance to those already employed and seeking to retain their jobs and acquire additional education. The cases on community partnerships focus on interagency collaboration for special populations as well as increased service coordination.

3. *Promoting agency restructuring:* The last set of cases captures multiple approaches to the restructuring of county social service agencies to better serve the community and the TANF population. Three of the cases are related to significant agency restructuring. One focuses on the merging of a social service agency and a workforce investment agency (formerly known as employment services or private industry councils drawing upon federal funding from the Department of Labor). Another case introduces high-level organizational development strategies and personnel to assist with significant organizational change processes (dealing with staff communications, resistance, and empowerment). A third case involves the extensive redesign of staff development programming by introducing a foundation curriculum for all staff engaged in client contact. Other aspects of agency restructuring can be found in cases that feature (1) the blending of multiple funding streams to provide greater responsiveness to changing community needs and (2) crossover services in which TANF services are linked to child welfare services to foster increased service coordination.

The final chapter features a discussion of the expanded set of managerial skills displayed by those in the leadership roles in many of the cases. The promising practices and programs emerging from the implementation of welfare reform resulted, in large part, from the leadership capacities of staff members at all levels of public and nonprofit agencies.

IMPLICATIONS AND LESSONS LEARNED

In conclusion, it is important to highlight some of the implications of this collection of case studies. Although several implications for service delivery, partnerships, and agency restructuring are described in Chapter 2, the focus here is on the implications for research, organizational change, and leadership.

BOX I.2. Supporting Low-Income Workers in the Twenty-First Century: An Evolving Vision Statement

Agency Philosophy

Social Service Agencies As Catalysts for Private Action: Social service agencies should develop their role as catalysts for change, in order to expand the social economy and to ensure that communities do not abandon the most needy families.

Building Community and Fostering a Civil Society: Social service agencies in a civil society need to work in multiple partnerships with the nonprofit and for-profit sectors as catalysts for change by mobilizing resources and building infrastructures in order to create healthy families and communities.

Agency Mission

Social Development Approach: Social service agencies guided by a social development approach focus on enhancing the capacity of the needy to participate in the economy, through an investment approach targeting communities and individuals.

Developing a Career-Resilient Workforce: Social service agencies have an important role to play in supporting workers and employers to ensure that skill development keeps pace with the rapidly changing economy.

Supporting the Family: Social service agencies must seek to help working families to move out of poverty, through a family-centered investment policy providing support for child care, transportation, housing, and health care.

Family-Focused, Neighborhood-Based Human Service Systems: Human service systems should be based on values of social inclusiveness, community development, and social investment.

Public Policy Directions: The unfinished business of welfare reform will require new, more targeted public policies (e.g., earned income tax credit, child or family allowances, and asset development or micro-investment programs) to increase the income and assets of low-income families and address the inequities of the private market for those who are working to support their families.

Agency Culture of Learning

Changing Staff Roles: In order to support workforce development and empower families, agency staff must assume new responsibilities, including assessment, counseling and referral, advocacy, program development, and social activism focused on employment, and must understand clients' work-related values and skills.

Source: Developed by members of the Bay Area Social Services Consortium in northern California in June 1999 in response to welfare reform and changing public attitudes about the role of government.

Implications for Future Research and Organizational Change

As is the case with most qualitative research that uses the case study method, more cases are needed from throughout the country in order to gain more confidence in generalizing from the experiences captured in this collection of cases. In particular, follow-up research is needed to assess the sustainability and institutionalization of the programs and practices described in these cases. Which programs expanded and in what directions? Which programs failed to sustain themselves and why? Which programs were so successful that they were incorporated into ongoing operations and no longer appear as distinct or separate entities? What are the crosscutting factors that explain expansion, contraction, incorporation, and demise?

With respect to organizational change, it is useful to identify the skills and values needed to foster and sustain change in agency operations. One factor that has emerged as critical in implementing welfare reform is agency leadership. Kotter (1990) makes an important distinction between leading and managing; leading involves coping with change (setting directions, aligning people, and motivating/inspiring others), while managing includes coping with complexity (planning and budgeting, organizing and staffing, and evaluating and problem solving). As noted in Chapter 1, the leadership activities of the county social service directors included *setting directions* for implementing welfare reform such as active outreach to the business community and statewide lobbying to influence legislative policy development. In addition to direction setting, the agency directors sought to *align various groups* such as supporting community planning forums, promoting the development of coalitions of nonprofits, engaging advocacy groups, and reaching out to provider agencies. The heavy emphasis on *motivation and inspiration* can be seen internally, as staff were empowered to develop new approaches to service delivery, and externally, as financial and human resources were made accessible to the community to develop shared ownership in reforming welfare. At the same time, agency directors were heavily involved in helping staff *manage the complexity* of implementing the new welfare reform legislation by reallocating resources, retraining staff, and upgrading information systems.

Welfare reform implementation represents one of the major events in the history of human service delivery, and it required immense leadership at the local level, paralleling the enormity of local-level implementation of the 1960s federal War on Poverty. One of the skill sets to emerge from implementing welfare reform is the complex process of "managing out." The development of partnering skills proved to be essential for effective middle and top management. This process is described in detail in the concluding chapter.

Public Policy Implications

This book of cases is going to press in early 2004 as Congress enters its third year of discussions about reauthorizing the welfare reform legislation. While the president advocated increased workforce participation of TANF participants (from 50 to 70 percent of the TANF caseload by 2007 and increased work activities by TANF participants from thirty to forty hours per week), there was increasing consensus, especially among the governors who oversee program operations, that the legislation should be reauthorized with some changes. However, most of the implementation issues will most likely be buried in the legislative details with respect to promoting marriage, determining immigrant rights, serving the hard to serve, providing child care benefits, foreseeing the future of sanctions and time limits, and understanding the impact of Medicaid changes.

The biggest unknown facing welfare reform is the direction of the American economy. The success of helping people to move off of welfare and into employment is based, largely, on the growth of the economy and the growth of jobs that pay on a living wage. The vast majority of TANF participants who have moved from welfare to work are employed in entry-level, low-skilled, service-sector jobs with limited opportunities for advancement. To address this reality, a combination of factors will be needed to promote self-sufficiency among the working poor: (1) job retention and job advancement opportunities based on economic stability and growth, (2) adequate child care and health care supports, and (3) a network of support services such as those described in this book.

While the economy and public policy debates capture newspaper headlines, the network of support services operates below the radar screen of the American public and policymakers. Because support services are designed to respond to the changing needs of the working poor, they need more attention with respect to funding, evaluation, and dissemination. This book seeks to address the need for increased understanding and dissemination of promising practices and programs.

REFERENCES

Austin, M. (2003). The changing relationship between nonprofit organizations and public social service agencies in the era of welfare reform. *Nonprofit and Voluntary Sector Quarterly,* 32(1), 97-114.

Austin, M., Martin, M., Carnochan, S., Berrick, J.D., Goldberg, S., Kelley, J., and Weiss, B. (1999). Building a comprehensive agency-university partnership: The Bay Area Social Services Consortium. *Journal of Community Practice,* 6(3), 89-106.

Carnochan, S. and Austin, M. (2002). Implementing welfare reform and guiding organizational change. *Administration in Social Work,* 26(1), 61-78.

Cherlin, A. (2000). *What Welfare Recipients Know About the New Rules and What They Have to Say About Them.* Policy Brief 00-1. Baltimore, MD: Johns Hopkins University.

Duncan, G.J. and Chase-Landsale, P.L. (Eds.) (2001). *Welfare Reform and The Well-Being of Children and Families.* New York: Russell Sage Foundation.

Edin, K. and Lein, L. (1997). *Making Ends Meet: How Single Mothers Survive Welfare and Low-Wage Work.* New York: Russell Sage Foundation.

Gais, T.L., Nathan, R.P., Lurie, I., and Kaplan, T. (2001). Implementation of the Personal Responsibility Act of 1996. In Blank, R.M. and Haskins, R. (Eds.), *The New World of Welfare* (pp. 35-69). Washington, DC: Brookings Institution Press.

Glazer, S. (2002). Issues, viewpoints, and trends. In Lin, A.C. (Ed.), *Welfare Reform* (pp. 1-53). Washington, DC: CQ Press.

Hagen, J.L. (1999). Public welfare and human services: New directions under TANF. *Families in Society: The Journal of Contemporary Human Services,* 80(1), 78-90.

Hagen, J.L. and Owens-Manley, J. (2002). Issues in implementing TANF in New York: The perspective of frontline workers. *Social Work,* 47(2),171-182.

Kingsley, G.T., McNeely, J.B., and Gibson, J.O. (1997). *Community Building: Coming of Age.* Washington, DC: The Urban Institute.

Kotter, J.P. (1990). What leaders really do. *Harvard Business Review,* May-June, 103-111.

Loprest, P.J. (2002). Making the transition from welfare to work: Successes but continuing concerns. In Weil, A. and Finegold, K. (Eds.), *Welfare Reform: The Next Act* (pp. 17-31). Washington, DC: The Urban Institute Press.

Lurie, I. (2001). Changing welfare offices. *Welfare Reform and Beyond,* Policy Brief No. 9. Washington, DC: Brookings Institution.

Meyers, M.K., Glasser, B., and MacDonald, K. (1998). On the front lines of welfare delivery: Are workers implementing policy reforms? *Journal of Policy Analysis and Management,* 17, 1-22.

Pavetti, L. and Bloom, D. (2001). State sanctions and time limits. In Blank, R. and Haskins, R. (Eds.), *The New World of Welfare* (pp. 245-269). Washington, DC: Brookings Institution Press.

Seefeldt, K.S. (2002). Politics and policy. In Lin, A.C. (Ed). *Welfare Reform* (pp. 54-101). Washington, DC: CQ Press.

Weil, A. and Finegold, K. (2002). Introduction. In Weil, A. and Finegold, K. (Eds.), *Welfare Reform: The Next Act* (pp. xi-xxxi). Washington, DC: The Urban Institute Press.

Weil, M. (1996). Community building: Building community practice. *Social Work,* 41(5), 481-499.

Zedlewski, S.R. (2002). Family incomes: Rising, falling, or holding steady? In Weil, A. and Finegold, K. (Eds.), *Welfare Reform: The Next Act* (pp. 53-77). Washington, DC: The Urban Institute Press.

SECTION I:
AN OVERVIEW OF WELFARE REFORM IMPLEMENTATION AND PRACTICE

Chapter 1

Implementing Welfare Reform and Guiding Organizational Change

Sarah Carnochan
Michael J. Austin

Following passage of the federal welfare reform legislation in 1996, California responded with enactment of its CalWORKs program in August 1997. Counties have spent the past several years engaged in the planning and implementation of welfare reform. Members of the Bay Area Social Services Consortium (BASSC), a coalition of county social service agency directors, social work deans, and foundation executives, have sought to capture the dynamic process of change occurring in county social service agencies in the era of welfare reform. This chapter identifies the core organizational challenges faced by the BASSC directors in implementing welfare reform along with the values and strategies employed to address these challenges. The ultimate goal was to document some of the preliminary lessons learned from implementing a work in progress.

The county directors had a specific interest in this exploratory study. In the early 1990s, they had challenged themselves to develop a vision of social services in the year 2000. That vision included such themes as fostering family self-sufficiency amidst extensive diversity, engaging clients and the community in neighborhood-based service planning and delivery, and fostering prevention-oriented integrated services utilizing blended funding. For many directors, the massive scope of welfare reform implementation seriously challenged their abilities to accomplish this shared vision. They wanted to use the findings of the study to update the previous vision statement by taking into account the impact of welfare reform on such internal

---

This chapter originally appeared in *Administration in Social Work* 26(1): 61-77. Copyright 2002 The Haworth Press, Inc.

operations as human resources (job redesign and expanded training) and fiscal and information systems (performance-based budgeting and outcome assessment) as well as external operations related to expanded community partnerships (see Appendix in this chapter).[1] This chapter includes the major findings related to the directors' description of organizational change and culture, the guiding values they articulated, and the lessons they identified in reflecting on implementing welfare reform.

ORGANIZATIONAL CHANGE AND CULTURE

In the area of organizational change, the directors identified five primary challenges. First, cultural change has been a fundamental goal in implementing welfare reform, as agencies move from determining eligibility to fostering employability and self-sufficiency. Second, the demands of delivering the new self-sufficiency-oriented services have required substantial organizational restructuring. Third, agencies expanded their partnerships and collaborations with a wide range of partners, including other county departments, community-based organizations, and for-profit businesses. Fourth, integrated services linked to the collaborations and interdisciplinary teams needed to be developed in a number of counties. Finally, the demands of welfare reform have increased the importance of data-based planning and evaluation for staff at all levels of the organization.

Cultural Change

Changing the culture of the organization emerged in the interviews as the dominant theme. The new culture was described in terms of a transition to a customer service orientation, a shift from people processing to fostering self-sufficiency, and transforming an insular bureaucratic organization into an open, community-based agency as reflected in the following comments from the interviews:

- "Our bureaucracy was seen in the county as an indifferent federally funded operation. When I first got here, the mission statement indicated that the primary goal of the agency was to administer state and federal programs in a legally efficient and ethical manner...."
- "The old routines that eligibility workers do, and do very well, are now totally out of place in the context of welfare reform.... In our business, you have long-term civil servants, and we can count on the union culture to clash with the new demands for systems change. For example, it's a big change to move someone from eligibility case pro-

cessing and regulation compliance to assessing employability, providing initial counseling, and developing a case plan to foster self-sufficiency."
- "The new agency mission indicates that we're here to improve the quality of life in the community through the services and programs that we provide, using strategies that include collaboration and partnership designed to handle the current wave and future waves of reform. . . ."
- "The organization had a history of being very punitive and dictatorial. . . . I would call the climate a 'fear-based environment'. . . . The new organizational culture needed to operate on mission-related principles, whereby (a) everyone needs to be treated with respect; (b) diverse opinions are to be valued; (c) the emphasis on customer services was nonnegotiable; and (d) risks are inherent in creativity and innovation. . . ."
- "First, I think I'm trying to create an organization that can learn as it functions. . . . Issue number one is trying to build a learning culture in the agency."

In many agencies, staff resistance to changing the organization's culture was a significant phenomenon, often appearing at all levels of the organization. One director noted that "resistance to change went from the top of the organization to the bottom." In contrast, others stated that their staff presented very little resistance to the redefinition of the agency's mission. A number of methods were used to address staff resistance, including the extensive use of staff training on customer service orientation (shifting from a recipient to a customer orientation) and the use of role modeling and coaching by senior managers to instill in staff a customer-friendly service philosophy.

Organizational Restructuring

Many directors were engaged in major restructuring of their agencies, including the creation of new departments, merging of old departments, integrating previously separate divisions, and redesigning job classifications. In some counties these structural changes preceded welfare. The primary goal of restructuring was to create agency structures more responsive to client and community needs. As with cultural change, extensive training was required to assist staff throughout the restructuring process.

Major restructuring in one urban county took the form of reorganizing two major departments, the Department of Economic Services (Aid to Families with Dependent Children [AFDC], General Assistance, Food Stamps, Medi-Cal) and the Department of Employment Services (the Greater Avenues for Independence [GAIN] program, Food Stamp Employment Training Program, and private industry council) into two new departments. The Department of Welfare to Work now integrates benefit determination and employment services to create a more holistic approach to serving families in need. The smaller Department of Workforce and Resource Development uses the recent workforce legislation to help the private industry council operate as a community resource department, working closely with community groups to promote early intervention and prevention programs, especially through the use of school-based services. The director noted that organizational restructuring helped to reduce the historic tension between employment services and economic services staff.

Community Involvement and Collaboration

All of the directors described a shift in the focus of their own work and the activities of their agency to fostering more community involvement. An extensive array of new collaborations and partnerships were being formed, with significant financial resources being contracted to community groups and outposting of agency staff into neighborhood-based service centers. These collaborations included new relationships with the business community, as well as with other county departments and community-based organizations. For example, one county social service director noted that

> In an effort to rally the management team to proactively respond to welfare reform, we engaged immediately in a joint planning process with the Human Service Commission, which was a new role for both them and us. . . . I had never undertaken a community planning process on this scale before, although I had chaired various task forces and committees on special projects. The effort was a success for both the management team in terms of supporting the agency goal of shared decision making and community members related to affirming a commitment to partnership. We're also working very closely with the community-based organization that provides paratransit services under a contract with the transit district. . . . We're working to develop some collaborative efforts around housing with other commissions and coalitions that frankly we've never worked with such as the Housing Commission that is advisory to the Planning Department and another commission that works with the Redevelopment Agency. . . . Our community college has been a major partner—I can't speak highly enough of our local community college. . . . We believe strongly in fostering open communication and in partnering with the community and the client. We try to involve clients in all aspects of our

work, including the community planning sessions, work groups, or task forces.

Service Integration and Teamwork

A central element of restructuring and culture change involves the integration of services, the use of interdisciplinary teams to deliver services, and efforts to consolidate and blend funding streams to support integrated services. A suburban county director described a comprehensive integration initiative as follows:

> We began working with neighborhoods, particularly those which had a high concentration of our clients. We created school-linked services by outposting our staff and working together with the health department and education systems, using multidisciplinary teams to work with at-risk families. . . . We weren't reforming just one thing, but were really trying to reform the entire system of services, using prevention and early intervention approaches to strengthen families and communities. . . . We were very clear that the family self-sufficiency teams had to work in a multidisciplinary environment, with a prevention and early intervention orientation. The changes for our eligibility workers were also significant because we created a comprehensive screening and assessment process and had to retrain staff to become effective in interviewing and assessment. . . . The way our eligibility workers had functioned had been quite fragmented, with workers responsible for either AFDC eligibility, Medi-Cal eligibility, or Food Stamp eligibility. We changed all this, creating a generic eligibility worker position, and offered training initially on a voluntary basis.

Data-Based Planning and Evaluation

A number of directors described the importance of data in the planning process as well as in evaluation. Data permit effective targeting of resources and development of predictors to guide interventions. Several directors pointed out the many problems associated with trying to use the data reported externally to the state and federal government for local internal decision making. One director noted,

> The planning wasn't driven from the federal or state level. It was grassroots work, building on what we had done through the community strategic planning process. Our strategic plan called for using data to inform the planning process . . . to ask, "What do we know?" and

then planning on the basis of information. Particularly with welfare reform issues, people take ideological positions, and that's not always helpful when you're trying to build common understanding and direction. There were a lot of stereotypes about the large sizes of families on welfare, when actually the majority of clients were moms with two kids, reflecting a real mix of race and ethnicity. People also had incorrect assumptions about the length of time families spent on welfare. What we found was that we had two populations: one group that wasn't on aid for very long and a second group that was on a long time, concentrated in about six communities. We also created a geo-map showing exactly where the families lived according to zip code that really was an eye opener for people. The use of this kind of data in the planning process allowed us to target resources and programs.

The core values guiding the implementation process can also be traced throughout these examples of organizational changes related to culture, restructuring, partnerships, teamwork, and data-based decision making.

GUIDING VALUES

The core values articulated by the directors as guiding their work in implementing organizational changes included social and economic justice; self-sufficiency; dignity and respect; equity; and building a learning organization. The values provided personal guidance to the directors and often became part of the agency's revised mission statement:

1. Promoting client self-sufficiency and moving away from dependence, blame, and people processing
2. Fostering community involvement, shared responsibility and outreach, outcome-based community control, and integrated partnerships
3. Demonstrating participatory management (respect, risk taking, collaboration, anticipatory cross-system thinking and planning, flexible and open communications and problem solving, dealing with diversity and conflict, fairness and honesty, and balancing creative chaos with structured implementation)
4. Empowering staff to participate in change processes, internalize change values, and build a learning organization
5. Valuing clients with a customer service orientation that invests in clients by treating clients and staff with dignity

6. Focusing on outcomes for adults and children using performance-based assessments
7. Advocating major social values related to equity and a living wage, adequate health care and child care, and social and economic justice

A number of directors also noted their desire to promote these values as a central feature of the agency's culture.

- "The core values guiding the agency, and my personal work, are *social and economic justice.*"
- "*Self-sufficiency* is a central value; I firmly believe that we need to hold people accountable and that parents ought to be expected to support their children and that self-sufficiency is a value that we should all be encouraging people to work toward."
- "I focus on *respecting the client* and I teach at all of the staff induction sessions that when people come to this agency for service, in the great majority of cases they have lost a great deal of self-respect to get to this point (of asking for help). We have it in our power to build on their strengths to help restore their sense of dignity. I also recognize that staff cannot treat clients with dignity if they are not also treated with dignity."
- "I'm really interested in *building a learning organization,* where we gain insights from our mistakes and develop a culture where individuals feel valued and take calculated risks, where honest dialogue is encouraged and respected, and creativity and innovation are the norm."

LESSONS LEARNED

The directors identified a number of lessons that they had learned from guiding the agency's change process:

1. *The nature and pace of change*
    - Massive and rapid change cannot be completely planned.
    - Change takes time and requires patience, incremental steps, and some agreement on the value of change.
    - Comprehensive change is very different from incremental change, especially in unfamiliar territory.
    - Change yields tension, as interests shift and stress levels rise.
2. *Adapting one's management style*
    - Control must be replaced by influence, featuring the participatory styles of negotiating, educating, and persuading.

- People have limits on the amount and pace of change they can tolerate.
- We need to set realistic expectations, internally and in the community.
- We need to get comfortable with the inability to accurately foresee all that will occur in the change process.
- We need to relinquish some management control in light of volume and pace of change in order to trust the collaborative process.
- Sometimes we need to be more direct in articulating and modeling core values.
- Relying on staff for information and delegation is important.

3. *Balancing internal and external relations*
   - Implementing change requires attention to internal operations, especially internal customers.
   - External and internal relations need to be balanced since they can no longer be separated.
   - It is important for senior managers to be out in the community.

4. *Dealing with the political environment*
   - Agencies are in a political environment which requires special skills.
   - The agency director's job is increasingly political.
   - The community leadership role goes beyond traditional human services.

5. *Handling the demands of leadership*
   - We need to persevere in order to effect massive change.
   - We need to exercise power with caution by being aware of perceived power.
   - We need a vision to help staff view the agency as a temporary way station for clients in order to avoid fostering dependency.
   - It is difficult to create climate conducive to change without generating fear among staff.
   - Value peer support, especially when it gets lonely at the top.

In describing the striking difference between the agency's traditional approach to incremental change and the new demands of strategic change, one director used the metaphor of a hurricane, an avalanche, a tornado, and an earthquake all rolled into one to describe the magnitude of change. He called for

> a new definition of change since we're not used to this depth and breadth of change. We're used to dealing with incremental change such as a new mandated program, a new classification of staff, or a

new child care contract. We really were not prepared to deal with the depth and breadth of concurrent change required in nearly all of our systems.

Although the directors generally thrive on promoting change, they recognized that many members of their staff had very different responses. The directors reported that some staff members expressed sadness at the change of old relationships following major restructuring, as well as doubts about their abilities to maintain good job performance in an environment which demanded new skills and responses. Some staff members feared that the new organizational changes were a response to their poor job performance in the past. In contrast to this kind of apprehension, several directors noted that staff members were excited and pleased about new job assignments because of the new flexibility to more adequately address client needs.

In order to guide agency staff through a massive change process, a number of directors noted that the exercise of restraint and patience has been essential, although not always easy to find. One director stated,

> I've learned to have much more patience, and it's probably a good thing that this is happening as I'm getting older and less driven. The slower pace of change is hard for me since I'm the type of person who really likes to see things get done sooner rather than later.

Directors often initiated small changes by allowing staff to engage voluntarily at their own pace rather than the pace that public policy seemed to dictate. It was also important for many to learn to set more realistic expectations for themselves and others. This was necessary to reduce stress levels among staff, as well as protect against the loss of credibility if unrealistically high expectations were not met. One director noted that

> one of the lessons I've learned is that more attention needs to be given to setting realistic expectations, internally and externally, in terms of significant change. We do a lot of staff education on what's coming and what we're going to be doing, but we do not develop realistic expectations on what we will get accomplished and by when.

In addition, the volume and pace of change led many directors to the realization that it was necessary to relinquish some control. This involved trusting partners in collaborations, delegating responsibility to staff, and embarking on initiatives without having fully completed the planning process. As one director stated,

> One of the biggest lessons I've learned is that welfare reform and related changes have helped me to put more trust in the collaborative process, where partnering is built on the values of true collaboration, which doesn't require a lot of management control. . . . The volume and speed of the changes related to new and modified programs makes it impossible to use the old command and control accountability model.

Another noted that

> An important aspect of my administrative style is that I don't expect to do it all myself and really have learned how to rely on staff. I try to select and hire staff who are self-starters, able to keep me informed, and comfortable handling delegated responsibilities.

However, some directors noted the importance of providing direction and modeling a changed management style. One director noted that at times she had to be far more directive than she really wanted to be, in order to ensure that implementation was successful.

For several directors, the rapid pace of change required endurance and skill, since the policy changes required numerous and extensive adjustments in both internal and external operations. Other directors focused on the need to take risks in decision making in the absence of clear data or relevant precedents. Several directors emphasized the complexity of the change process in terms of the ability to thrive in chaos or engage in multitasking. Finally, several directors relied heavily on their experience and seniority to draw upon an extra dose of steadiness amidst uncertainty as they negotiated among competing interests, unraveled the complexity of the change process, or engaged in strategically planned change initiatives.

REFLECTING ON THE ORGANIZATIONAL CHANGE PROCESS

As noted previously, this study was undertaken to explore and describe the change process from the unique perspective of the agency directors. The learning organization model developed by Senge (1990) provided a useful framework for analyzing the findings. While some directors made explicit reference to their interest in "building a learning organization" or to "trying to build a learning culture in the agency," other directors described the concrete staff skills and knowledge required by new agency roles which represent another approach to building learning organizations.

The study findings are analyzed from a learning organization perspective by identifying examples in which the changes described by the directors of these ten agencies reflect Senge's (1990) five learning organization principles:

1. *Systems thinking* refers to a process in which people identify complex interrelationships and underlying patterns of causation, rather than simple linear cause-and-effect relationships.
2. *Mental models* include the internal images we hold about how the world works; in a learning organization, these mental models are continually surfaced, tested, and reformulated.
3. *Shared vision* is created through the integration of the visions of all members in an organization and is based on individual choice rather than compliance or persuasion.
4. *Personal mastery* refers to an ongoing process involving the juxtaposition of an accurate picture of one's current reality and a clear vision of a desired future.
5. *Team learning* describes a process in which team members become aligned and function as a whole with a common direction, achieved as a result of operational trust, insightful thinking about complex issues, and dialogue and discussion (Senge, 1990).

Agencies' Views of Organizational Principles

Systems Thinking

A number of the directors described the importance of data in planning and evaluating their programs, especially to base decisions on information rather than ideology or stereotypes. It is important to be able to identify underlying patterns of relationships when the organizational mission involves the complexity of helping human beings make changes in their lives. The process of systems thinking requires agencies to look at the numerous factors related to client outcomes, including economic, service, and personal characteristics, and explicitly engage in identifying patterns that result in particular outcomes.

Mental Models

All the directors emphasized the importance of cultural change taking place in their agencies. Intentional cultural change involved a change in staff's mental models about clients, the role of the agency, and community support. However, as one director noted, this process continues to evolve:

"It's still hard to get some staff to think differently . . . to get them to conceptualize work in a different way and to build something new." Although Senge (1990) notes that systems thinking is the central principle defining a learning organization, the directors in this study described the changing of mental models as the key element in the organizational changes required by welfare reform:

> The most significant change in this agency is the change in culture. I stress culture because I think welfare to work or CalWORKs is synonymous with changing the culture of the organization to make it more adaptable and flexible to handle the current wave and future waves of reform, such as child welfare and adult protective service reform.

Shared Vision

The importance of vision in effective leadership is a persistent theme in much of the organizational change literature (see, e.g., Tichy and Devanna, 1990; Schein, 1986). Senge (1990) argues that vision in a learning organization must be a shared vision which integrates the perspective of all members. The directors in this study described a number of initiatives directed at developing a shared vision for the agency. One director described a process in which internal planning groups that included staff from all levels of the organization "came together to help define the challenges and what we're going to do about them . . . to get common understandings of where we're going." Many of the agencies went beyond the boundaries of the organization to include the community in developing a shared vision through collaborative community planning processes. However, it is also clear that the directors brought a clearly articulated set of personal values to the process of vision development. Without interviewing a representative sample of staff members, it is difficult to determine the extent to which the perspectives of staff were integrated into the agency's vision.

Personal Mastery

A number of directors described the increased demands placed on staff by the shift from eligibility to employability services. Personal mastery on the part of workers responsible for client services takes on added meaning. The employment and self-sufficiency goals of welfare reform depend, in large part, on the ability of line staff to master new service delivery functions. It was clear to the directors that achieving such personal mastery would take time and require special training supports. As a result, staff development and human resource managers began to recognize the need to help staff develop personal goals for career development as well as education pathways involving training resources outside the agency, including community colleges. It remains to be seen whether the demand for the personal mastery of new skills and knowledge will translate into more effective services for those served by the agency.

Team Learning

As part of the organizational restructuring process, many of the agencies developed service delivery models that included multidisciplinary teams at the managerial, supervisory, and line staff levels. These teams offer an opportunity for team learning that generalizes learning across agency boundaries. However, teamwork also presents challenges, as senior members are called upon to listen to new perspectives and line staff assume new responsibilities for generating ideas rather than simply relying upon directives from above.

CONCLUSION

The directors participating in the study identified a number of lessons learned related to guiding organizational change processes. First, fundamental organizational change often requires a change in the organization's culture. The directors noted the importance of identifying and addressing resistance to these changes through extensive training, mentoring, and role modeling. Second, traditional managerial "command and control" processes need to be examined and changed through the use of participatory management, delegation, and teamwork. Third, without the use of current data in the planning process, new programs and services are likely to be based upon limited and/or biased information about clients and communities. Finally, the ability to tolerate chaos is essential to helping staff function in an environment of uncertainty. This involves the simultaneous processes of searching for accurate data and articulating values and vision while, at the same time, implementing changes without sufficient data and using an evolving vision.

As the directors sought to transform their agencies into learning organizations, the principles developed by Senge (1990) became useful tools for analysis. The directors described their ongoing efforts to uncover and change mental models about clients, organizations, and communities. Many engaged in developing a shared organizational vision for the agency. In using data to identify the actual characteristics of the clients and communities they serve, directors and their staff members used systems thinking to identify complex factors and relationships that relate to service outcomes. Implementing the significant organizational changes stimulated by welfare reform clearly reflect the core principles of a learning organization.

However, welfare reform is neither the first nor the last major policy initiative requiring significant change on the part of public social service agencies. These organizations are subject to an ongoing stream of reforms, generated by policymakers, that often require changes in organizational goals, structures, and operations. It remains to be seen if the learning organization framework offers a sufficiently robust model for assisting agencies in addressing mandates for continuing change. The directors in this study identified the need to become "more adaptable and flexible to handle the current wave and future waves of reform." The learning organization principles involve constant reflection and learning, key ingredients in developing flexibility and adaptability to changing environments.

A number of questions remain about the value of the learning organization model for public agencies. First, although this study begins to identify some examples of learning organization processes, can the learning organization framework be applied to public social service agencies over time? Second, although many agencies have created team-based structures to deliver services, can these teams effectively coordinate and sustain trust and open dialogue over time? Third, although agencies have begun to identify the complex range of variables relevant to assessing client outcomes, can outcome data truly lead to service improvements and enduring organizational change? Fourth, with regard to personal mastery, it remains to be seen if the individual abilities of staff members can be accurately assessed and ultimately addressed through a continuum of educational opportunities (in-service training, certificate programs, and college degree programs). Finally, as organizational goals and operations are subject to repeated external pressures related to changes in public policies, there is continuing demand for public agencies to develop new shared visions using new mental models. It is not clear how much time is needed to stabilize the focus on new visions before being challenged to come up with another set of new directions.

However, it is clear that the benefits of learning organization initiatives for public agencies need to be evaluated over time in terms of their impact on client and staff satisfaction, staff recruitment and retention, and relationships with community stakeholders. The ultimate test of the application of learning organization principles is the impact they may have on the service outcomes for the individuals, families, and communities served by public social service agencies. The chapters that follow provide further evidence of staff investment in experimentation and learning as a way to identify innovative programs and practices.

APPENDIX: SUPPORTING LOW-INCOME WORKERS IN THE TWENTY-FIRST CENTURY: THE EVOLVING BASSC VISION STATEMENT

Introduction

In 1993, the Bay Area Social Services Consortium (BASSC) developed its first vision statement, *Human Service—2000: An Evolving Vision Statement,* to serve as a framework for agency and community discussions about implementing a neighborhood-based human service system. The statement included a vision of a community service system that serves all families in need by fostering self-sufficiency, based on a collaborative community approach to meeting human needs and achieving tangible positive outcomes for family and community well-being.

This updated version of the vision statement is titled *Supporting Low-Income Workers in the Twenty-First Century.* As social service agencies take on new roles in response to welfare reform and changing public attitudes about the role of government, they are assuming unprecedented responsibility for assisting individuals to enter the workforce in order to provide economic support for their families. In this work, directors are leading dedicated staff committed to clients' dignity. This updated vision statement is based on an analysis of workforce development and incorporates a social development perspective that involves partnerships to support the growth and development of community and family well-being.

The Eight Principles of the Vision Statement

The vision statement is organized into eight principles. The first principle outlines the social development approach to meeting social needs. The second principle addresses the goals of building community and fostering a civil society. The third principle describes the essential role social service agencies need to play in developing a career-resilient workforce. The fourth principle addresses the need for family supports to help low-income working families become economically self-sufficient. The fifth principle outlines the original BASSC vision for family-focused, neighborhood-based human service systems. The sixth principle identifies the changing professional roles that social service workers are taking on in helping families enter the workforce. The seventh principle addresses the changed role of the agency in becoming a catalyst for private/public action. Finally, the eighth principle includes public policy directions that can help to support low-income families.

The Social Development Approach

The social development model is built on the premise of enhancing the capacity of needy individuals, families, and communities to participate in the economy. Participation in the productive economy is the preferred, primary means of meeting social needs. Social development shifts the emphasis from consumption-based, maintenance-oriented services to a focus on creating opportunities and enhancing capacities. It proposes an investment approach targeting communities as well as individuals, with a closer integration of economic and social policy and programs to enhance economic growth and the welfare of the entire population. Social development theory also recognizes that a minority of individuals will not be able to participate in the productive economy and will require long-term or indefinite social supports.

The role of government. In the social development model, the government intervenes appropriately to promote development. The model assumes that the free market is not adequate to meet all social needs. Government initiates and facilitates, using public expenditures combined with individual, family, and community efforts. It has a key role in ensuring people have the skills, knowledge, and opportunity necessary for effective participation in the economy. This means that employment and self-employment opportunities are maximized, the benefits of economic growth are equitably distributed, and the vulnerable are protected from economic exploitation.

Implementation/strategies. A number of strategies are being developed to implement the social development model, including the following:

- investment in cost-effective programs (to prevent unnecessary transfer of resources out of a productive economy);
- human development and human capital investments (education, job training);
- investments that promote employment and self-employment (job placement, job creation, self-employment, wage support);
- social capital investments (community economic development, community building);
- investments in individual and community assets (individual asset accounts); and
- investments that remove barriers to economic participation (lack of transportation, child care, asset limits, discrimination).

Building Community and Fostering a Civil Society

Upon entering the twenty-first century, it is clear that the well-being of low-income workers and families involves complex community issues requiring collaboration through multiple partnerships. Social service agencies are no longer islands in communities of poverty. They are catalysts for change working together with clients and community organizations to create healthy communities and families. In a broader context, we are talking about promoting the growth of a strong, vibrant civil society. Civil society describes that network of private, voluntary associations that provide essential services and support to families and individuals in our communities.

Traditionally, the debate over addressing poverty in this country has polarized around two ideological positions. The first position, typically espoused by liberals, argues that government must provide protection for disadvantaged individuals and families to mitigate the destructive competition that rules the marketplace. The second position, advanced by conservatives, holds that government suppresses the natural, voluntary activities of private organizations and associations, supplanting local, targeted, and effective voluntary programs with ineffective, unresponsive government programs for the poor. The debate is characterized by ideological rigidity; individuals in either camp rarely listen to each other or engage in actual dialogue out of which productive policy might be developed. In order to move beyond this ideological divide, it will be essential to envision a new model for government and community responsibility and relationship.

The proponents of a civil society offer an alternative vision. They assert that although the private, voluntary sector plays an essential role in addressing community needs, it cannot survive without the support of government. Although government may not be the most effective provider of services in all cases, it has the ability to organize broad initiatives, mobilize resources, and build infrastructure.

The role of public social service agencies in a civil society is to help build and strengthen communities by linking the valuable services and functions of nongovernmental agencies with government resources and capacity to catalyze others inside and outside of government. They must help to develop opportunities for members of a diverse community to engage in candid, open debate about the kind of society we choose to create and support.

Developing a Career-Resilient Workforce

Upgrading workplace skills is essential in helping workers to meet the challenges of a high-skill labor market. As social service agencies form partnerships with employers and training programs, they need to foster and implement the following values and goals:

1. Continuously assess the current and future workforce demands of the local economy by
   - identifying sectors where job growth is predicted;
   - working with business to identify the skill sets that are required to perform jobs in those sectors;
   - working with educational institutions to develop a curriculum that provides the foundation for those skill sets; and
   - assisting students at the secondary and higher education levels by encouraging high schools and community colleges to form links with employers to ensure the relevance of curriculum and the development of an employable workforce.
2. Encourage training programs to reflect the abilities/goals of workers and the needs of the workplace by
   - seeing that specific occupational training programs are linked to specific employers;
   - seeing that successful training programs are integrated with job placement programs and ongoing job retention services; and
   - ensuring that training program quality and intensity are high.
3. Foster collaboration between employers and employees to upgrade workers' skills so that workers remain competitive in the labor market by
   - helping employers move beyond minimum wage entry-level jobs, which do not provide income adequate to support a family;
   - helping employees upgrade their skills to ensure continuing employability; and
   - helping employers recognize how they will benefit from the development of a well-trained labor force.

A career-resilient worker is one who is able to succeed and thrive in the current economy in which fast-paced change is the norm. Because workers make transitions in and out of jobs at an increasingly rapid pace, it is essential that they keep their skills current, those skills demanded in the broader employment market as well as those required by their own jobs. They must also be prepared for the challenges they face in job transitions, by developing job search and interview skills, financial reserves, and emotional resilience in the face of uncertainty. The responsibility for maintaining employability should be jointly shared between the employer and the employee. Social service agencies must find new ways to promote career-resilient workers by seeking to establish a new covenant between employers and employees so that career advancement can lead to a living wage.

Supporting the Family

The central goal for our human service agencies is the achievement of economic and social well-being for all families. It is not enough to simply assist parents to get a job; our goal is to assist families to move out of poverty, especially given the rising costs of living. Essential to this goal will be the development of a family-centered investment policy, which includes a comprehensive system of social supports provided by the community and employers in the following areas: child care, transportation, housing, and health care.

1. *Child care:* In order for parents to work, they must be able to arrange child care for their children. Adequate child care is not enough; child care must be high quality, safe, affordable, and sufficiently flexible to meet the needs of families regarding work schedules, family obligations, and other needs. Child care plays an essential role in early education and learning readiness, facilitating improved educational outcomes and successful participation in the workforce of the future.
2. *Transportation:* Transportation must be affordable, comprehensive, and responsive to work and child care schedules. Transportation services are an important step toward addressing the imbalance of jobs and housing that exists in many counties and bridging the distances between housing and jobs in rural areas.
3. *Housing:* The rising cost of housing prevents many families from being able to survive in high-cost counties. Housing for families should be affordable and safe. A range of permanently affordable housing models should be promoted, including housing that is privately owned as well as publicly subsidized housing. The nonprofit sector is an important partner with government in creating and maintaining affordable housing. Private developers and the business community should also contribute to the development of affordable housing for low-income families.
4. *Health care:* As nonstandard work arrangements have become more common, the availability of employment-based health insurance has declined. Health care should be universal; workers should not have to choose between a job and health care. In addition, health care can play an important role in assisting individuals in succeeding in the workplace, through provision of adequate mental health and substance abuse services, family planning services, and preventive care for adults and children.

Family-Focused, Neighborhood-Based Human Service System

Ten major service delivery values underlie the advancement of an outcomes-oriented community approach to family-focused, neighborhood-based human services. These values are organized into the following three areas:

1. Resource distribution: Social inclusiveness
   - *Equality of access and opportunity* (including geographical, physical, temporal, legal, informational, and linguistic and cultural access)
   - *Fairness and equity* (the fair distribution of societal resources, power, status, and opportunities)
   - *Adequacy of income and economic support* (redistributed resources must provide a minimal level of health and decency to individuals and families)
2. Decision making and authority: Community development
   - *Community approaches to problem solving* (concerning questions of economic development, community institutions, physical integrity of the community, physical health of the community, and constructive interaction among community groups)
   - *Consumer ownership* (community must determine which needs have priority, the appropriate means of addressing needs, and the criteria for measuring success)
   - *Decentralized neighborhood-based service delivery system* (people interact most effectively with systems that are near their place of residence and that reflect the characteristics of their living environment)
3. Service design and delivery: Social investment
   - *Proactive prevention-oriented services* (reflecting a strategy of investing in the community to address human needs)
   - *Deep commitment to racial and cultural diversity* (at the core of the principles of equity, access, and community participation)
   - *Comprehensive and noncategorical services* (to ensure the most effective and appropriate use of resources)
   - *Universal family investment policies* (to avoid stigmatizing recipients and to develop a broad, politically stable constituency)

Changing Professional Roles

Just as the role of the agency in the community has expanded and grown to help families become self-supporting, the roles played by public social service staff are changing. These roles now encompass a dual perspective in which the worker acts to empower the family and support workforce development. In order to support workforce development, agency workers are assuming roles as job developers, job coaches, employment advisors, retention support workers, and job-placement advisors. Their new responsibilities will include work-focused assessment, counseling, and referral; work-focused advocacy; work-focused program development; and work-focused social activism. Assessment will require understanding a client's attitudes and values relating to education and work, work-related skills and challenges, and access to work opportunities and information. In order to support family empowerment, staff need to be organizers and brokers for a range of supportive services, including child care, transportation, health care, and housing.

In order to ensure that our policies and programs for families are responsive and effective, we need to work toward a set of family-focused professional practices and policies, including the following:

- Family-accountable professional services and policies (fully taking into account family members' perceptions of needs and solutions)
- Family-partnered service approaches and policies (treating families as experts and collaborators in goal setting and in the mobilization of solutions)
- Family-led services and policies (families participating in the design and convening of their own case staffing, summits, and congresses)
- Family-delivered services (delivered by families, one to another)
- Family-organized service systems and policies (developed by families to meet needs and address aspirations, involving culturally competent and resource-based mobilization)

Public Social Service Agencies As Catalysts for Private Action

Responsibility for the poor is now being shared between public agencies and the broader community. Community organizations are playing a much more active role in supporting and aiding families. Public social service agencies no longer simply provide cash and in-kind benefits; they are now called upon to catalyze private activity, providing funding for projects and creating an environment that supports families and individuals in need. Catalysts are agents of social change who foster interactions between people and/or forces and thereby promote important and sustained changes in the ways we do business. Our goal should be to develop this role as catalyst, to ensure that the community does not abandon needy families.

We can serve as catalysts to promote community action in a number of ways, including the following:

- identifying social problems affecting neighborhoods through our work in the community;
- providing targeted funding (time-limited rent subsidy programs working with private landlords, community-based paratransit services);
- promoting tax incentives (enterprise zones, tax credits for employer-based child care programs);
- creating partnerships (collaborations with government, business, nonprofit, and voluntary organizations); and
- fostering community leadership and community problem solving (community advisory boards, commissions, and task forces).

An important role for public sector catalysts is to expand the social economy providing support for people living in poverty through a community network of family support services, including youth-based organizations, nonprofit agencies, and voluntary associations. These networks need to reflect extensive collaborative partnerships in such areas as housing, health, child care, and transportation.

Public Policy Directions

The increasing income disparity in the United States demands comprehensive approaches to improve the economic status of low-income and poor families. The competitive labor market is no longer able to provide income levels adequate to support the family of low-skill workers. Government needs to act to address the inequities of the private market for individuals who are fulfilling their obligation to work to support their families. The unfinished business of welfare reform will require new, more targeted public policies to increase the income and assets available to low-income families. The earned income tax credit may prove to be an effective mechanism for increasing the income available to working families. Similarly, child or family allowances, as used in a number of European countries, may provide targeted assistance to children. Asset development and microinvestment programs are being implemented in this country to make capital available to individuals historically excluded from access to capital due to racism, poverty, and disadvantage.

NOTE

1. This exploratory study focused on the experiences of ten county social service directors in the San Francisco Bay Area of northern California. The data were collected in spring 1999. The primary goal of the study was to identify the first set of perceptions and impressions emerging from the early phase of implementing federal and state welfare reform legislation. The following research questions served as

the foundation for in-depth interviews of one to two hours with each director conducted by the first author:

1. How have your prior work experiences and education impacted your efforts as the agency director to implement welfare reform?
2. What are the major organizational changes in your agency that are emerging from welfare reform implementation and how would you describe the implementation processes?
3. What are the major values which underlie these organizational changes and guide your actions?
4. What are some of the lessons learned from implementing welfare reform as you reflect on your role as director?

These general questions, with follow-up probes, were developed in collaboration with the ten directors prior to the interviews, resulting in increased clarity and focus. The interviews were recorded, transcribed, and edited. The editing process included input from each director to check on the accuracy of each case description and to capture the "voice" of each director. The cases were then content analyzed by using the four categories reflected in the major questions and a cross-case matrix was developed to facilitate data analysis.

The primary themes identified in the content analysis are illustrated with quotes from the interviews with the directors. The findings are then interpreted with the use of Senge's (1990) learning organization framework as the directors sought to transform their agencies into learning organizations. Although the study did not originally seek to assess the change process with reference to learning organization principles, the learning organization framework emerged as a useful tool for interpreting the findings.

It is important to note the several limitations to this exploratory study. First, it reflects only the perceptions and views of the social service agency directors. The views of senior management, middle management, line staff, elected board members, contract service providers, clients, and local opinion leaders are not included in this study. Although efforts to triangulate these multiple perspectives would have made an interesting study, it would have resulted in a much larger investigation. Second, this study captures only one point in time (January 1999), namely twenty-eight months following the August 1996 passage of the federal welfare reform legislation and twelve months following the implementation of California's welfare reform legislation (passed in August 1997 for January 1998 implementation). Although there is value in reflecting on a change process in midstream, there are significant limitations given the fast pace of change and the absence of documented staff reactions to implementing major change. Third, it is difficult to generalize from the perceptions of ten county social service directors in northern California. Although their experiences may parallel those of directors in other counties or states, the variability in local economic, political, social, and population characteristics greatly limits the ability to generalize. Despite these limitations, this study captures the rarely documented perceptions of busy administrators in order to add to our knowledge base of public-sector organizational change and program implementation.

REFERENCES

Schein, E. H. (1986). *Organizational culture and leadership*. San Francisco: Jossey-Bass.
Senge, P. (1990). *The fifth discipline: The art and practice of the learning organization*. New York: Doubleday.
Tichy, N. M. and Devanna, M. A. (1990). *The transformational leader*. New York: Wiley.

Chapter 2

Overview of Innovative Programs and Practices

Jonathan Prince
Michael J. Austin

The 1996 federal welfare-to-work program (Temporary Assistance to Needy Families, or TANF) contains a variety of policy measures designed to reduce dependency and promote self-sufficiency. Within these policy constraints and opportunities, social service agencies and their community partners are transforming themselves as they make the change from eligibility determination to employability enhancement. The shared goal is to build a more comprehensive social service system that enables low-income individuals and families to become self-sufficient.

The passage of TANF legislation required social service organizations to engage in a substantial reassessment of their mission and organizational structure. As noted in Chapter 1, the major outcomes of this assessment included the following findings:

1. cultural change is a fundamental goal in implementing the family self-sufficiency model;
2. the demand of delivering new services requires substantial organizational restructuring;
3. agencies are engaging in partnerships with a wide range of partners, including other county departments, community-based organizations, and for-profit businesses;
4. integrated services and interdisciplinary teams are being developed in a number of counties; and
5. the demands of welfare reform have increased the importance of data-based planning and evaluation.

Most of this chapter originally appeared as "Innovative Programs and Practices Emerging from the Implementation of Welfare Reform," in *Journal of Community Practice* 9(3): 1-14. Copyright 2001 The Haworth Press, Inc.

One way to describe this process of organizational change is to use the concepts of Cameron and Quinn (1999), namely a shift from a hierarchy culture (characterized by rules, impersonality, and accountability) to a clan or ad hoc culture (characterized by cohesiveness, participation, flexibility, and creativity). Social service agencies are becoming less bureaucratic and isolated from the community as they seek to evolve into "learning organizations" that are able to develop and implement new structures and services in response to changing client needs and new policy mandates.

The case studies in the following chapters represent some of the first reports from the front line of organizational change. They describe innovative programs and practices that were chosen by county social service directors based on one or more of the following criteria: (1) a new approach to delivering social services, (2) practices that enhance public/private community partnerships, and/or (3) a unique administrative process or change. This chapter provides an overview of the twenty-one cases in order to identify several crosscutting themes and challenges as well as lessons learned from innovations emerging during four years of welfare reform implementation (January 1998 to December 2001). The case study method was used to describe the programs and practices emerging in the implementation of welfare reform.[1]

NEW APPROACHES TO SERVICE DELIVERY

The ten cases on service delivery innovations are divided into two categories: removing barriers to workforce participation and promoting self-sufficiency through support services.

Removing Barriers to Workforce Participation

In the booming post-welfare reform economy of the 1990s many TANF recipients were able to find work without help or with limited vocational assistance. It became clear, however, that in order to participate more actively in the labor force, a significant percentage of hard-to-place TANF participants (about 20 to 30 percent) needed services which addressed barriers to employment such as low basic work skills, mental health problems, chemical dependency, medical problems, and lack of child care or transportation (Danziger et al., 1999; Kramer, 1998; Olson and Pavetti, 1996; Pavetti, 1996; Pavetti et al., 1997; Loprest and Acs, 1996). This section describes several new programs and practices designed to address obstacles to self-sufficiency.

Connections Shuttle

Lack of transportation is one of the most common employment barriers for TANF participants (Edin and Lein, 1997; Loprest and Acs, 1996). To address this issue, Santa Cruz County created a TANF-funded Connections Shuttle which provides about 133 free rides per day to family members who can prove that they are unable to commute to and from work, job training, school, or child care using existing public transportation (see Chapter 3). It is designed as a temporary solution until participants are able to find permanent solutions linked to self-sufficiency. The shuttle program includes a seven-month training experience for interested TANF participants with clean driving records and negative drug tests to become paid drivers and dispatchers. As a result, the shuttle program provides both publicly supported employment and responsive transportation needed to remove, temporarily, a major barrier to labor force participation.

Guaranteed Ride Home Program

Also designed to address the transportation needs of TANF participants, Santa Clara County's Guaranteed Ride Home Program (launched in 1999) offers car rides to and from the workplace and home, including necessary stops (e.g., child care facilities, schools, medical centers) (see Chapter 4). In addition, transportation is provided in situations that include the following:

1. nonscheduled overtime requests from employers,
2. car breakdowns,
3. when the participant or his or her dependents become ill and must leave work,
4. household emergencies,
5. when a carpool is unexpectedly not available, or
6. when a change in schedule makes alternate transportation unavailable.

Participants are eligible to receive a total of forty-eight rides over a six-month period, and the service is always available (twenty-four hours per day, 365 days per year) in all of the fifteen Santa Clara cities. In the first eight months of operation, over 900 people have been able to get to work despite the lack of a vehicle or alternate transportation, resulting in the increased job placement and retention of TANF participants. Furthermore, participants have become educated about travel options and have learned to develop effective transportation plans.

Training Child Care Providers

In addressing the widespread lack of affordable child care for low-income working parents (Edin and Lein, 1997), the Exempt Provider Training Program in San Mateo County helps to build the capacity of high-quality child care providers in the community by encouraging TANF participants and others to launch and improve their own child care business (see Chapter 5). The training program focuses on the promotion of healthy infant and toddler development by recruiting, training, and supporting unlicensed (exempt) providers who care for their own children, the children of relatives, and/or the children of only one other family. After the learning needs of providers are assessed, they participate in a sixteen-hour English- or Spanish-speaking training session (four Saturday sessions of four hours each) and can access home visits, support groups, referrals, educational literature, mentors, child care (for their own children during sessions), and transportation to and from sessions. The project offers incentives (twenty dollars) to encourage attendance at the training sessions, scholarships (forty dollars) to attend CPR/first-aid training, and other financial assistance (as needed) for obtaining licensure and/or registering with Trustline to assure parents that their child care provider does not have a criminal conviction. The program has grown tremendously since its inception in 1997, with class sizes increasing from three or four people in the first class to as many as sixty arriving to participate in later classes. Each year the program assists hundreds of providers in delivering quality as opposed to custodial child care. The ultimate goal of the program is to increase the amount of affordable and accessible child care which can assist low-income working parents to maintain labor force participation.

Colocating Support Services

In addition to the societal barriers of child care and transportation, several studies have found that personal issues such as mental health problems or substance abuse can interfere with employment (Bush and Kraft, 1998; Grayson, 1999; Young and Gardner, 1997). Until recently, support services that address these issues were not a formal part of the welfare-to-work program (Pavetti et al., 1997). Sonoma County has responded to this need by colocating mental health and substance abuse services for TANF participants near the social services agency (see Chapter 6). This colocation makes it possible for a consumer in a single visit to apply for aid, get program information, set up child care services, get a child support order, check out an array of county employment services, and access community resources through an information and referral service. The county also provides cross training for social service, substance abuse, and mental health staff which is critical to the success of colocated services. The colocation of these services

1. makes access more convenient for consumers,
2. improves the show rate for appointments,
3. enables staff to communicate efficiently,
4. allows consumers to receive support services for up to one year after they are no longer eligible for TANF,
5. increases the use of services,
6. contributes to a declining unemployment rate, and
7. facilitates job retention.

Sheltered Workshop

Building upon the success of a traditional vocational rehabilitation facility, the San Mateo County Human Services Agency utilizes its WorkCenter (founded in 1967 on a two-hundred dollar grant) to address the work skill deficits of hard-to-place TANF participants by employing them to assemble, package, and ship products while they look for permanent employment (see Chapter 7). Personal problems relating to substance abuse, health, mental health, literacy, or domestic violence are assessed by human service agency staff, and if necessary referrals are made to other county departments. Additional assistance includes the following:

1. a weeklong job-seeking skills class and a ten-day work assessment (if indicated);
2. access to a network center that is staffed by job-search specialists and equipped with computers, telephones, job listings, and other resources that assist in seeking employment;
3. availability of home visits to help resolve issues that interfere with attendance; and
4. ongoing case management.

The WorkCenter offers on-the-job training to hard-to-place welfare recipients and provides them with a temporary income while they address personal barriers to workforce participation.

Self-Sufficiency Support Services

After TANF participants have addressed barriers to workforce participation and have found employment, Edin and Lein (1997) have demonstrated that they (1) continue to be underpaid, (2) have little chance of promotion, (3) have increased expenses, and (4) have almost as much difficulty balancing their budgets as they had on welfare. Social service agencies are helping TANF participants to maintain self-sufficiency through family loans, mentoring, job-retention telephone hotlines, special access to training and employment, and individual development accounts.

Family Loan Program

With the support of the McKnight Foundation's (Minnesota) Family Loan Program, in 1998 San Mateo County launched a program for working families to help them deal with large or unexpected one-time expenses (see Chapter 8). It provides loans of up to $3,000 to eligible low-income individuals to help temporarily with vocational or educational expenses which typically include car purchase, car repair, work or school uniforms, tools for a trade, and child care. The loans are serviced by one of three local banks that are able to qualify for low-interest federal funds under the Community Reinvestment Act of 1977. Of the first 203 applications received, eighty-nine (44 percent) were approved, and 91 percent of these were repaid. In addition to benefiting from the financial assistance, consumers learn how to apply for, obtain, and repay a bank loan, and they report (1) a 90 percent decrease in work absenteeism, (2) a 93 percent reduction in travel time to work, and (3) a 26 percent increase in attendance to job-related educational activities.

Adopt-A-Family Program

In addition to material support to help families make the transition to self-sufficiency, the Adopt-A-Family Program in San Mateo provides mentoring to low-income families over a period of one year by matching consumer families with "godparents" who are carefully screened individuals and/or employees of local businesses (see Chapter 9). Godparents are encouraged to develop a relationship with the family and, in the tradition of holiday donation programs, contribute needed secondhand items (typically pots, pans, toys, clothing, bedding, and cribs). In the first eighteen months, the program matched approximately 100 families with godparents; it has the advantage of being easy to replicate and expand, as it is based exclusively on donations of time and materials and requires only one quarter-time employee. Furthermore, as the poorest families are at a high risk for social isolation (Wilson, 1996), the program can increase low-income family interaction with the larger community.

Helping Participants Stay on the Job

Designed to help TANF participants retain their jobs and help the unemployed gain access to needed resources that may help them find a job, the

Santa Clara County JobKeeper Hotline provides round-the-clock counseling, crisis intervention, and referral services (see Chapter 10). When calling JobKeeper, recipients reach trained, volunteer phone counselors who can actively listen and provide linkage to a network of community resources, including child care, employment services, education and training programs, legal services, and transportation. JobKeeper is developing a "seamless system" in that individuals calling with child care questions, for example, are transferred directly to a child care coordinating agency, and callers seeking employment are transferred directly to job-search professionals. The hotline is utilized widely (between forty-five and sixty-five calls per month, totaling almost 800 calls between July 1998 and June 1999) by people who are transitioning from cash assistance yet are able to retain support services (for a period of up to one year) that help them to maintain long-term employment and self-sufficiency.

Hiring Your Own Clients

Although businesses have been encouraged to hire former welfare recipients, it is equally important for social service agencies to demonstrate employer responsibility (see Chapter 11). As an example, the San Mateo County Human Services Agency offers jobs to TANF participants by employing them as welfare eligibility workers and support staff. In the Medi-Cal Benefits Analyst I position, for example, former TANF participants process applications for public health insurance and provide ongoing monitoring of individuals' eligibility for benefits. Applicants for the Analyst I position complete seven weeks of on-the-job, classroom, and computer training in groups of ten to twelve individuals. Out of the training group approximately six are offered positions (others do not pass training tests, have poor attendance, or elect not to continue). The recipients who are hired and then assisted in passing the civil service test are offered full-time, permanent employment with comprehensive benefits. This practice enables the agency to address staffing shortages, set an example for the larger community, and assist former welfare recipients with work experience, training, and becoming self-sufficient.

Individual Development Accounts (IDA)

Working one's way out of poverty requires special attention to the process of building a savings account through regular deposits. This is a program of community-based organizations designed by the San Mateo County Human Services agency using TANF incentive funds to assist low-income families with establishing special savings accounts to build assets over time (see Chapter 12). In collaboration with twenty-three banks and a local foundation, the program includes a money-management course, individual tutorials to establish and monitor savings objectives, and investor support groups. The minimum monthly savings by program participants are matched by investors (foundations and TANF funds) on the basis of a two-to-one matching formula. The flexible and supportive program results in not only increased savings but also healthier lifestyles (e.g., money saved from reduced smoking), increased self-confidence, and improved family relationships often affected by the tensions related to managing scarce resources.

PARTNERING WITH THE COMMUNITY

The next set of cases features social service agency practices that enhance public-private community partnership. In order to address more comprehensively the needs of low-income individuals who are transitioning from welfare to work, several Bay Area counties have begun to develop partnerships with local organizations to better provide housing, education, training, and a variety of social, health, and behavioral health services. The following six partnership cases are divided into two categories: neighborhood partnerships, including self-sufficiency centers and a jobs program, and community-wide partnerships, including a coalition to address homelessness, a transitional recovery community, a coalition of nonprofit agencies, and community college collaboration.

Neighborhood Partnerships

Neighborhood Jobs Program

The first illustration of partnerships responding to welfare reform is the Alameda County public-private Neighborhood Jobs Pilot Initiative (NJPI) (see Chapter 13). The NJPI was launched in 1997 with a Rockefeller Foundation planning grant to develop one-stop employment resource centers in three low-income neighborhoods. The primary goal was for all the centers to be self-supporting within two years through membership dues, community volunteer time, public and private job service contracts, contracts with corporations, and space rental from local colleges for job skills and basic education classes. Currently the county provides welfare-to-work funding while most of the services are delivered by community-based organizations. These one-stop centers are located in ethnically diverse neighborhoods characterized by poverty, low educational attainment, and high numbers of welfare recipients. The unique characteristics include the following:

1. a common intake form and computerized database which facilitate service referrals,
2. the inclusion of linguistic and cultural experts along with assessment tools in five languages,

3. an on-site community living room with comfortable furniture, television, videos, reading materials, and emergency child care,
4. assistance to individuals who are ineligible for county funds, and
5. information and referral assistance available from collaborative partners.

Neighborhood Self-Sufficiency Centers

To increase the access of low-income working parents to the resources they need to care for their children, Santa Clara County businesses, community groups, public and private agencies, and public assistance recipients began to collaborate with the county social services agency (SSA) in 1996 to develop one-stop, single-point-of-entry neighborhood centers (six) (see Chapter 14). In order to receive SSA funding, the centers need to provide TANF recipients with

1. vocational skills training, skills upgrade training, case management, job-placement services, job-retention assistance, and a variety of support services;
2. age-appropriate educational and recreational child care activities so that parents have time to receive assistance and pursue self-sufficiency; and
3. specialized classes on topics of interest to TANF recipients.

Furthermore, all centers must demonstrate a collaborative partnership with a minimum of three providers and be able to leverage additional revenues or in-kind services; the centers' ability to maximize funding has been a major success. For example, in addition to receiving $175,000 in SSA welfare-to-work funding, one center leveraged an additional $722,000 from several organizations for housing, family, and employment services. In relation to service delivery, the collaborative partnerships have increased the continuity of care received by TANF participants and are promoting interagency dialogue about service effectiveness and improvement.

Community-Wide Partnerships

Coalition to Address Homelessness

A community mobilization effort rarely has much influence on resource allocation decisions made by county social service staff. Typically funding constraints directly influence community service providers. In Napa County, however, a community coalition developed a proposal and received funding from the federal Department of Housing and Urban Development (HUD) to support an integrated network of services for the homeless, including TANF participants (see Chapter 15). The homeless were not being adequately served by existing local programs, especially to address the needs of domestic violence survivors and their children as well as individuals with substance abuse issues. While the county human services department served as the lead agency, community-based nonprofits provided the outreach services related to rental subsidies for transitional housing, case management, and referrals. The success of the new program is due, in large part, to its ability to effectively capitalize on the strengths of each of its partners, namely the ability of community-based agencies to reach the homeless and to effectively provide services along with the county's ability to assist in the leveraging of federal funds.

Building a Transitional Recovery Community

In order to assist homeless families recovering from substance abuse, a fourth unique partnership was undertaken in 1998 by several Monterey County human service agencies (see Chapter 16). The directors of housing, health, behavioral health, and social services developed "Pueblo Del Mar," a transitional recovery community offering eligible substance-abusing homeless families (including TANF participants) a variety of transitional support services (up to eighteen months). The services include substance abuse treatment, child protection, job training and employment, counseling, child care, independent living services, and parent education. In addition to assisting with program planning and development, community-based organizations deliver all of the direct services while the county housing authority is the property manager, property owner, and grant recipient of HUD funds earmarked for the maintenance of fifty-six housing units on a former military base (Fort Ord). Clinically, the program has been a success, as indicated by a low relapse rate (12 percent, or six relapses among the forty-nine families served in 1999). Administratively, the county directors found that bureaucratic opposition decreases substantially when all potential stakeholders, especially local government officials, participate actively in program planning meetings.

Coalition of Nonprofit Agencies

Another unique partnership which anticipated welfare reform is seen in the formation of the Napa County coalition of nonprofit agency directors (see Chapter 17). The coalition sought to develop a comprehensive human service system for all individuals (including TANF participants), regardless of their ability to pay, that addressed the multiple service gaps and fragmentation resulting from program closures. The Napa coalition of social, health, and behavioral health service representatives obtained foundation support to subsidize a variety of needed services including the following:

1. outpatient psychotherapy,
2. paraprofessional lay counseling and crisis counseling,
3. crisis hotlines,
4. in-home support services,
5. group counseling,
6. psychological assessments and evaluations,
7. family and play therapy,
8. youth development services, and
9. school-based supportive services.

As a result, these services have all become much more accessible, and the coalition has newfound political and economic power in the community. It has grown in membership and is increasingly called upon to provide input on a range of city and county issues.

Community College Collaborations

In addition to an increased number of partnerships with community-based organizations, county social service agencies are also working more closely with community colleges. Before the passage of TANF and Workforce Investment Act (WIA) legislation, the San Mateo County social services agency had recognized the merits of increased partnership with community colleges in order to help educate and train low-income individuals for employment as well as assist social service staff with skill enhancement. To address these shared objectives, local community colleges collaborated with the county departments of social service, health, and rehabilitation in order to develop a human services certificate program (see Chapter 18). The program prepares current human services staff, service consumers, and other interested individuals for entry-level occupations (e.g., mental health case manager, job coach/employment specialist, community health worker, and social service intake specialist). It includes five core courses and four electives related to case management and employment assistance. Each course includes forty-eight to fifty-four hours of instruction (three hours per week) that is completed in sixteen to eighteen weeks, and more than 150 employees of the social services agency and about 200 other adults have attended within the first three years of the program.

SOCIAL SERVICE AGENCY RESTRUCTURING

The last set of cases reflects some of the organizational changes brought about by the implementation of welfare reform in county social service agencies. They include (1) the hiring of an organizational development specialist to assist with changing the agency's culture, (2) the development of a new training program for staff serving TANF participants and other clients, (3) merging a workforce investment board and a social service agency into an employment and human services agency, (4) blending multiple funding streams into county welfare-to-work programs, and (5) restructuring agency programs to foster intra-agency collaboration between child welfare services and welfare-to-work programs.

Introducing Organizational Development

For assistance in managing organizational changes related, in large part, to welfare reform, social service agencies rarely recognize the value and capabilities of an internal organizational development (OD) specialist. However, as early as 1996, it became apparent that transforming an agency's culture would require an internal OD function in the San Mateo County Human Services Agency (see Chapter 19). A department-wide staff assessment indicated that personnel were struggling to keep up with the myriad of recent policy, organizational, and personnel changes, including the emergence of welfare reform. Top management supported the hiring of an OD specialist to help improve the agency's problem-solving and learning processes, particularly through a more effective and collaborative assessment of the organizational culture (McLagan, 1989). OD in public agencies can work particularly well with modest goals that relate to reducing conflict and improving communication and can tackle manageable issues, but not an entire system at one time (Golembiewski, Proehl, and Sink, 1982; Stupak and Moore, 1987). The agency found OD to be especially helpful in the implementation of welfare reform and in addressing staff issues arising from partnerships with a variety of community-based organizations.

Family Development Credential

One of the biggest challenges facing social service agencies implementing welfare reform was the need to retrain line staff who needed to make the transition from the job functions of individual eligibility determination to family-focused employability enhancement. This case study (see Chapter 20) describes the efforts of a county human services agency to train line staff (high school and college graduates) in collaborative case management to deliver strength-based services within a new interdisciplinary service system. It focuses on the start-up and implementation of the family development credential (FDC) in San Mateo County, California. The FDC is a comprehensive training program that enables paraprofessionals from a wide range of human service agencies to help families solve problems and achieve enduring self-sufficiency. The curriculum addresses the following topics: family development, worker self-empowerment, relationship building with families, communication skills, culturally competent practice, ongoing assessment, home visiting, accessing specialized services, facilitating family conferencing and support groups, and promoting interagency collaboration. All these skills are designed to enable TANF participants and other clients to become more self-reliant, become their own "case managers," develop informal support networks, and engage more successfully with other community resources.

Merging Employment and Social Service Agencies

Currently the California one-stop employment centers are managed and operated jointly by workforce investment boards (WIBs were formerly called private industry councils) and the county social service agencies to promote universal access to welfare-to-work services. The Workforce Investment Act of 1998 created new Department of Labor funding and functions for the WIBs that overlapped with TANF funds and services. In some locations, such as Contra Costa County, the two organizations actually merged into a single employment and human services agency in which the CalWORKs funding continues to flow through the newly restructured social service agency (see Chapter 21). In a break from tradition, the WIB executive director directly oversees CalWORKs policy instead of the social services director. Although it has been a challenge to blend the different staff perspectives (e.g., WIB staff tend to be more employer centered and CalWORKs staff tend to be more employee centered), the merger has increased the communication, cooperation, and resource sharing between the two program areas.

Blending Funding Streams

In addition to the restructuring processes related to organizational development and agency mergers, Bay Area social service organizations have utilized the flexibility of the TANF block grants to creatively pool funding streams in order to design more client-responsive programs. The Sonoma County social service agency, for example, pooled financial resources to support community-based service programs (e.g., the Summer Youth Conservation Corps and Social Advocates for Youth) (see Chapter 22). Although some funds are kept by the county to offset administrative expenses, the majority of funds are distributed through cost reimbursement service contracts based on specific eligibility criteria. For example, in keeping with CalWORKs funding guidelines, 40 percent of children in the youth programs must be TANF eligible. To satisfy WIB funding requirements, 30 percent of total funds to each program must address the needs of out-of-school youths aged fourteen to twenty-one. One advantage of pooling CalWORKs and WIB funds is that social service consumers can receive WIB services after their eligibility has expired for the CalWORKs program. In addition, the social service organization can ensure the survival of programs that are struggling financially by blending funding streams. The ultimate value of using alternate methods of funding services is reflected in situations in which the state funding formula does not always fit the needs of the local residents.

Linking TANF to Child Welfare Services

In addition to restructuring their administration and funding, social service agencies are finding new ways to increase their intradepartmental collaboration. For example, to meet the needs of social service consumers who are involved with both child welfare programs (designed to protect children from maltreatment) and welfare-to-work programs (designed to facilitate economic self-sufficiency), there is a growing recognition that 40 to 60 percent of the consumers are participating in both programs. This percentage is referred to as the crossover rate (Riverside County, 1998; Zeller, 1999). The necessity of addressing the needs of this crossover population becomes very apparent when a single parent must be in court or parenting class at the same time he or she is required to participate in employment activities to maintain welfare-to-work benefits. Failure to fulfill child welfare responsibilities could result in the drastic decision to place a child in foster care. Similarly, the failure to meet welfare-to-work requirements could result in the loss of financial benefits. After a crossover case has been identified, Contra Costa social services agency staff deliver crossover services by connecting the workers in both programs, promoting a dialogue about the consumer's program needs, and collaborating with the consumer to develop a coordinated plan of action (see Chapter 23). This method of crossover service delivery helps to resolve conflicting consumer obligations. In addition, the increased communication between divisions helps to prevent the inefficient use of resources and the duplication or fragmentation of services.

THE CROSSCUTTING THEMES OF INNOVATIVE PROGRAMS AND PRACTICES

Using the comparative case study method to assess this array of innovative programs and practices emerging during the era of welfare reform implementation, the following themes emerge: (1) the cases cluster into the three categories of innovative service delivery, new community partnership, and organizational restructuring, (2) the cases reflect a new service delivery model that can be assessed using a social development framework, (3) the cases provide an array of implementation challenges, and (4) a variety of lessons can be learned from the development of innovative programs and practices.

Innovative Service Delivery

Several common themes in service delivery have emerged. Social service organizations are *ensuring universal eligibility* to employment services (e.g., Alameda County's Neighborhood Jobs Pilot Initiative), behavioral health services (e.g., the Napa County coalition of nonprofit organizations), and services for the substance-abusing homeless population (e.g., the Napa County Transitional Residential Alliance). The scope of services has also expanded, as social service organizations are *more actively assisting community residents with transportation* (e.g., the Connections Shuttle in Santa Cruz County and the Guaranteed Ride Home in Santa Clara County) and *child care* (e.g., the Exempt Provider Training Program in San Mateo). In addition, the personal obstacles to labor force participation such as low basic work skills, mental health problems, chemical dependency, or medical problems are more easily addressed when they are *colocated in a single facility* (e.g., integrating mental health and substance abuse services into the Sonoma County welfare-to-work program). Services are frequently colocated in one-stop employment centers to increase consumer access, service utilization, staff communication, employment in the community, and job retention.

Furthermore, social service organizations are *actively engaged in promoting the employment of welfare participants* by providing them with jobs and training, addressing public agency staffing shortages, and setting an example for the larger community (e.g., hiring TANF participants to work in the San Mateo County Human Services Agency). Publicly supported job creation often *combines business with rehabilitation,* such as the San Mateo County WorkCenter where participants are employed to satisfy the job demands of private industry (e.g., packaging and shipping) and at the same time receive support services and assistance with job training, placement, and retention.

New Community Partnerships

Social service organizations are *increasingly involved with community-based organizations and coalitions* in building partnerships as seen in the neighborhood-oriented approaches to service delivery. County social services agencies often serve as the lead administrative agencies due to their access to resources and their ability to leverage funds. In a similar way, community-based nonprofits take the lead in delivering many of the services because of their more intimate understanding of local needs and neighborhoods. In working more closely with community-based organizations, social service agencies are *increasing their partnership with community residents,* as is evident in San Mateo County's Adopt-A-Family Program that recruits godparents to provide material and social assistance to TANF participants.

Furthermore, social service agencies are expanding collaboration within their organizations, as seen in the coordinated case planning in Contra Costa County's child welfare and welfare-to-work crossover service programs. In addition, social service agencies are increasing internal collaboration between all programs and staff members when they involve organizational development specialists to improve staff collaboration in order to prevent the fragmentation of services.

Increased collaboration between agencies is also evident in Contra Costa County's comprehensive one-stop employment centers, Monterey County's Pueblo Del Mar wraparound services program, and the San Mateo County community college human services certificate program.

Organizational Restructuring

As part of helping low-income working individuals find employment and become self-sufficient, social service agencies are finally able to design and implement innovative employment and training programs. This change emerges, in part, as a result of the increased flexibility of federal TANF and workforce legislation which allow for *combining funding streams in order to be more responsive to the needs of local residents.*

Social service organizations are also finding more effective ways to deliver services by *merging* with other organizations such as workforce investment boards, housing organizations, and health departments. Mergers frequently increase communication, cooperation, and resource sharing between two organizations despite the complexity of the process. In addition, the combined expertise of personnel in merged organizations can increase the quality of service planning and delivery, especially when funding streams are blended.

Finally, social service organizations are *improving problem-solving and learning processes* by actively using organizational development techniques (e.g., staff feedback and self-assessment tools) to address such issues as increasing cultural competence or feedback on implementing strategic plans. The techniques are also used to increase attention to program outcomes as well as increase staff capabilities in fostering teamwork. New training programs are also increasing the problem-solving capabilities of staff members.

A Synthesis of Crosscutting Themes

It is helpful to examine the underlying forces fostering unique programs and practices in order to understand the crosscutting themes of innovative service delivery, new partnership, and organizational restructuring. The restructuring of social service agencies can be viewed as part of an ongoing process of increasing public accountability. The accountability process incorporates private-sector principles (e.g., organizational development and a greater emphasis on accountability and cost-effectiveness) that are needed to foster increased flexibility (e.g., the combination of funding streams and crossover services) to address a wider range of human needs (e.g., in health, housing, transportation, and child care). In addition, social service organizations are restructuring in order to improve services by focusing on the removal of barriers to labor-force participation (e.g., mental health or substance abuse problems) in order to promote job training, placement, and retention. Service availability and effectiveness are enhanced through partnerships with other county or state public agencies (e.g., the housing authority or the department of transportation), community coalitions (e.g., the Alameda County Neighborhood Jobs Partnership Initiative), and community service providers (e.g., the San Mateo County Exempt Child Care Provider Training Project). Typically community-based organizations deliver many of the services while county social service agencies provide financial, supervisory, or technical oversight along with seeking the continuous input and involvement of local residents.

THE SOCIAL DEVELOPMENT MODEL FOR CROSS-CASE ANALYSIS

In addition to describing the cases in relation to service delivery, partnership, and organizational restructuring, the innovative programs and practices can be analyzed in relation to current concepts of social development. Midgley (1997) defines social development as "a process of planned social change designed to promote the well-being of the population as a whole in conjunction with a dynamic process of economic development" (p. 181). The model is based on the following four principles: (1) participating in a productive economy is the preferred mechanism for meeting economic and social needs, (2) investing in individuals and communities can create opportunities and enhance capacities, (3) the free market is not adequate to meet all social needs and government is needed to promote and facilitate self-sufficiency in partnership with individuals and communities, and (4) a minority of individuals require long-term social and economic supports.

Midgley (1997) describes three types of social development programs that promote economic growth by investing in social welfare. *Programs that emphasize employment* (labor-force attachment) help low-income individuals and welfare recipients participate more fully in the labor force, thereby reducing welfare dependency and increasing tax revenues. *Social capital programs* enhance the volume and intensity of cooperative networks and social relationships in communities, social and economic infrastructure (e.g., clinics, schools, housing), and individual asset accumulation (e.g., matched savings accounts). Third, *human capital programs* promote economic growth by investing directly in individual welfare (e.g., education, health care, nutrition). The cases can be clustered according to these three types of social development programs as follows:

1. Programs/practices that emphasize employment (Labor-force attachment)
   - The JobKeeper Program
   - The Neighborhood Jobs Pilot Initiative
   - Neighborhood self-sufficiency centers
   - The merging of workforce investment boards and social service agencies
   - The blending of multiple funding streams into welfare-to-work programs
   - The hiring of TANF recipients in social service agencies
   - The family loan program
   - The colocation of support services in welfare-to-work programs
2. Programs/practices that invest in social capital
   - The Connections Shuttle
   - The Guaranteed Ride Home Program
   - The Transitional Residential Alliance and Integrated Network
   - Wraparound services for homeless families
   - The Adopt-A-Family Program
   - Coalition of nonprofit agencies
   - Introducting OD principles within social service agencies
   - Crossover services between child welfare and welfare-to-work services
   - Family development credential

3. Programs/practices that invest in human capital
   - The WorkCenter
   - Child care provider training
   - Collaboration between community colleges and social service agencies
   - Individual development accounts

Within this framework, most of the cases reflect an investment in employment and social capital related to the self-sufficiency emphasis of the TANF legislation. As a result, there appears to be a greater need for investment in human capital. In other words, the first wave of work-first strategies has been successful in reducing welfare caseloads, promoting employment, and building community networks, yet future efforts are needed to help the low-income working population (1) further their general education, (2) advance in their careers, and (3) access community supports that are needed to maintain long-term family self-sufficiency.

THE CHALLENGE OF SUSTAINING INNOVATIONS

Underlying these crosscutting themes are continuing challenges that impact the ability of innovative programs and practices to be sustained over time. They reflect the three themes of service delivery, partnerships, and organizational restructuring. With respect to service delivery, one of the biggest challenges relates to the hard-to-place TANF participant who must contend with a very competitive workforce environment in the job search, let alone sustain employment by managing new work-related expenses (i.e., transportation, child care, medical care, and work clothes). Another service delivery challenge is to maintain client confidentiality in integrated service environments which rely on interagency communication, resource sharing, and collaborative case planning.

With respect to creating and sustaining collaborative partnerships, a major challenge involves the time it takes to build and maintain coalitions, especially dealing with diverse political perspectives and personalities. Furthermore, when relying on several different agencies for service delivery, it is often difficult to maintain consistency across the agencies in terms of the services that clients receive, staff responsibilities, and organizational objectives. Finally, sustaining a collaborative vision is a challenge when program implementation is often seen as more difficult than program design.

Several challenges also relate to organizational restructuring. First, when new policies and procedures have not yet been fully operational and staff positions are changing, considerable confusion can ensue. For example, when social service staff who had engaged primarily in client screening and eligibility take on new client employability mandates, it is not surprising to find role confusion and skill deficits. Second, maintaining highly qualified staff members is a challenge for most social service agencies, especially when new employees must be trained in the new family self-sufficiency service delivery model. Third, it has been difficult to structure multifunctional service delivery teams to present a wide range of employment and social services within the guidelines of welfare-to-work policies.

LESSONS LEARNED

Dealing with these challenges requires consensus building, motivation for organizational reform, and maintaining momentum. These case studies illustrate several lessons learned.

1. In relation to client services, social service agencies implementing welfare reforms need to *provide extra staff support and transitional time to assist individuals making the transition from welfare to work*. This support contributes significantly to job retention and career advancement, especially through mentoring relationships and expanded work internship opportunities. In addition, social service agencies need to *build strong working relationships* with local businesses, landlords, transportation agencies, and child care programs in order to better *assist consumers with these common obstacles to labor-force participation*.
2. With respect to staff, social service agencies implementing welfare reform need to use *teams of staff members to effectively promote significant change* based on clear organizational mandates. They have also learned to *anticipate and proactively address personnel issues* related to merging organizational functions in order to help staff understand that complex issues can be resolved over time and that change and risk are inevitable. Furthermore, social service agencies have learned to *schedule a substantial number of staff meetings to clarify changing roles in an evolving system and provide information to all levels of staff at the same time*.
3. With respect to developing partnerships, social service agencies that implement welfare reforms need to identify and *include all potential stakeholders* (especially local government officials whose support is needed for implementing new practices) *in program planning meetings* in order to decrease bureaucratic opposition, facilitate project investment, and strengthen working relationships. It is equally important to *promote team-building opportunities* for different public and private agency representatives in order to enhance partnerships, pursue common community goals, and build the high level of communi-

cation and trust that is necessary for collaborative partners with different values or cultural practices.
4. Finally, in relation to community building, social service agencies implementing welfare reform need to *assess in a comprehensive manner the needs of the community* and balance these needs with programs or services that funders will support, especially *locating unrestricted funding* to cover administrative and start-up costs for pilot projects and services. It is also important to expand their media relations capacities in order to *increase public awareness of new services* through the use of flyers, phone calls, Web sites, and presentations to reach a greater number of needy individuals and enhance community support. Social service agencies also need to expand their capacity to *provide outreach efforts that are culturally and linguistically appropriate* to address the needs of local residents (self-referral is not always effective in reaching socially isolated, low-income community members) and to *minimize bureaucratic procedures* and costs in order to facilitate consumer access to services.

CONCLUSION

This collection of case studies describes programs and practices that were selected for their innovative contribution to welfare reform implementation. The cases cluster into three categories. Most of the cases involve new approaches to service delivery, including the removal of barriers to workforce participation and self-sufficiency support services. The support programs include vocational rehabilitation, transportation, child care, loans, and other temporary assistance which facilitates self-reliance. The crosscutting themes include ensuring universal eligibility, more actively assisting community residents with transportation and child care, colocating services in a single facility, and actively promoting the employment of welfare recipients.

The cases related to community partnership often involve local interorganizational relationships that address employment, housing, income, education, mental health, and substance abuse. The emerging partnerships are usually with community-based organizations, neighborhood coalitions, other agencies (state, county, and city), and community residents.

The third set of cases describe social service agency restructuring, including the introduction of organizational development, a new staff training program, the merging of employment and human services, the blending of funding streams, and the linking of TANF to child welfare services. Organizational restructuring themes relate to program funding, program integration, intra-agency collaboration, and organizational learning processes.

These case studies of innovative programs and practices represent works in progress. Some will grow and become permanent, some will struggle and become integrated with other services, and others will phase out. Predicting the sustainability of innovations is difficult. However, several lessons have been learned to date. With regard to service delivery, social service organizations engaged in implementing welfare reforms need to

1. provide extra staff support and time to assist individuals in making the transition from welfare to work,
2. build strong collaborative interorganizational relationships, and
3. assist TANF participants with obstacles to labor-force participation.

In relationship to community partnerships, social service agencies need to

1. use teams to promote significant change,
2. proactively address collaboration-related personnel issues,
3. schedule a substantial number of staff meetings to clarify changing roles in an evolving system, and
4. carefully identify and include all potential stakeholders.

Finally, in relation to organizational restructuring, social service organizations implementing welfare reform need to

1. promote team-building opportunities,
2. assess comprehensively the needs of the community,
3. creatively use unrestricted funding,
4. expand their media relations capacities in order to increase public awareness of new services,
5. expand their capacity to provide outreach efforts that are culturally and linguistically appropriate, and
6. minimize bureaucratic procedures.

NOTE

1. According to Yin (1992), a case study represents an empirical investigation of a contemporary phenomena within its real-life context using multiple sources of evidence (agency documents, staff perceptions, and client perceptions). The purpose of a case study is to analyze in detail an individual, a situation, or a single phenomena in order to identify new understandings and/or lessons learned (Dufour and Fortin, 1992).

Karbo and Beasley (1999) describe four types of case studies. The first type is an atheoretical study that *holistically* describes a phenomena but is not guided by hypothesis testing or theory building. The second type is an *interpretive* study that uses concepts to understand the case. The third type (the *heuristic* study) investigates a case in order to build a theory, and fourth, the *plausibility* study determines whether the phenomena is consistent with existing theory. The cases in this book are both descriptively holistic (type one) in that the innovative programs and practices are fully described with lessons learned. This overview chapter provides the interpretive dimension (type two) whereby conclusions are drawn by comparing the cases with one another. Karbo and Beasley (1999) refer to this interpretive process as the *comparative case study method* that is designed to systematically examine patterns within and across cases in order to trace change over time and offer an interpretation of the findings.

Each case study is based on information obtained from interviews with Bay Area social service agency staff and consumers as well as written documents (along with a brief literature review) relevant to each program or practice. Data were collected by social welfare graduate students from June 1999 to June 2001 using such questions and follow-up probes as the following:

1. How did the program get started?
2. What have been some of the difficulties or barriers to implementing the program?
3. How would you describe some of the program success as well as lessons learned from implementing the program?

The cases are clustered into three areas. The first set features new approaches to service delivery that help low-income working individuals find employment and become self-sufficient. The second group includes neighborhood and community-wide partnerships that help to provide low-income individuals with affordable housing, education, job training, and a variety of social, health, and behavioral health services. The third cluster involves organizational changes inside social service agencies brought about by implementing welfare reforms.

REFERENCES

Bush, I.R. and Kraft, M.K. (1998). The voices of welfare reform. *Public Welfare, 56,* 11-21.

Cameron, K.S. and Quinn, R.E. (1999). *Diagnosing and changing organizational culture: Based on the competing values framework.* Reading, MA: Addison-Wesley.

Danziger, S., Corcoran, M., Danziger, S., Heflin, C., Kalil, J., Levine, J., Rosen, D., Seefeldt, K., Siefert, K., and Tolman, R. (1999). Barriers to the employment of welfare recipients. University of Michigan Poverty Research and Training Center. Available at <http://www.fordschool.umich.edu/poverty/publications.htm>.

Dufour, S. and Fortin, D. (1992). Annotated bibliography on case study method. *Current Sociology, 40*(1), 167-181.

Edin, K. and Lein, L. (1997). *Making ends meet: How single mothers survive welfare and low-wage work.* New York: Russell Sage Foundation.

Golembiewski, R., Proehl, C. Jr., and Sink, D. (1982). Estimating the success of OD applications. *Training and Development Journal, 36*(4), 86-95.

Grayson, M. (1999). Kicking habits: Preparing welfare recipients for the work force. *Spectrum: The Journal of State Government, 72*(1), 5-7.

Karbo, J. and Beasley, R.K. (1999). A practical guide to the comparative case study method in political psychology. *Political Psychology, 20*(2), 369-391.

Kramer, F.D. (1998). The hard-to-place: Understanding the population and strategies to serve them. *The Welfare Information Network, 2*(5), 1-16.

Loprest, P.J. and Acs, G. (1996). Profile of disability among AFDC families. The Urban Institute. Available at <http://www.urban.org/periodcl/26_2/prr26_2d.htm>.

McLagan, P. (1989). *Models for HRD practice.* Alexandria, VA: American Society for Training and Development.

Midgely, J. (1997). *Social welfare in global context.* California, London, and New Delhi: Sage Publications.

Olson, K. and Pavetti, L. (1996). Personal and family challenges to the successful transition from welfare to work. The Urban Institute. Available at <http://www.urban.org/welfare/report1.htm>.

Pavetti, L.A. (1996). Time on welfare and welfare dependency. Testimony before the House Ways and Means Committee, Subcommittee on Human Resources. The Urban Institute. Available at <http://www.urban.org/url.cfm?ID=900288>.

Pavetti, L., Olson, K., Nightingale, D., Duke, A., and Isaacs, J. (1997). Welfare-to-work options for families facing personal and family challenges: Rationale and program strategies. The Urban Institute. Available at <http://www.urban.org/url.cfm?ID=410337>.

Riverside County (1998). Child welfare services—CalWORKs interface. Unpublished internal document.

Stupak, R. and Moore, J. (1987). The practice of managing organization development in public sector organizations: Reassessments, realities, and rewards. *International Journal of Public Administration, 10*(2), 131-153.

Wilson, W. (1996). *When work disappears: The world of the new urban poor.* New York: Alfred A. Knopf.

Yin, R.K. (1992). The case study method as a tool for doing evaluation. *Current Sociology, 40*(1), 121-137.

Young, N. and Gardner, S. (1997). *Implementing welfare reform: Solutions to the substance abuse problem.* Washington, DC: Children and Family Futures and Drug Strategies.

Zeller, D.E. (1999). Welfare reform impacts on child welfare caseloads: A research agenda. The Arkansas Department of Human Services, Division of Children and Family Services. Available at <http://www.state.ar.us/dhs/chilnfam/nawrs/wriocwc.html>.

SECTION II:
REDEFINING SERVICE DELIVERY

REMOVING BARRIERS TO WORKFORCE PARTICIPATION

Chapter 3

Connections Shuttle: Transportation for CalWORKs Participants

Debbie Downes
Michael J. Austin

The Santa Cruz County Connections Shuttle is a transportation option for California Work Opportunity and Responsibility to Kids Program (CalWORKs) welfare-to-work participants. The Connections Shuttle consists of a small fleet of vans with drivers and dispatchers who work together to bring people from their homes to work and work-related destinations, including child care and job training. The primary purpose of the Connections Shuttle is to respond to the great need for transportation among CalWORKs families whose jobs are often far from their homes. Public transportation in Santa Cruz and adjoining counties is often insufficient for travel to work, school, child care, and errands from outlying areas. The Connections Shuttle provides temporary aid in the transition from welfare to work. The secondary purpose of the Connections Shuttle is to train welfare-to-work participants to become drivers and dispatchers. They are hired for a seven-month training period, during which they receive a Class B license, allowing them to drive commercial, fifteen-passenger vehicles.

BRIEF LITERATURE REVIEW

Transportation is a major obstacle for welfare recipients seeking work. Harbaugh and Smith (1998) found that public transit does not serve many rural areas, which is where many low-income families choose to live because housing is more affordable than in urban areas. Twenty-six percent of families below the poverty level do not own cars and must rely on public transportation. They often make multiple transfers to travel a relatively short distance. Harbaugh and Smith (1998) concluded that innovative, collaborative transportation options are necessary to help CalWORKs participants find and maintain employment.

Blumenberg and Ong (1997) studied a random sample of Aid to Families with Dependent Children (AFDC) recipients who worked in Los Angeles in 1992. They found that those who travel the farthest from home earn the least amount of money because actual travel expenses and opportunity costs reduce their take-home earnings. The cost of private transportation and availability of public transportation make it more desirable for recipients to seek employment close to their homes. For some welfare recipients, it is cheaper to stay at home and receive aid than it is to travel to work. Creating jobs in poor areas benefits those who live there by reducing their job-related expenses. However, as Blumenberg and Ong (1997) point out, it is difficult to create an adequate supply of jobs in inner cities and rural areas. They concluded that accessible and affordable transportation is necessary to cut job-related expenses for welfare recipients.

Kaplan (1998) calls attention to the multiple transportation needs of CalWORKs participants. Often they need to travel to and from work, child care, health care, shopping, and an assortment of other services. She recommends that vehicles used to transport senior citizens, people with disabilities, Head Start participants, and schoolchildren be shared with CalWORKs recipients. Many organizations use their vehicles only at certain times of the day. CalWORKs programs could operate the vehicles when they are not in use.

In summary, transportation is a major barrier for CalWORKs participants seeking and maintaining employment. Many low-income families live in rural areas without access to a car, and public transportation routes do not provide adequate transport to work, home, child care, or a variety of other necessary errands. If CalWORKs participants are to find and maintain employment, they need a transportation option that provides for their needs.

HISTORY

CalWORKs legislation (Assembly Bill 1542) requires counties to assist CalWORKs welfare-to-work participants with transportation, child care, and job training. Assembly Bill 2454 requires county welfare departments and local and regional transportation agencies to work together to develop and implement a plan that identifies transportation options for CalWORKs participants. In 1997, the Transportation Task Force of the Santa Cruz County Coalition for Workforce Preparation was created to develop a plan that would meet CalWORKs' requirements. The Coalition for Workforce Preparation is an informal consortium consisting of representatives from local school districts, community colleges, transportation associations, child care organizations, environmental organizations, employers, business organizations, training providers, employment agencies, job seekers, and social services. The coalition works with the business community in Santa Cruz County to help CalWORKs participants find employment and to develop collaborative solutions for transportation problems that do not increase traffic or degrade air quality. Through the Transportation Task Force, the coalition helps to provide transportation for CalWORKs participants.

In 1997, there were over 6,000 adult CalWORKs recipients, with another 6,000 children in Santa Cruz County; the Transportation Task Force surveyed them. Box 3.1 provides some highlights of the findings. CalWORKs families indicated that transportation was the second most significant barrier in the search for employment, after child care. They were seeking safe, reliable, flexible, and affordable transportation. Many survey respondents noted that the fixed route system of public transportation did not work for them because they needed to make multiple stops on the way to and from work to pick up and drop off their children. In addition, many CalWORKs recipients live in rural areas, where public transportation is often inadequate for low-income families. In order to help them become self-sufficient, CalWORKs families in Santa Cruz County needed a supplement to public transportation. Many of the available jobs are in adjoining counties and the bus system within Santa Cruz County and between counties was often insufficient for regional job search or employment.

With the survey findings, the Transportation Task Force began to develop an array of ideas including multiple stops, midday service, transport in rural areas, and transport in emergency situations such as picking up a sick child from school. In January 1998, they produced a plan for what they called the Connections Shuttle. By Fall 1998 they had identified $412,700 in funding from the county social services agency in the form of CalWORKs (Temporary Assistance for Needy Families), a governor's discretionary 15 percent

> **BOX 3.1. Transportation Needs of CalWORKs Participants in Santa Cruz County**
>
> Currently, children travel to and from school and child care in the following ways:
>
> - 43 percent get rides with a parent
> - 37 percent take the bus
> - 36 percent walk
> - 15 percent get a ride with another relative
> - 12 percent ride bicycles
> - 11 percent get a ride with a neighbor
>
> Once a CalWORKs recipient finds work, his or her children will travel to and from school and child care in the following ways:
>
> - 41 percent will get rides with the parent
> - 36 percent will take the bus
> - 28 percent will walk
> - 19 percent will get a ride with a relative
> - 9 percent will ride bicycles
> - 9 percent will get a ride with a neighbor
> - 3 percent will receive transportation from their day care agency
>
> CalWORKs parents run errands in the following ways:
>
> - 53 percent drive themselves
> - 37 percent take the bus
> - 34 percent walk
> - 27 percent get a ride with a relative
> - 12 percent ride bicycles
> - 12 percent get rides with neighbors
> - 9 percent ask others to run errands for them
>
> Of the CalWORKs recipients who responded:
>
> - 76 percent would be very likely to use a shuttle service for themselves and their children if it were available
> - 40 percent would be willing to pay $1 to $2 per ride
> - 36 percent would pay less than $1 per ride
> - 17 percent would ride only if it were free
> - 58 percent own a car
>
> Among car owners, when their vehicles are not working:
>
> - 50 percent walk to complete their errands
> - 47 percent take the bus
>
> *(continued)*

(continued)
- 37 percent ride with a relative
- 26 percent borrow a car
- 24 percent ride with a neighbor
- 18 percent ride a bicycle
- 15 percent ask someone else to run the errand for them

When traveling to work:
- 71 percent of participants must stop one to two times to drop off children or run other errands

On the way home from work:
- 80 percent of participants must stop one to three times to pick up children or run other errands

If conveniently available, respondents preferred the following travel alternatives:
- 55 percent bus
- 48 percent carpooling
- 45 percent walking
- 34 percent bicycling
- 28 percent telecommuting
- 23 percent vanpooling
- 16 percent train

The following factors would encourage participants to use a travel alternative:
- emergency ride home (67 percent of participants)
- extra compensation for using an alternative (62 percent)
- child care at the work site (59 percent)
- discounted bus passes (58 percent)
- convenient bus routes (54 percent)
- fast bus routes (54 percent)
- employers subsidizing commute costs (51 percent)

welfare-to-work grant, and Job Access/Reverse Commute organization funds from the Federal Transit Administration.

Job trainers, job seekers, and employers take an active part in transportation planning so that the shuttle responds to the changing needs of its clients. Planning for transportation, child care, and workforce preparation involved consideration of transportation issues for low-income job seekers, trainees, and their children.

PROGRAM OPERATIONS

The first goal of the Connections Shuttle is to meet the immediate transportation needs of CalWORKs participants in order to help them make the transition from welfare to work. The shuttle is not meant to be a permanent source of transportation for low-income workers but a temporary aid to help welfare-to-work participants find and retain jobs. The primary goal of the shuttle program is to remove transportation as a barrier to employment, workforce preparation, and/or child care programs by making transportation available to job seekers, students, workers, and their children.

The second goal of the Connections Shuttle is to provide job training for CalWORKs participants, qualifying them to receive the Class B license needed to operate commercial, fifteen-passenger vehicles. CalWORKs recipients are trained for seven months as dispatchers and drivers for the Connections Shuttle. Topics covered in training include employee policies, workplace conduct, licensing requirements, driving skills, emergency procedures and protocol, passenger assistance, passenger policies, and dispatch and scheduling procedures. Box 3.2 reproduces the table of contents of the training manual. Trainees are also given the opportunity to be trained as mechanics or school bus drivers.

Food and Nutrition Services, Incorporated (now known as Community Bridges), a community-based organization, operates the Connections Shuttle. The following list shows the partners that support the Connections Shuttle and their roles:

- Food and Nutrition Services: Consolidated Transportation Services Agency, service provider for shuttle service
- Human Resources Agency/CareerWorks: CalWORKs provider and welfare-to-work formula and competitive grant recipient; operates Job Training Partnership Act program
- Santa Cruz County Regional Transportation Commission: planning
- Association of Monterey Bay Area Governments: planning
- Private Industry Council: oversees welfare-to-work services
- Santa Cruz Metropolitan Transit District: coordinates bus routes
- Employment Development Department: provides labor market information
- Santa Cruz Area/Pajaro Valley Transportation Management Associations: educate business owners and managers about shuttle services and transportation subsidy programs; train welfare agency and human resources agency staff

- Service Workers International Union Local 415: support for the program
- United Transportation Union Local 23: support for the program

Since 1979, this agency has contracted with multiple county, state, and local jurisdictions and the local transit district to provide child care, child food programs, adult day care, meals-on-wheels, and paratransit services to residents of Santa Cruz County. In 1982, the State of California required each county to designate a Consolidated Transportation Services Agency (CTSA) to oversee specialized transportation to county residents. Santa Cruz County designated Food and Nutrition Services as the local CTSA. They focus mainly on serving elderly and disabled county residents, although the Connections Shuttle qualifies as a CTSA program. In the fiscal year 1998-1999, they provided over 165,000 rides to county residents.

The Connections Shuttle contract was signed in February 1999, and Deana Davidson became the shuttle project supervisor. She immediately instituted the training program for shuttle drivers. In March 1999, the first

---

BOX 3.2. Components of the Connections Shuttle Training Manual

Section A—Orientation

Part 1: Welcome
Part 2: Employee Policies
Part 3: Workplace Conduct
Part 4: Training and Licensing Overview

Section B—Driver Training

Part 1: Basic Driving Skills
Part 2: Defensive Driving
Part 3: Emergencies
Part 4: Driver Procedures
Part 5: Emergency Protocol
Part 6: Accident Procedures
Part 7: Passenger Assistance

Section C—Office Training

Part 1: Passenger Policies
Part 2: Office Staff
Part 3: Dispatch Procedures
Part 4: Scheduling Procedures

group of four were hired and trained to be drivers and dispatchers. During the seven-month training period, all trainees are paid and taught both driving and dispatching skills in order to qualify them for as many jobs as possible. The first group worked in pairs, one driver and one dispatcher for the morning and evening shifts. In April 1999, the shuttle began operation and recruited the next four trainees. After three months, the shuttle had fourteen drivers and dispatchers and six vans. Three vans were purchased with state welfare-to-work matching funds, and three were taken from the Food and Nutrition Services vanpool and reconditioned. Eventually, the Federal Transit District provided funds for four additional vans.

In July 1999, the Connections Shuttle hired a temporary CalWORKs trainee to work in the office, and in November of that year they hired a permanent assistant staff trainer to conduct the driver and dispatcher trainings. In February 2000, a trainee was hired as a permanent office assistant. The Connections Shuttle currently runs five routes. The most frequent routes are between Watsonville and Santa Cruz, with many stops to drop off and pick up children at various places. The initial goal was to provide 100 one-way rides to individuals per day. In the first week of service, the Connections Shuttle provided seventeen individual rides. They are now providing over 133 individual rides per day, and they have difficulties adding new passengers because the vans are full to capacity. Given the high demand, the shuttle staff plan to expand services and provide rides for everyone who requests the shuttle.

In Santa Cruz County, CareerWorks operates under the human resources agency, which is the county social service agency. CareerWorks encompasses both CalWORKs assistance and the work training and employment services. CareerWorks staff refer their clients to the Connections Shuttle driver training program. Every six weeks, the shuttle announces openings in a training class. CareerWorks staff are constantly searching their caseloads for qualified driving trainees. Trainees must be in the welfare-to-work formula grant program designed for people with special barriers to work. Some of the major barriers include receiving welfare for over thirty months, lack of a high school diploma, receiving low scores on reading and math competency tests, recovering from substance abuse, being homeless, and having a poor work history. Trainees are also required to have clean driving records and to have passed a drug test.

The Connections Shuttle provides low-income families with the transportation that they need to enter the workforce and become self-sufficient, as well as training for those who are seeking work. "When I started having something to look forward to, I started to feel good about myself and my life," says Anita, a former driver/dispatcher.

It's a job, but there's a lot of support. If you can't find the support you need from the other drivers, you can turn to the administration. Drivers and administration give a lot of emotional support so that no one feels intimidated in asking for help.... What you get out of the job is what you put into it. People who invest in the program tend to move on to bigger and better things.

PROGRAM SUCCESSES

One of the employment and training specialists for the Human Resources Agency, CareerWorks Division, who recommends clients to the Connections Shuttle training program, reports an increase in self-esteem through participation in the program. "They are part of a team, they're treated well, and they have an important job," she explains. "The drivers help others get to work as they themselves find work, and they feel good about that."

A state labor market analyst and member of the Childcare Task Force includes in his list of Connections Shuttle successes, "Raising the consciousness of the community and getting people from different agencies to work together." The Transportation Task Force pulled together people from many community and government organizations and encouraged them to find the best solution for the lack of transportation for CalWORKs recipients. In line with the temporary nature of the Connections Shuttle, only twenty of the original clients are still using the shuttle. Most of the riders have found other solutions for their transportation needs.

The Connections Shuttle has helped thirty-three drivers to obtain their Class B licenses. Of those, ten are still employed by the shuttle. Three were unable to complete the training due to illness or difficulties and three have moved to unknown locations. The other seventeen drivers successfully transitioned into outside jobs, using the skills they learned from the Connections Shuttle.

Morale among drivers and dispatchers is also an integral part of the shuttle's success. The shuttle drivers have formed a morale committee which focuses on managing conflicts and maintaining high morale. Each month, two volunteers serve along with the shuttle project supervisor on the committee. They address all recommendations from the suggestion box and plan staff parties.

Sammy, a former Connections Shuttle driver and dispatcher, finished his training and was hired as a driver at a nonprofit agency. He is grateful for the opportunity that the shuttle offered him:

> Connections Shuttle gives you confidence. Working in the lettuce fields, I felt I was missing something, wasting away, not using my po-

tential. When I came to Connections, I found total support. I learned from my mistakes. I feel confident that I can compete in the job market now. . . . We [drivers] help others break out of the welfare cycle by driving them to work. We give them freedom.

Anita, another former Connections Shuttle driver and dispatcher, is the Connections Shuttle permanent office assistant. She says,

I'm living proof that the shuttle has a lot to offer. I got experience in all aspects of the company. I took advantage of every aspect so I would have a nice résumé when I left. I did most of the scheduling, stats, and office work in all of my spare time between dispatching and driving. There is a lot of incentive to come to work and do your paperwork on time. We reward drivers with "Driver of the Month" awards. It builds up their confidence.

In 1999, Deana, the shuttle project supervisor, and Joanne, who was one of the drivers, received the outstanding employer and outstanding employee awards from CareerWorks. One of the Connections Shuttle's biggest successes was making the case to improve existing public transportation to serve a wider range of people, especially low-income workers.

PROGRAM CHALLENGES

Some of the difficulties that the Connections Shuttle planners faced were related to the time frame for the project. For example, the program was designed to have five vehicles and one backup. The county had only enough money for three new vans, but the county money did not come through in time to purchase the three vans by the project start date. The shuttle then borrowed vans from other Food and Nutrition Services programs to start on time. Finally, the Federal Transit District came through with funds for four additional vans.

Transporting children posed another challenge for the Connections Shuttle. In order to transport children to and from school, drivers normally need a school bus driver's license. For six months, Scott Bugental, director of the Transportation Division for Food and Nutrition Services, searched for the legislation and laws related to school bus license requirements. He discovered that a driver must operate a large school bus in order to require a school bus license. However, an adult driver can transport children to and from school in a vehicle that carries less than ten people. So, the drivers modified their vans by removing seats so that the carrying capacity was less than ten in order to transport children.

The final hurdle that Connections Shuttle planners cleared was convincing the unionized public transit drivers that the shuttle drivers would not compete with them for passengers. It was important to secure the support of the public transit drivers for the Connections Shuttle so that it could operate. Although Transit District management was involved in the task force from the beginning, the unionized transit drivers were not involved in the planning meetings, so they did not understand the need for the shuttle. When the shuttle planners explained that the shuttle passengers would be allowed to ride only after proving that they could not use public transportation, the United Transportation Union signed off in support of the program.

The Connections Shuttle drivers face a challenge as trainees in searching for a permanent job. The drivers know that their training time is limited to seven months, and ideally they would like to secure a job that starts as the training period ends. However, they often end up with job offers with starting dates either before their training period ends or long after the training period is over. The shuttle program suffers when drivers leave prematurely to take permanent jobs. Drivers would like more coordination between the Connections Shuttle training and local companies who hire drivers so that the training dates are in accord with hiring periods.

LESSONS LEARNED

Connections Shuttle planners and implementers learned the following lessons:

1. It is important to invite all relevant participants to engage in the planning process, including local officials, public transit drivers, and affected union leaders, in order to identify potential sources of resistance and address all problems as soon as possible. It is also important to allow for enough planning time. As a member of the Santa Cruz Area Transportation Management Association notes, "Make sure everyone is at the table from the start. It prevents misunderstanding. Our short time frame made the process less than ideal. We focused on getting the program going, then addressing problems. Give your program enough time to plan it all out."
2. A clear and comprehensive protocol for the driver and dispatcher training is essential, along with the establishment of a morale committee for drivers.
3. The human resources workers who recommend CalWORKs participants to the Connections Shuttle training must continuously recruit and screen for appropriate participants in order to maintain a steady

stream of applicants while carefully screening out participants who should not be in the training program.

4. Although the Connections Shuttle staff let clients know from the beginning that the shuttle is a temporary solution, it is important to provide additional assistance to help riders find more permanent solutions as soon as they become more self-sufficient.

REFERENCES

Blumenberg, E. and Ong, P. (1997). Can welfare recipients afford to work far from home? *Access, 10,* 15-19.

Harbaugh, C. and Smith, T. (1998). Welfare reform and transportation: There is a connection. *TDM Review, 6*(2), 15-16.

Kaplan, A. (1998). Transportation: The essential need to address the "to" in welfare-to-work. *Project ACTION Update, 3,* 4-9.

Chapter 4

The Guaranteed Ride Home Program: Transportation Services for Welfare-to-Work Participants

Christine M. Schmidt
Michael J. Austin

Welfare reform, as set forth in President Clinton's 1996 Personal Responsibility and Work Opportunity Reconciliation Act, includes welfare-to-work policies designed to address barriers to work and propel welfare recipients into sustained employment, through block grants to the states for Temporary Assistance to Needy Families (TANF). In California, the CalWORKs legislation is a response to federal standards and authorizes the counties to institute welfare-to-work programs. Because transportation is viewed as an important barrier to obtaining and maintaining long-term employment, counties have been encouraged to address transportation issues as an important obstacle to self-sufficiency.

To address the many challenges involved in defining local issues, strengths, needs, and strategies in Silicon Valley, the Santa Clara County Social Services Agency (SSA), along with the Santa Clara Valley Transportation Authority (VTA), and the state-funded Bay Area Metropolitan Transportation Commission (MTC) initiated the Santa Clara County Welfare-to-Work Transportation Planning Project. The overall objectives of this project were to assess transportation requirements and identify strategies to increase availability, affordability, and effectiveness of existing services. In addition, the county social services agency hoped to establish agreements with transportation providers and employers to ensure the availability of transportation options. This is a case study of how the Santa Clara County Social Services Agency collaborated with key organizations throughout the county to design and implement the Guaranteed Ride Home Program (GRHP) to address the transportation needs of its CalWORKs participants.

BRIEF LITERATURE REVIEW

For the poor, the single largest obstacle to getting and keeping a steady job can be the lack of adequate transportation. Few welfare recipients own cars, and in fact, 26 percent of below-poverty-level households are without a vehicle (Harbaugh, 1998). For those who do own a vehicle, depending on the state, assistance may be reduced or even denied when the cost of the vehicle is calculated as an asset. In addition, many welfare recipients live in areas with no public transportation systems or systems that do not operate during evening hours. Welfare-to-work transportation services such as the Guaranteed Ride Home Program can increase access to employment for those without a car or with limited transit options, as well as for persons with emergencies.

Increasing access to employment, however, is not a simple process. Although jobs in some areas may be plentiful or easy to access, they often do not match the skills or experience of the people attempting to transition from welfare to work. The effect is a gradual separation of low-income workers and the job opportunities for which they are qualified (Hughes, 1995). In addition, employment suburbanization can dramatically reduce job opportunities for those who rely on fixed-route public transportation to reach their work destinations. In a study of low-skilled commuters in ten U.S. cities, Taylor and Ong (1995) found that reduction in access to employment was affected more by dependence on public transit than by any other factor, including residential location.

Although middle- and upper-income workers can often increase their earnings by accepting jobs that demand a longer commute, research has shown that this is not generally possible for low-income workers. In fact, the result is just the opposite. Ong and Blumenberg (1998) found that among welfare recipients in Los Angeles County who were employed in 1995, those who worked within four miles of home had median incomes of $634 per month. Those who worked between four and ten miles of home earned $620, and those who commuted more than ten miles to their jobs earned only $433 per month (in Wachs and Taylor, 1998, p. 15). Because of the nature of the low-skilled jobs and the fact that employers generally do not reimburse workers for travel expenses, workers who accept jobs farther from home must expect to see both their income reduced monetarily and their work days lengthened.

In order to increase access to available jobs for low-skilled workers, states and counties need to create more transportation options by allocating more welfare-to-work dollars to transportation support services. Some of the options include the following (Reichert, 1997):

- Make transportation part of the recipient's responsibility contract. Detail a recipient's obligations and specify services the department will provide.
- Do not penalize workers for owning a car. Many states have raised the asset limit to accommodate the value of a car, while Michigan and Arkansas disregard its entire value.
- Help recipients buy a car.
- Find ways to connect workers with suburban areas.
- Mandate collaboration between human services and transportation departments to reduce barriers and afford better solutions.
- Provide transitional transportation for those leaving welfare.

Recognizing the need for a viable transportation plan, Santa Clara County created transportation options through a collaborative effort called the Welfare-to-Work Transportation Planning Project.

WELFARE-TO-WORK TRANSPORTATION PLANNING PROJECT

To begin the process, Santa Clara SSA, together with VTA and MTC, launched a planning process that brought together social services staff, transportation professionals, and county supervisors. Consultants from Moore Iacofano Goltsman (MIG), Inc., and RIDES for Bay Area Commuters collaborated with an advisory board of agency representatives to design a planning process which included four phases: needs assessment, inventory of county transportation options, strategy/action plan development, and implementation (Moore Iacofano Goltsman, Inc., 1998).

In the Phase 1 needs assessment, the transportation needs of Santa Clara's CalWORKs participants were documented through interviews with both CalWORKs participants and the SSA staff who work with them on a regular basis. In addition, a series of meetings were held with transportation providers, education and job training providers, and employers. Some of the key findings of the assessment reflected issues of coordination, access, and availability.

In terms of *coordination,* some CalWORKs participants must juggle and coordinate many different trips, including drop-off and pickup at child care, education, and job training. For transit-dependent persons, these trips can be costly, time consuming, and require multiple transfers. Transit delays may cause CalWORKs participants to be late for work, which may eventually contribute to loss of employment.

Access to reliable transportation can also be a problem. While many CalWORKs participants live in the eastern part of the county, a large number of jobs being created are in the northern areas. This lack of significant job concentrations in the neighborhoods where participants live can make public transit access and ride sharing difficult. In addition, the costs associated with owning and operating an automobile are prohibitive for many lower-income people, and mechanical breakdowns are a frequent problem for those who do own autos.

In addition, many job opportunities involve swing, night, and weekend shifts when public transit is not readily *available,* and rail and bus services are often located some distance from work and home. CalWORKs participants and support programs have difficulty getting comprehensive information on the range of transport options; much of this transportation service information is available only in English, but only 51 percent of CalWORKs heads of households speak English as their primary language.

Phase 2 included the development of an inventory of existing programs and services, which could be used for improving transportation services. Through interviews with staff from VTA, Caltrans, RIDES for Bay Area Commuters, MTC, Bay Area Air Quality Management District, and others, information on bus, light rail, carpool, and public/private shuttle services was collected. The inventory information was used to identify service gaps that may be barriers to CalWORKs participants in finding or keeping steady employment. The information was also assembled into a comprehensive transportation resource guide for use primarily by SSA staff, community service providers, and others who assist CalWORKs participants in determining transportation options.

Phases 1 and 2 of the Transportation Planning Project helped to identify a number of transportation-related gaps and barriers that impede a CalWORKs participant's ability to obtain and maintain employment. These barriers were organized into the following three categories:

1. gaps in service (availability, convenience, reliability, and safety),
2. gaps in necessary information and skills (language, literacy, and navigational competency), and
3. gaps in affordability (cost).

Phase 3 of the project identified specific strategies to address the three types of barriers, through the involvement of community representatives including local transportation providers, education and job training providers, child care specialists, CalWORKs, and those that participated in Phases 1 and 2.

Members of the planning group were organized into four strategy teams: (1) ride sharing, trip planning, and information, (2) transit, (3) automobile, and (4) taxi, bicycle, paratransit, and kids' shuttle. Team members were encouraged to think creatively, to build on existing resources, to identify potential partnerships, and to be strategic and selective. After brainstorming opportunities and solutions related to their areas, they prioritized the most promising ideas and developed action plans along with key partners to assist in implementation (Phase 4). The final plans consisted of a series of strategies to be carried out in two stages. The first strategies were to be initiated in the first year and included the following:

- developing a trip planning test,
- compiling a transportation resource guide,
- hiring a transportation program coordinator,
- developing a guaranteed ride home program,
- improving transit stop security and amenities,
- expanding lending capacity of the family loan program,
- developing an auto repair program participant list,
- developing emergency skills training, and
- subsidizing emergency roadside assistance.

Out of these planning sessions the idea for the Guaranteed Ride Home Program was developed: a strategy for meeting the immediate transportation needs of CalWORKs participants in getting to work.

THE GUARANTEED RIDE HOME PROGRAM

Getting Started

When the county needs assessment indicated that additional transportation options for CalWORKs participants were needed, a collaboration was formed between Santa Clara County SSA, VTA, and OUTREACH, a nonprofit transportation service agency, to develop a plan. Because paratransit services are required for all federally funded public transportation, and therefore were already in place, the three organizations saw a way to utilize the existing paratransit system, mainly serving the elderly and disabled, for a program that could assist CalWORKs participants in obtaining a reliable means of getting to and from work. The Guaranteed Ride Home Program began as a pilot program in November 1999.

OUTREACH is an independent, private nonprofit transportation agency which operates with a state-of-the-art Intelligent Transportation System that utilizes high technology such as automatic vehicle locators and global positioning satellite technology to provide superior paratransit service throughout the Silicon Valley area. The agency had an available fleet of cars, empty seats on a daily basis, and the technological means to support the operation of a program that would coordinate rides for CalWORKs participants in need of transportation to sustain employment.

To institute such an operation, it was necessary to obtain approval from both the VTA which owned the fleet and the county which had access to funding from the Federal Transit Authority (FTA). The county was required to match the $500,000 in funding that came in from the FTA, giving the project a total operating budget of $1 million for the year. Following approval of the pilot program, intensive training was initiated to help staff learn about GRHP, general transportation issues, and the needs of the new population they would begin serving. Over 750 CalWORKs employment services staff and community partners received three hours of in-depth training from professional transportation consultants. The notion was that agency staff and community partners would support clients by not only making referrals to the program, but also by assisting them in completion of written individual transportation self-sufficiency plans. Staff and community organizations were provided with forms labeled "My Transportation Plan" in three languages and asked to disseminate them widely in the course of case management and other means. County staff keep track of persons they assist with transportation issues using a transportation information and referral tracking form which lists client name, date assisted, and type of service provided.

Enrollment

Enrollment in the program is limited to CalWORKs-eligible participants. The program offers same-day transportation to work, home, education, child care, and other approved locations for eligible enrolled participants, and it is limited to those situations when notice of more than twelve hours is not possible for alternate transportation. Referrals to the program come from county CalWORKs employment services staff, social workers, district office receptionists, staff at community-based organizations, or from the clients themselves.

Enrollment is a simple process that can be completed by faxing the enrollment form or simply by calling OUTREACH, and a client is generally enrolled and able to receive rides within twenty-four hours. The eligible GRHP participant is one who is entering employment or engaging in job-readiness activities, with priority given to a single head of household with custodial responsibility for one or more young children (up to thirteen years) or other dependent adults unable to care for themselves. Santa Clara

SSA determines the clients' eligibility for the program and then refers them to OUTREACH who enrolls them and begins processing ride requests. At the time of enrollment, participants are required to develop a plan for continued self-sufficiency when GRHP is no longer available. "My Transportation Plan" outlines destinations, usual trips, backup plans, cost, stops, transfers, and other details relating to getting to and from work and any other related trips. The document also includes tips on getting maps and directions, information on various types of travel, and numbers that clients can call if they need more information on services. Forms are also available at Transportation Resource Centers, located in the Employment Connection sites, along with transportation forms, GRHP enrollment forms, and bus maps.

Features of GRHP

The GRHP offers transportation for eligible enrollees in situations that include, but are not limited to, the following:

- Nonscheduled overtime requests from employers
- Car breakdowns
- When the participant or participant's dependents become ill and must leave work
- A household emergency
- When a carpool is unexpectedly not available
- When a change in schedule makes alternate transportation unavailable

In general, transportation is provided to and from the workplace or home, including necessary multiple destination stops at child care locations, schools, or other sites where dependents might be located. At times, OUTREACH will also transport the rider and dependent, if ill, from home to a health care provider, although emergency medical transportation is prohibited.

A client is eligible to receive a total of forty-eight free guaranteed rides home over a period of six months, and the transportation service is available twenty-four hours a day, 365 days a year. The GRHP is available in all fifteen cities in Santa Clara County, spanning an area of over 342 square miles. Rides with multiple stops still count as one ride, and riders may schedule multiple same-day rides with one call to OUTREACH. As remaining rides approach ten or less, calls are made by staff to inform clients in order to give them time to make alternate arrangements as soon as possible.

When calling OUTREACH, clients need to provide a program identification number, the time of desired pickup, and the exact name and address of the drop-off or pickup location. Riders inform the dispatcher if they intend to take a dependent with them, as well as any other pertinent information relating to the ride. Although riders are free to bring along car seats for young children, car seats are available through a generous donation to the program by California State American Automobile Association (AAA). OUTREACH dispatchers then inform the rider if the pickup or drop-off location is within the OUTREACH service area and provide him or her with transfer locations for alternate transportation. Currently, OUTREACH schedulers/dispatchers are available who speak English, Spanish, Vietnamese, Chinese, French, and Russian.

By August 2000, over 1,000 CalWORKs participants were enrolled in the program, and the number is steadily increasing. The program is featured prominently in the Santa Clara County Transportation Resource Guide (another product of the planning project) that was mailed upon its completion in October 1999 to 12,000 CalWORKs recipients throughout the county. The guide is available in English, Spanish, and Vietnamese and is a comprehensive outline of all available transportation services in Santa Clara County.

In addition, the project has developed laminated posters, available in several languages, that describe the program and are widely distributed among social service offices and community-based nonprofit organizations. The number of participants is rapidly increasing due to these efforts as well as word of mouth among riders and county staff. Rides for GRHP participants average nine miles per ride, with many rides including two or more stops.

PROGRAM EVALUATION

Throughout the first eight months of operation (November 1999 to July 2000), ongoing evaluation was an important feature of the Guaranteed Ride Home Program. The process included phone calls to regular riders (10 percent of riders selected at random) to inquire about the quality of services, and county employment centers collected survey feedback from clients to be delivered to VTA. A comprehensive customer survey was prepared to give feedback from the first year of operation. In addition, clients leaving the program complete exit interviews with county staff to obtain further information about their levels of satisfaction and recommended areas for improvement.

In terms of updating and improving services, OUTREACH is mapping the location and destinations of program participants by utilizing GIS software to geocode addresses of participants and their frequent destinations, such as work sites and child care facilities. In the future, this database will include geocoding scheduling and routing information as well, using factors such as time of day, size of street, and destination to increase safety and efficiency. In using this type of technology, OUTREACH is in a unique position to increase the efficiency of existing services and the effectiveness of future services.

PROGRAM SUCCESSES AND CHALLENGES

The successes of the Guaranteed Ride Home Program have been many. More and more people (over 1,000 to date) are able to get to work despite the lack of a vehicle or alternate transportation, resulting in increased job placement and retention of CalWORKs participants. Participants have been educated about travel options and given the tools for developing effective transportation plans. Due to increased usage, OUTREACH has doubled their existing phone system and added automated push/speech recognition functions. The demonstrated successful collaboration among agencies can also serve as a catalyst for future partnerships and further progress.

Although challenges have been relatively few, some are significant. First, rush hour is a challenge for any transportation system. Getting drivers and riders to destinations during peak hours requires careful planning and knowledge of alternate routes. Second, many riders become aware of their need for rides without much advance notice, making the situation even more complex given time constraints. Although program staff encourage participants to engage in preplanning whenever they can, it is not always possible. Third, trips with multiple stops can often require more time than can be predicted due to unforeseen factors such as waiting at schools or health centers, or assisting elderly persons or small children. Fourth, although data are collected on a monthly basis, usage tends to fluctuate from month to month, and it is difficult to project utilization rates for the system.

A future challenge involves the county's attempts to get state funds earmarked for future operations. Building on the success of the pilot program, the county would like to offer additional services to address the needs of more of its county residents. For example, there is a proposal to expand services for low-income women, which would include not only CalWORKs participants but also the working poor (who are currently not eligible), the homeless population, and children only, who could be taken to school, day care, health appointments, and other necessary destinations.

LESSONS LEARNED

The following are some of the lessons learned from launching the Guaranteed Ride Home Program:

1. Implementing transportation services for welfare-to-work participants can be a difficult process. Service delivery agencies must commit large amounts of existing resources to planning before hiring staff and providing services. It is important to use existing systems whenever possible.
2. When instituting pilot programs, it is often difficult to predict usage patterns. It was unforeseen that so many GRHP participants would need multiple stops. In programs such as this, it may not be prudent to count multileg trips as one ride.
3. It is sometimes difficult to collect the feedback that is necessary to evaluate the program. It is important to train both social services and transportation staff to be proactive in seeking feedback from clients on a regular basis.
4. It is important to develop contingency plans for clients whose needs exceed program services. Some clients need more than their allocated forty-eight rides due to emergency situations, while others do not use all of their forty-eight rides. Criteria are needed to address under- and overutilization.
5. It is important to attempt to leverage resources for noneligible clients who are in need of services. Currently no sponsors support services to the working poor or children, although efforts are being made to secure funding.
6. When creating new transportation programs, it is important to secure the commitment of top leadership of local agencies and government. Local match in funding plays a major role in supporting long-term sustainability of state and federal funds.

REFERENCES

Harbaugh, C. (1998). Welfare Reform and Transportation: There Is a Connection. *Public Roads,* 61(4), 38-43.

Hughes, M.A. (1995). A Mobility Strategy for Improving Opportunity. *Housing Policy Debate,* 6(1), 271-297.

Moore Iacofano Goltsman, Inc., in association with RIDES for Bay Area Commuters (1998). *Santa Clara County Welfare-to-Work Transportation Planning Project: Summary of Project Findings.* Oakland, CA: Metropolitan Transportation Association.

Ong, P. and Blumenberg, E. (1998). Job Access, Commute, and Travel Burden Among Welfare Recipients. *Urban Studies,* 35(1), 77-91.

Reichert, D. (1997). On the Road to Self-Sufficiency. *State Legislatures,* 23(10), 32-33.

Taylor, B.D. and Ong, P.M. (1995). Spatial Mismatch or Automobile Mismatch? An Examination of Race, Residence, and Commuting in U.S. Metropolitan Areas. *Urban Studies,* 32(9), 1453-1473.

Wachs, M. and Taylor, B.D. (1998). Can Transportation Strategies Help Meet the Welfare Challenge? *Journal of the American Planning Association,* 64(1), 15-19.

Chapter 5

Training Exempt Providers to Deliver High-Quality Child Care Programs

Jonathan Prince
Michael J. Austin

In meeting the child care needs of low-income working parents, child care advocates have recently discussed the urgent need to increase the capacity and training of infant and toddler child care providers (Carnegic Corporation of New York, 1998; Annie E. Casey Foundation, 1998; Kahn and Kamerman, 1998; Modigliani, 1994). One way to increase the capacity and quality of these providers is to recruit, train, and support exempt providers in the community.

Providers are considered *exempt* from licensure when they care for their own children, the children of relatives, and/or the children of only one other family. This case study describes and analyzes the Exempt Provider Training Project sponsored by the Child Care Coordinating Council in San Mateo County which provides outreach, training, and other forms of assistance to child care professionals. The study includes a brief review of literature on child care training, a description of the project's dramatic growth since its establishment in 1997, a description of the project's goals and services, and the experiences of a project participant. It concludes with lessons learned and future challenges.

BRIEF LITERATURE REVIEW

Training of providers has been shown to increase the quality of child care as well as help providers view child care as a profession (Debord and Sawyers, 1996; Kendrick, 1994; Kontos, Howes, and Galinsky, 1996; Mueller and Orimoto, 1995; Pence and Goelman, 1991). In California, license-exempt providers that care for children in their own homes are called *home care providers.* Because they are not monitored by local regulators, license-exempt home care providers are typically viewed as being a hidden child care resource in the community, operating with limited outside support (Bailey and Osborne, 1994; Fiene, 1995; Pence and Goelman, 1991). Once trained and licensed, these formerly exempt providers become *family child care homes* (California Child Care Resource and Referral Network [CCCRR], 1999) and thereby increase the availability of licensed child care in the community.

Despite the lack of licensure, many parents prefer exempt providers because (1) they tend to be more affordable and convenient than licensed professionals (Pence and Goelman, 1991), (2) there are usually fewer children in exempt-provider homes, resulting in a greater potential for individual attention (CCCRR, 1999), and (3) they are seen as a valuable hidden community resource for working parents (Pence and Goelman, 1991).

Providers have their own reasons for choosing unlicensed over licensed child care as a vocation. Almost all are female (Mueller and Orimoto, 1995), and most have children of their own and limited education and family income (Bailey and Osborne, 1994). They tend to have a traditional view of the family in that the father is seen as the primary wage earner while the wife cares for the children (Bailey and Osborne, 1994). Becoming a home care provider allows these women to (1) care for their own young children at home, (2) provide companionship for their children, and (3) earn extra income as a provider.

Many home care providers intend to change careers once their own children enter school (Mueller and Orimoto, 1995), thus viewing child care as a temporary occupation, which often acts as a disincentive for seeking licensure. Other disincentives include (1) the lack of substantial increase in compensation for providing licensed care and (2) the lack of career development in the child care profession (Bailey and Osborne, 1994).

It is generally agreed that the training of license-exempt providers will increase the quality of child care in the community. Improving the recruitment and training of license-exempt providers is necessary because exempt child care providers may have less access to training (and other resources) than their licensed counterparts (Bailey and Osborne, 1994). Second, research has demonstrated that, compared with licensed providers, exempt providers spend less time with young children in planned activities related to shared tasks that facilitate healthy development (Pence and Goelman, 1991).

Most child care training is offered on evenings and weekends, when providers are most likely to be available (Bailey and Osborne, 1994). Three types of training are available for providers (Kendrick, 1994). Before entering the profession they can receive *preservice training,* or they can receive *orientation training* that highlights essential skills when they first begin the job. *Ongoing training* is provided periodically during the child care provider's career. Typical training needs include child development, health and safety, food and nutrition, discipline, educational methods, activity planning, collaboration with parents, and business practices such as record keeping and business contracts. In addition, Bailey and Osborne (1994) found that many providers desire training in stress management. Most providers complete training once they have started (Mueller and Orimoto, 1995). Those that do not complete training have somewhat less experience as providers and tend to use fewer business and safety practices (Kontos, Howes, and Galinsky, 1996).

Several authors have made the following recommendations to improve the quality of training offered to child care providers:

- Trainers need to learn the context in which child care providers work every day and use terminology that is relevant, nontechnical, and easily understood (Kendrick, 1994).
- Trainers need to encourage participants to learn from one another by fostering active participation and interaction among people with different experiences and backgrounds (Bailey and Osborne, 1994; Kendrick, 1994).
- Administrators need to reimburse or provide vouchers to child care providers who wish to receive additional training in their homes or at colleges, conferences, seminars, or workshops (Fiene, 1995).
- Scholarships are needed to help unlicensed providers afford the cost of training (Fiene, 1995).
- Training needs to be linked to the ongoing monitoring of child care, such as monitoring child immunizations (Fiene, 1995).
- More training and support to people who have been providing child care for longer periods of time are needed in order to increase provider retention and decrease turnover (Mueller and Orimoto, 1995).

As these recommendations suggest, provider training is generally accompanied by a variety of other services which include home visits, support groups, financial assistance, assistance obtaining licensure, ongoing consultation, and the opportunity to observe and interact with an experienced child care mentor (Mueller and Orimoto, 1995). Financial assistance can be offered to pay for business start-up costs that include licensing fees, the purchase of safety devices, and the construction of fences around backyards. In addition, trainers often help providers coordinate with local zoning departments, insurance companies, and other community agencies.

This combination of training and support activities typically produces very positive outcomes, including (1) success in recruiting providers, (2) significant gains in knowledge and skills, (3) increases in confidence, commitment, patience, interest, and job satisfaction, and (4) a better awareness of children's abilities and needs (Mueller and Orimoto, 1995). Kontos, Howes, and Galinsky (1996) found that training increases both the amount of planned, daily activities shared with children and financial accountability, with increased reporting of incomes and expenses on tax returns. Finally, training has been shown to increase compliance with health standards (Kendrick, 1994).

Despite these positive findings, at least two major challenges are noted in the literature with respect to the recruitment and training of child care providers: (1) retaining providers after they have been trained, where it is estimated that only about half of all family child care providers remain in the field twelve to eighteen months after they receive training (Mueller and Orimoto, 1995) due, in part, to low status, long hours, and limited financial rewards (Bailey and Osborne, 1994), and (2) ensuring that training reaches those providers that need it most. Kontos, Howes, and Galinsky (1996) point out that providers who seek out training are more motivated and middle class than those that do not attend and may provide a higher quality of care to begin with.

With this brief literature review in mind, it is clear that many of the issues are reflected in the Exempt Provider Training Project in San Mateo County. It provides outreach, training, and support to a population of child care providers that would not otherwise receive these services. Almost 75 percent of participants are Latina women with limited English-speaking abilities. Without the help of this training project, many of these women would have remained in the hidden child care community as a result of language barriers, lack of time, transportation issues, and other factors which reduce access to services. Most live in close proximity to one another, and, as illustrated in the next section, the program has grown significantly by word of mouth in its first two years of operation.

A HISTORY OF THE EXEMPT PROVIDER TRAINING PROJECT

The Exempt Provider Training Project of San Mateo County, California, was established in June 1997 to provide training and support to child care providers to increase the overall quality of care. The project's original plan was to offer training to licensed or exempt providers whom low-income working parents selected to care for their children. In other words, an employed woman receiving health services from Medi-Cal's Prenatal to Three program could choose any local provider to care for her children and the project would train the selected provider.

This original goal needed to be modified, as the project staff (at the time composed of one and a half full-time employees) quickly found that most mothers in the Prenatal to Three program were not working outside the home. They had instead decided to become exempt providers themselves by staying at home, caring for their own children, and caring for the children of friends or relatives to earn extra income. They chose themselves, therefore, to receive training and support from the project instead of designating a provider in the community. Despite this departure from the original goal, staff agreed to train them and help with licensure, if desired, to provide high-quality child care in the community. Project staff even began to train stay-at-home mothers who did not care for other children. They simply expressed an interest in providing high-quality care to their own children and possibly taking care of children in the future.

The dramatic early growth of the program can be understood, in part, by examining the child care services that are provided for the participants in the training program. Within the first year of the project, the informal child care service for less than six children had grown into a structured program for twenty-four to thirty children during each provider training session. To accommodate these children, a pool of child care providers were recruited and trained, and the program was relocated to larger space in schools and community-based organizations.

Program growth was not spontaneous. In fact, staff members were concerned in the first two months of operation because there were so few participants. Initially, it was planned that parents would refer themselves to the project after learning of it from staff at the Prenatal to Three Initiative. When this resulted in fewer referrals than expected, project staff called interested parents directly after obtaining their names and telephone numbers from the staff at the Prenatal to Three Initiative. In addition, project staff sent flyers about the program to collaborative organizations such as Head Start and WIC (Women, Infants, and Children). Finally, individuals that had received training recommended it to friends and relatives, and shortly thereafter a snowball effect occurred and referrals arrived at increasing rates.

In the second year of operation, the number of project staff increased from one and a half to two full-time members, and class sizes increased from three or four people in the first class to as many as forty in later classes. To preserve the individualized attention offered to trainees drop-ins were no longer accepted and all participants were required to register for the program in advance. In addition, many parents interested in becoming a provider were placed on a waiting list for as long as two months. Project staff began to increase their training emphasis on economic development and the advantages of licensure. More and more providers became interested in pursuing their license and receiving technical assistance.

As the project entered its third year of operation, as many as sixty people would arrive at a single training. While about forty people stayed for training, others were told to register and are placed on the waiting list. The essence of the training experience can be found in the program's goals, services, participants, and outcomes.

PROJECT GOALS AND SERVICES

The project has five major purposes:

1. increase the quality of care offered by exempt child care providers,
2. promote the healthy development of infants and toddlers served by exempt providers,
3. increase the availability of child care for low-income parents receiving services from Medi-Cal's Prenatal to Three Initiative and other community services,
4. educate providers about the economic benefits of family child care as a profession, and
5. evaluate the effectiveness of outreach services and education to exempt child care providers.

Staff members continuously encourage providers to promote healthy child development, such as reading to the child rather than letting the child watch television alone all day.

Staff provide extensive outreach in Spanish and English through flyers, phone calls, presentations at community-based organizations, and the media. These efforts yield referrals from Prenatal to Three Initiative staff members, human services agency staff members, community-based programs such as Healthy Start and Head Start, family resource centers, previous program participants, and self-referrals. When they first began the training program, the participants were mostly interested in learning about

1. physical and social development related to ages and stages of walking, talking, and other aspects of child development,
2. nutrition, such as what is a normal lunch for a two-year-old,
3. appropriate and fair discipline,
4. neatness, and
5. child safety.

Training needs are assessed as part of a sixteen-hour training program that is organized into four four-hour sessions. Classes are conducted in Spanish and English and are usually held on Saturdays to meet the needs of working providers. Topics include

1. how quality child care experiences can facilitate healthy early child development,
2. the importance of self-assessment in providing patient and consistent care,
3. teamwork and relationship building with children and their parents, and
4. creating an environment for infants and toddlers that fosters healthy child development.

Incentives are used to encourage attendance at the training sessions. Initially all participants were paid twenty-five dollars for each session they attend and another twenty-five dollars for coming to all four, but these payments were reduced to twenty dollars after class sizes became larger. In addition, the project offers forty-dollar scholarships to attend CPR/first aid training and ninety dollars for becoming Trustlined. Trustline is a registry of child care providers that have submitted fingerprints, and parents use this registry to ensure that their provider of choice does not have a criminal conviction. Incentives such as toys and books are also given to participants that agree to informal, voluntary home visits by project staff. In these visits, staff members assess the living and child care environment of providers and offer feedback which supplements classroom training. Much of this feedback concerns household safety issues, the licensing process, and community resources. Staff use these opportunities to strengthen their rapport with participants and to model appropriate and nurturing interaction with children. Other support staff, including nurses and mental health clinicians, may be contacted to visit the home of families in the Prenatal to Three Initiative if needed. Home visits may also be requested by providers who are unable to attend classroom instruction but plan to attend in the future.

The project offers many other services, in addition to trainings and home visits, including the following:

- *Support groups:* These groups are scheduled informally by participants. Initial efforts to establish a set time and place for support groups were abandoned after the diversity of provider schedules became apparent.
- *Transportation:* Participants are encouraged to carpool, reimbursed for public transportation, or provided with taxi vouchers if no other means of transport is available.

- *Child care:* The children of participants are cared for during training sessions and other project events.
- *Referrals:* Participants are referred to licensing orientations, Trustline, CPR/first aid classes, a technical assistance hotline, other training and educational forums, seminars, and workshops such as the Family Child Care Conference.
- *Mentors:* The opportunity to talk with licensed providers is offered to participants who wish to learn more firsthand information about operating child care programs.

Primary sources of revenue for the Exempt Provider Training Project are annual grants from the Peninsula Community Foundation (PCF) and a contract with the San Mateo County Human Services Agency. During fiscal year 1999-2000, the project expected to receive $110,000 from PCF and $90,000 from the county human services agency. These funds would cover annual expenditures of about $200,000 for child care during training sessions, participant transportation, books and program literature, incentives and scholarships, food, home health and safety repairs/additions, and other necessary items. In addition, the project receives about $30,000 from Bank Street College in New York for participant support groups. Information obtained from these groups is used to inform research (sponsored by the Packard Foundation) on the training needs of exempt providers.

The sections that follow provide a closer look at project participants, their progression toward licensure, and other project outcomes, as well as lessons learned and future challenges. Introducing these sections is a description of a single participant's experience in the program.

PROJECT PARTICIPANTS

At the age of forty, Marta began providing child care ten years ago after migrating to the United States from Mexico. She is married and has two teenage children. With halting English she describes her experience as a project participant: "I found out about the training from a friend that had attended. She told me, 'I know you do a very good job with the children, but you should go to these meetings. They really teach you a lot.' I decided to attend because I like to do the best job that I can at baby-sitting. They help me when I have many questions and nobody tells me how to do things. I was thinking the other day that I have been in this area for ten years but there is no one who speaks my language who can help when I have stress, or problems with my own children, or the children that the parents drop off. My boys are older now and I feel really comfortable with them. But when they were little—I wish

I could have had somebody to help me at that time. [Staff at the project are] the only people I know that are working with this community.

"Every Wednesday I go to baby-sitting school. They teach us many things, such as how to be very patient, very alert to all the signs with the baby, to connect with the baby, and how they change from six months to twelve, eighteen, twenty-four, and so on. Ana, the other day she taught us how to use *Sesame Street* to connect with the baby. The teachers, they speak Spanish and they explain everything and ask us many questions. I enjoy it a lot. Every time I go to these meetings I meet more persons in the community. It's really important.

"They also give out information in papers and books, books that tell you how to take care of children—not just babies but older kids too. This one book tells you how to prepare your house when you are about to start caring for a new baby. It is just terrific. I also go to a support group and they give you invitations to go to different things, different events.

"I plan to get licensed. Last year—before this class—I thought, 'I don't think I can get my license because of the ladies who come by my house every day to bring the kids. I don't have enough time to shop, or do other things, or things you have to do before the license.' But two months ago I did the CPR class, so I have started already. Just a few things I have to do before I get my license. When I went to the first meeting with Ana, she asked us how many years have we been doing this job, and she asked us 'Who is taking care of children in your own home?' I said 'me,' and she asked me how many kids I take care of and I told her. Ana, she said, 'that's illegal—you can't take care of all those kids in your house without a license.' So they are helping me to get one.

"When I first moved here I started taking care of kids in my friends' houses for two or three years. Then we got our own house and they dropped off the kids. But I didn't know I needed a license. I never worked for many families. Maybe two at a time. My husband and my brothers try to convince me to get another kind of job, but I am not interested in another job. I like babies and kids. I don't know if it's because when I was very young I always say, 'I want to be a teacher.' Baby-sitting kids right now I feel like I am a teacher. I really want to get my license, so that when I get it, it's like 'Yes, I am ready. I am a teacher.' I will feel like I have something very legal. They say I do a very good job right now, but I don't have the paper where they say I am approved for being a baby-sitter.

"I know a lot of persons—my neighbors—that say, 'When you have your license maybe you can take care of my kids part-time.' I know many mothers that don't work because they haven't had very good experiences at the places where they leave their kids. They come to visit my house and ask, 'Can you take care of my kids?' And I say, 'Let me get my license first please.' Right now I only care for one baby full-time and a little boy part-time. When I go to the meetings I hear many struggles of other baby-sitters, maybe because they are taking care of many, many kids or many different families. But with me it's only two kids. It's really easy.

"I work from seven in the morning to six at night, but I am very flexible. Other places open at seven or seven-thirty, but you have to come pick up the kids by five p.m. I don't have exact hours. They come before seven sometimes or on weekends. In the future I want to care for four or five every day. I want one baby and three or four others between one and a half and four years old."

In their second year of operation project staff developed a questionnaire to learn more about the participants. Initially used as a screening form, the completed questionnaires yielded a great deal of data about participant characteristics, employment outside the home, and provider business practices. Information from this questionnaire and from staff observation provides the following description of participants:

- About 75 percent of the first-year participants were Spanish-speaking immigrant women. Most of their children were born in the United States. Some are undocumented and are concerned about involvement with public services. As a result, staff do not ask questions about documentation but will refer them for help with the citizenship process when the subject is broached by the participant.
- Many women were educated in their country of birth in professions such as teaching and nursing but were unable to continue their professions in the United States.
- Most are married or live with a partner or one or more adult relatives. There is usually another working adult in the home in addition to the exempt provider, and many homes contain two families. Usually the women work inside and the men work outside the home.
- About 63 percent of last year's participants were parents of children under the age of four. Most are not first-time mothers and their ages vary. Some grandmothers participate as well.
- Most homes have low combined incomes from work, resulting in difficulties finding affordable, adequate housing and providing for the needs of children. Men often hold down two or three jobs simultaneously.

Although not typical, participant difficulties include custody battles, child abuse or neglect, marital problems, and substance abuse. As a result of their cultural beliefs, some men do not support their wives in pursuing child care as a profession because they do not believe their wives should work, while others are very supportive and bring their wives to the training sessions. Most men do not participate in home visits, and only two have attended training since the project began.

Many women in training have remarked that obtaining a child care license and starting a business offers them an opportunity to elevate their own economic and social status. While many participants choose this path, others face serious obstacles to obtaining their license. The next section describes these obstacles as well as successes in pursuing licensure. In addition, other project outcomes are highlighted.

PROJECT OUTCOMES AND PROGRESS TOWARD LICENSURE

Project outcomes are difficult to quantify, but the following staff observations provide some highlights:

- an increase in attention paid to children in care instead of primarily completing household chores,
- an increase in the safety and utilization of child care environments such as covering electrical outlets and clearing more space for the children to play,
- an increase in provider patience and a decrease in overprotectiveness (as well as improved parenting abilities displayed by husbands/partners),
- an increased connection between participants and public services, leading to increased utilization of support services, and
- an increased connection among participants leading to continued support of one another personally and professionally.

Participants face many serious barriers in progressing toward licensure. These barriers include the following:

1. the scarcity of local Spanish-speaking licensing classes (e.g., CPR/first aid), orientations, paperwork, or staff,
2. the requirement that participants be citizens to advance to licensure when many are not documented,
3. housing that often does not meet licensing requirements because too many adults and children are sharing a residence,
4. the requirement that all residents of the child care home be fingerprinted when some residents may have criminal backgrounds,
5. the requirement that participants must let the owners of their homes know about their child care business when too many people, families, or children are living there that are not on the lease or known by the owner,

6. a lack of support from some husbands of participants, and
7. a lack of money that participants need to furnish the home with child care supplies (e.g., cribs, latches, fire extinguishers) which are required for licensure.

Despite these barriers, a significant number of participants have received their pediatric CPR certificate (33 percent), have gone to a licensing orientation, or have completed a licensing application. Seventeen percent have completed the licensing process. Still others have had project staff come to their homes for a prelicensing visit to prepare them for the State Department of Social Services licensing visit.

With a description of program operations, it is now important to note the lessons learned as well as future challenges.

LESSONS LEARNED AND FUTURE CHALLENGES

In addition to the barriers to obtaining licensure, a few organizational challenges have presented themselves in the first two years of the project's operation. First, some child care professionals disagree with the goal of providing training to exempt providers. They believe that such training undermines the professionalism of licensure by devoting limited resources to unregulated providers. Licensed providers may attempt to limit project growth to protect their own access to public resources (i.e., "gate-keeping"). Second, the explosive growth of the program has required project staff to explore the possibility of adding more staff time and resources. For example, there are over 300 participants who can request home visits from only two full-time project staff. Finally, the diverse needs of participants have generated many ideas for additional supportive services. Although these ideas would improve the quality and scope of the program, they tend to require increased funding.

Several lessons have been learned by project staff in the first two years of operation:

- Most low-income women with infants and toddlers that receive health services from Medi-Cal's Prenatal to Three Initiative do not plan to leave their children in child care but instead choose to care for their own children at home while providing exempt care to the children of friends or relatives. Most choose this form of self-employment instead of finding work in the community in accordance with welfare reform legislation.

- When self-referral was not effective in reaching this hidden community of exempt providers, staff greatly increased participation through phone calls, flyers, and community presentations. Participation increased even more rapidly after the first few groups of participants spoke positively of the project to friends and family members.
- Parents that care for only their own children (i.e., they are not child care providers) are also interested in attending project trainings. The program uncovered a general need for public child care training that goes beyond the realm of professional providers.

Having identified these lessons, staff members suggested several courses of future action that include the following:

1. contracting to hire a Spanish-speaking instructor to facilitate licensing orientations in San Mateo,
2. hiring additional staff (especially support staff) to accommodate program expansion,
3. making efforts to involve more men in training to improve the child care they provide and to enlist their support in their wife/partner's child care business,
4. increasing the quality of child care provided during classes by training the providers of care and increasing the availability of space and resources (e.g., toys, games, books),
5. expanding outreach to other communities that need project services, and
6. placing training classes in locations that are more accessible to low-income individuals with limited transportation.

Although there is no shortage of ideas, project staff members are limited by the availability of resources. In the future, program administrators hope that the program will be seen as a model for exempt provider training and become funded by the Department of Social Services and/or the state Department of Education. These sources of revenue are more stable and flexible than grant funding, enabling project staff to continually deliver a wide range of supportive services that enhance the quality and quantity of child care in the community.

REFERENCES

Annie E. Casey Foundation (1998). Confronting the child care challenge. *Governing,* 12, June, 44-52.

Bailey, S. and Osborne, S. (1994). Provider perspectives on the content and delivery of training for family day care. *Child and Youth Care Forum,* 23(5), 329-338.

California Child Care Resource and Referral Network (1999). Tips on finding child care that works best for your family. Available at <http://www.rrnetwork.org>.

Carnegie Corporation of New York (1998). Guarantee quality child care choices. In *Starting Points: Meeting the Needs of Our Youngest Children*. Available at <http://www.carnegie.org/starting points>.

Debord, K. and Sawyers, J. (1996). The effects of training on the quality of family child care for those associated with and not associated with professional child care organizations. *Child and Youth Care Forum,* 25(1), 7-15.

Fiene, R. (1995). Utilizing a statewide training system to improve child day care quality. *Child Welfare,* 74(6), 1189-1201.

Kahn, A. J. and Kamerman, S. B. (1998). *Big Cities in the Welfare Transition.* New York: Columbia University School of Social Work.

Kendrick, A. S. (1994). Training to ensure health child day-care programs. *Pediatrics,* 94(6), 1108-1110.

Kontos, S., Howes, C., and Galinsky, E. (1996). Does training make a difference to quality in family child care? *Early Childhood Research Quarterly,* 11, 427-445.

Modigliani, K. (1994). *Promoting High Quality Family Child Care: A Policy Perspective for Quality 2000.* Boston: Wheelock College.

Mueller, C. W. and Orimoto, L. (1995). Factors related to the recruitment, training, and retention of family child care providers. *Child Welfare,* 74(6), 1205-1221.

Pence, A. R. and Goelman, B. (1991). The relationship of regulation, training, and motivation to quality of care in family day care. *Child and Youth Care in Forum,* 20(2), 83-101.

Chapter 6

Integrating Mental Health and Substance Abuse Services into a County Welfare-to-Work Program

Christine M. Schmidt
Michael J. Austin

Sonoma County's welfare-to-work program (SonomaWORKS) opened its doors to the public on February 2, 1998, based on the California Work Opportunity and Responsibility to Kids Act (Assembly Bill 1542). The new welfare-to-work program is designed to assist CalWORKs recipients in transitioning as rapidly as possible from dependency on public assistance to self-sufficiency through unsubsidized employment. Under the CalWORKs program, adult recipients who are not exempt are required to meet work requirements by participating in welfare-to-work activities in order to maintain their eligibility for cash assistance. The current work requirement in Sonoma County is thirty-two hours of weekly participation, which may be met through a variety of activities.

Support services are available to help individuals participate in program activities or to accept work. These include but are not limited to child care, transportation, work-related or training-related expenses, and mental health and substance abuse support services that focus on removing barriers to employment. This case study is an analysis of best practices in Sonoma County with regard to substance abuse and mental health services for SonomaWORKS.

Figure 6.1 illustrates the client flow for individuals applying for CalWORKs benefits. Not all clients receive the same array of services. Some may already be working or going to school; others may be exempt from work requirements or eligible to receive a one-time lump-sum payment in lieu of monthly cash assistance.

During an orientation to SonomaWORKS, applicants receive information about the welfare rules and expectations and the types of services avail-

92   CHANGING WELFARE SERVICES

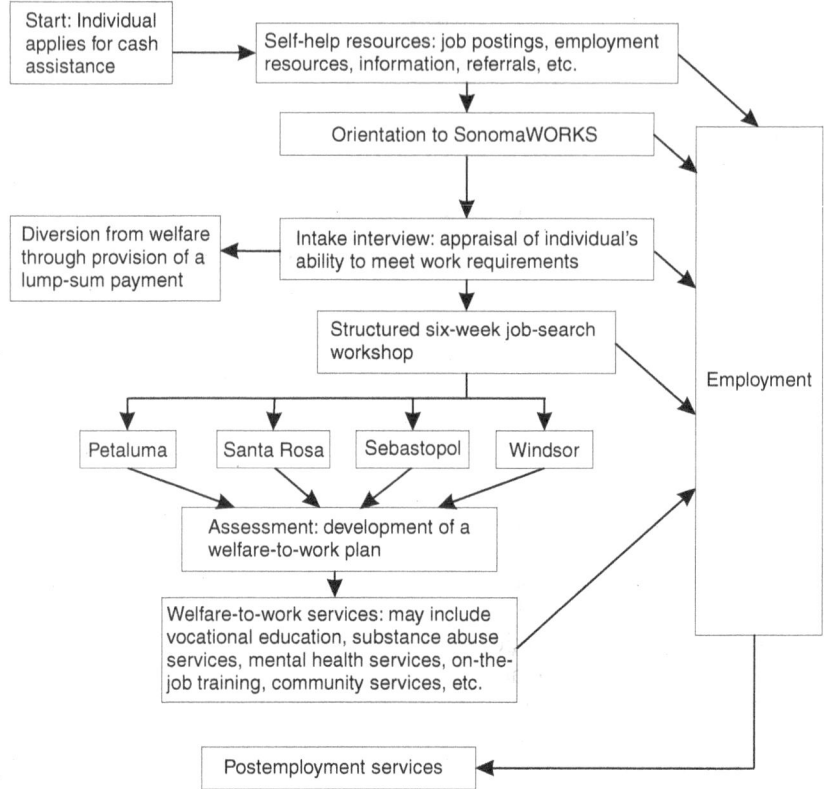

FIGURE 6.1. Client Flow in SonomaWORKS

able. If they are eligible for cash assistance and do not meet exemption criteria, they are then referred to job-search activities. Job-search workshops are conducted by contracted service providers at various locations throughout the county. During these initial activities known as the Preassessment phase, an eligibility worker serves the client's needs.

Clients who complete the job-search process and remain unemployed (or underemployed) are scheduled for a vocational assessment used in the development of a welfare-to-work plan related to education, training, and other services needed to achieve economic self-sufficiency. This assessment that follows the job search process involves a team of staff working with the client, including the eligibility worker, a social worker, and a vocational counselor. It may also include an employment services specialist from one of the job-search providers and/or a specialist from substance abuse services or mental health services (Sonoma County Human Services Department, 1999).

LITERATURE REVIEW HIGHLIGHTS

Although there is no shortage of information regarding substance abuse and mental health populations, treatment models, and statistics on outcomes, very little is written on strategies for implementing these services within welfare-to-work programs. Until recently, support services related to mental health and substance abuse programs were not a formal part of the welfare-to-work program (Pavetti et al., 1997). Current studies generally agree that substance use and/or abuse is a significant barrier to successful employment. Young and Gardner (1997) state that "providing treatment for alcohol and other drug problems is a necessary step toward job readiness" (p. 5). Grayson (1999) noted that between 5 and 39 percent of welfare recipients "use alcohol and other drugs in ways that impair their ability to secure and keep jobs, as well as their ability to be effective parents" (p. 5). As of 1998, projections of the number of substance-abusing welfare recipients exceeded 1 million (Bush and Kraft, 1998).

Young and Gardner (1997) note that treating chemically dependent welfare recipients not only produces more productive, employable persons, but also provides huge savings for government, especially the health and corrections systems. Studies show that for low-income persons, within two to three years of completion of treatment, the benefits of treatment far outweigh the costs. A recent study of substance abuse treatment in California showed that the results of providing treatment can be seen in savings to taxpayers, mostly through decrease in arrests and medical costs (Young and Gardner, 1997).

In addition to substance abuse, welfare recipients often face a broad array of mental health problems. Mental health problems or substance abuse may prevent recipients from being able to undertake the tasks necessary to find employment, or they may lack the self-confidence needed to take on new challenges. Others may be able to find employment but be unable to sustain it over time (Olson and Pavetti, 1996). The most basic argument in favor of providing counseling and therapeutic treatment and other supportive services for families seeking to move from welfare to work is that such services are enabling mechanisms. They enable people to cope with the personal difficulties that interfere with achieving goal-oriented success (Polit and O'Hara, 1989).

It is now relatively well known that a significant number of substance abusers suffer from serious mental impairment and that depression is widely prevalent among women (Woolis, 1998). This depression is often linked to feelings of low self-esteem and self-efficacy that are a result of being a welfare recipient (Nichols-Casebolt, 1986; Popkin, 1990; Pavetti, Holcomb, and Duke, 1995; Kunz and Kalil, 1999). It is now more important than ever to institute services in welfare-to-work programs that address the complex needs of these recipients, by addressing some of the following service activities (Steisel, 1999):

- Screening applicants
- Hiring qualified substance abuse professionals
- Integrating substance abuse education into job-readiness programs
- Teaching welfare clients about addiction and how to recognize it
- Providing screening and treatment for persons with mental health problems
- Providing transportation and child care for those who need treatment
- Addressing the needs of the entire family through a comprehensive approach to treatment
- Beginning pilot programs that provide financial incentives to businesses which hire welfare recipients

Sonoma County has developed some innovative approaches to address these needs. This is evident in their utilization rates, declining unemployment rates, and increased numbers of persons remaining in employment for significant periods of time. The following section describes how the county devised an integrated mental health and substance abuse service system into their welfare-to-work program.

SONOMAWORKS

Getting Started

When it became apparent in 1996 that Congress had passed legislation which would make drastic changes in the federal welfare system, Sonoma County leaders were concerned that many low-income people would become ineligible for various types of aid and thereby denied access to the skills and/or resources to fend for themselves. The community envisioned that community-based organizations would be inundated with persons seeking help and that these agencies would be ill equipped to handle such a crisis. The focus, then, was to find a way to put additional services in place before the need became emergent.

Sonoma County Human Services Department and Sonoma County Department of Health Services got together before CalWORKs was signed into law in 1997 to develop a plan to implement substance abuse, mental health, and domestic violence services into their welfare-to-work program. When word came that additional money would be set aside through CalWORKs to fund these special services, all that remained was hiring staff and getting started. Although the state-provided statistics of Aid to Families with Dependent Children (AFDC) clients who utilized substance abuse and/or mental health services proved to be unreliable as a gauge for estimating the number of staff needed, the county moved ahead and hired a full-time substance abuse specialist and a full-time and a half-time mental health specialist in the Department of Health Services to work specifically with SonomaWORKS clients.

Before long the rising caseload demanded hiring additional staff in both departments. As of spring 2000, two full-time and one part-time substance abuse specialists were on staff at Substance Abuse Services (SAS), and four full-time and one part-time mental health staff members comprise Mental Health Services (MHS). A psychiatrist is also available fourteen hours per week to assist with medication management for the more profoundly mentally ill clients.

In order to build a successful program, the county provided cross training for SonomaWORKS staff, contracted providers, and substance abuse and mental health staff. SonomaWORKS staff received training in identifying and referring clients with a need for substance abuse or mental health services. Substance abuse and mental health staff members were trained to focus on helping clients remove barriers to employment so that they could enter the workforce by concentrating on only those specific issues that stood in the way of employment. This was a difficult adjustment for some staff as well as for clients who expected to engage in long-term treatment.

The Screening and Referral Process

When a person applies for cash assistance, he or she is sent to a SonomaWORKS orientation session where he or she is given information about the program, including both the client's rights and responsibilities and information about support services. Immediately following this orientation, the prospective client meets with an eligibility worker who may give assistance in filling out the application and can often give the client a sense of whether his or her application for aid will be granted.

An advantage of the SonomaWORKS program is that clients are often able to take care of a number of tasks when they first come in to apply for aid. The colocation of CalWORKs mental health and substance abuse services makes it possible for a client to apply for aid, get program information, set up child care services, get a child support order, and investigate the array of county employment services. The client also has access, at this time, to the I&R (information and referral) service that offers an extensive listing of community resources. Part of the purpose of colocating these services is for the clients' convenience and efficient use of time. Because welfare is now time limited, the county sought to demonstrate to the client a sense of urgency in setting the job-search process into motion. This approach relates to the government's priority on getting clients to work as soon as possible and a human service value of assisting clients with their needs as effectively and efficiently as possible.

Despite a desire of the staff to quickly identify substance abuse and mental health needs of clients, eligibility staff did not directly assess these needs during the job-search orientation process. Staff decided, early on, that applying for assistance was difficult enough for most clients without asking more intrusive questions. So unless a client demonstrates a definite need for mental health or substance abuse services at intake, questions about these needs are left until their participation in the job-search process raises concerns or until a postemployment assessment.

Clients may be referred for alcohol and other drug (AOD) or mental health (MH) assessment at any point in the process, and any agency person who has contact with the client may refer for the assessment. Most referrals come from welfare-to-work staff who receive ongoing training on recognizing substance abuse or mental health issues. Some substance abuse referrals come from job coaches, social workers, or the clients themselves, but most come from eligibility workers. In MHS, most referrals come from social workers and vocational counselors. Clients are sent to AOD assessment first and then given a mental health appointment if necessary. Staff members believe that this process helps to reduce the no-show rate that may occur when clients are given too many appointments at one time.

In an average month, SAS receives approximately twenty to twenty-five new referrals, while MHS averages about thirty to forty new referrals. At any given time throughout the year, SAS may have approximately 170 open cases, with 115 to 120 clients in treatment each month, and MHS may have approximately 300 open cases with 150 completed appointments each month.

Client Assessment and Treatment

The referral process for AOD assessment generally takes less than a week, while a mental health assessment may take two weeks. Clients are assessed as to the extent to which they are capable of employment and under what conditions. SAS and MHS are colocated, making appointments easier for clients who utilize both services and easier for staff in consulting regarding client needs. Attendance records and AOD tracking summaries are kept by staff and utilized by the Department of Human Services to monitor clients and used in reporting on CalWORKs clients. AOD tracking summaries are monthly and include information on treatment hours, treatment participation, substance use and testing, and treatment progress.

SAS and MHS staffs assist clients in preparing individualized weekly plans for SonomaWORKS participation. These include time spent on work, supportive services, and treatment services. For mental health services, clients are allowed one hour biweekly for individual therapy and/or two hours per week to participate in group therapy, which counts toward their thirty-two-hour per week work requirement. Individuals may also receive credited time for family counseling services and/or services at outside agencies.

For substance abuse services, clients are allowed to count varying amounts of hours toward their work requirement based on their individual treatment plans. While some may count only one hour per week, others, such as those in residential treatment, satisfy their thirty-two-hour work requirement through hours of treatment. When clients begin working with SAS or MHS, they are informed of their rights to confidentiality and their right to bring disputes to the Sonoma County Human Services Department. Staff also provide ongoing case management for clients.

When clients do not show up to an assigned activity, good cause must be identified. If a good cause cannot be found, then clients are notified that unless they comply, their cash grant will be reduced. For some clients, threat or actual imposition of financial sanctions may not be a sufficient incentive to elicit compliance, and therefore the county may authorize a home visit. At the time clients become noncompliant, they are sent to postassessment services. At this time, staff may assist clients and/or other workers in preparing an agreement that describes a plan for future compliance. This may, in fact, be the first time a client is referred for substance abuse or mental health issues. For failure to comply with the conciliation agreement, the client may be officially sanctioned and sent a lowered monthly cash grant.

PROGRAM SUCCESSES

The success of these programs is evident in utilization rates. From the outset, the numbers of persons using these services has increased, as has number of persons exiting SonomaWORKS due to paid employment. The current show rate for Substance Abuse Services is an impressive 89 percent. There are high levels of communication in and among Human Service Department employees, Substance Abuse Services, Mental Health Services, and community treatment providers. Training between county staff, contracted staff, and specialists is ongoing in an attempt to understand the changing needs and difficulties facing clients. All clients are seen by county mental health staff unless clients are eligible for outside services or have more specialized service needs.

The goal of SonomaWORKS is to be client friendly and welcoming, as demonstrated by staff members who respect clients and work hard to maximize the physical and mental well-being of clients. Clients are viewed as customers and treated as whole persons. Staff members are committed to their focus on identifying and working through barriers to employment and not providing traditional, long-term therapy. Colocation of services makes access convenient, and the show rate for clients of MHS continues to improve. Postemployment services also provide continuing support for up to one year after a client leaves SonomaWORKS in order to assist that client in remaining in steady employment.

Clients seen in MHS feel supported and encouraged and feel that they have been given the tools to develop positive ways of coping with life stresses. SAS clients say that the program gives them hope and the self-confidence and motivation to seek self-sufficiency. Holding clients accountable for their behaviors as well as monitoring their progress are seen in a positive way. For many clients, it is the first time they have truly felt supported, and they see MHS and SAS as key factors in turning their lives around.

PROGRAM CHALLENGES

Although client utilization and compliance rates are comparatively high, substance abuse and mental health staff agree that client compliance continues to be the number-one problem. The client goal is to keep an appointment and take an active role in the treatment process, but a significant population of mental health clients repeatedly miss appointments and fail to follow up with treatment goals. Clients sometimes experience difficulty in navigating systems effectively and efficiently, due to numerous requirements to learn and large amounts of information to absorb.

Seeing clients in a timely manner is an ongoing struggle for MHS staff, who have decreased appointment wait times from six weeks to two weeks, but they still contend with large numbers of no-show appointments. One way staff has achieved some success with this problem is by overbooking appointments, allowing for a certain number of no-shows throughout the day. High monthly referral numbers make it difficult to accommodate client need. Although colocation may be convenient, it puts space at a premium, making it difficult at times for staff to find private space to meet with clients. There is also a joint waiting room for SAS and MHS, which may contribute to a client's sense of decreased confidentiality.

Although the clients' assessments of the services have been overwhelmingly favorable, they see the need for the increased availability of one-on-one counseling, which is currently limited by the availability of staff. Other client suggestions include a desire for more female staff, more parenting and family counseling, longer sessions, and possible coordination with legal services.

LESSONS LEARNED

In looking back on its past two years of services, SonomaWORKS employees along with SAS and MHS have identified some lessons learned along the way. Some items are issues staff wished they had known before the programs got started, while others are unexpected outcomes of new ventures. In either case, these issues have been learning experiences for all involved and opportunities to effect change within the system. The lessons include the following:

1. It is an ongoing challenge for management to convey to staff the importance of administrative tasks for maintaining the continuous flow of funding. Constant documentation, monitoring, and adjusting are crucial to maintaining state and federal funding. Staff members need to be educated about the reasons for collecting and reporting certain types of information.
2. Initial orientation and ongoing staff training are important to early detection and identification of treatment placement needs. Not providing the proper amount of programmatic structure may lead to disparity in treatment approaches and a lack of team decision making.
3. There is an ongoing need for an integrated family system and a staffing contingency plan to promote continuity of care. Continuity of service may suffer when systems assisting parents do not work cooperatively with systems assisting their children. For best results, case managers for both groups need to communicate on a regular basis. Staff turnover may lead to longer wait times for client appointments and decreased success in terms of no-show rates and client compliance with treatment.

4. In spite of clear advantages to group therapy with regard to efficiency and clients' shared experience, it may be difficult to implement in mental health services. There may be some resistance on the part of staff and clients in using group as opposed to individual therapy. In the mental health field, traditional therapy models regard individual counseling as highly effective, and some staff may hesitate to use group models, which they believe may not produce the same results. Clients often prefer individual therapy because it feels more personal and may allow them the space to express more complex issues. Special attention needs to be given to helping staff make the transition from traditional treatment approaches to short-term welfare-to-work approaches designed to help clients remove barriers and get back to work.
5. In spite of adequate funds to pay for services, it may be difficult to spend budgeted money. Although funds are budgeted for outpatient mental health and substance abuse services, the county does not expend the funds when the service is billable to Medi-Cal. This may create a situation wherein funds are not used according to budget and may result in decreased funding the following year.

REFERENCES

Bush, I.R. and Kraft, M.K. (1998). The Voices of Welfare Reform. *Public Welfare,* 56(1), 11.

Grayson, M. (1999). Kicking Habits: Preparing Welfare Recipients for the Work Force. *Spectrum: The Journal of State Government,* 72(1), 4-10.

Kunz, J. and Kalil, A. (1999). Self-Esteem, Self-Efficacy and Welfare Use. *Social Work Research,* 23(2), 116-124.

Nichols-Casebolt, A. (1986). The Psychological Effects of Income Testing Income-Support Benefits. *Social Service Review,* 60, 287-303.

Olson, K. and Pavetti, L. (1996). *Personal and Family Challenges to the Successful Transition from Welfare to Work.* Washington, DC: Urban Institute.

Pavetti, L., Holcomb, E., and Duke, A. (1995). *Increasing Participation in Work and Work-Related Activities: Lessons from Five State Demonstration Projects.* Washington, DC: Urban Institute.

Pavetti, L., Olson, K., Nightingale, D., Duke, A., and Isaacs, J. (1997). *Welfare to Work Options for Families Facing Personal and Family Challenges: Rationale and Program Strategies.* Washington, DC: Urban Institute and the American Institutes for Research.

Polit, D.F. and O'Hara, J.J. (1989). Social Services. *Welfare Policy for the 1990s.* Cambridge, MA: Harvard University Press.

Popkin, S. (1990). Welfare: Views from the Bottom. *Social Problems,* 37, 64-79.

Sonoma County Human Services Department (1999). *First Annual SonomaWORKS Report.* Santa Rosa, CA: Author.
Steisel, S. (1999). Leaving Addiction Behind. *State Legislature,* 25(4), 20-28.
Woolis, D.D. (1998). FamilyWorks: Substance Abuse Treatment and Welfare Reform. *Public Welfare,* 56(1), 19-27.
Young, N. and Gardner, S. (1997). *Implementing Welfare Reform: Solutions to the Substance Abuse Problem.* Washington, DC: Children and Family Futures and Drug Strategies.

SELF-SUFFICIENCY SUPPORT SERVICES

Chapter 7

Combining Business with Rehabilitation in a Public Work Center for Disabled and Low-Income Participants

Jonathan Prince
Michael J. Austin

Work centers represent a true partnership that benefits the business community, the recipient of public assistance, personnel in social services, and the taxpayer. The business community benefits by contracting with work centers to complete low-cost, high-quality jobs that include assembly, packaging, and shipping. The participant benefits by receiving job training, work experience, and possibly competitive mainstream employment while having access to a wide variety of rehabilitation services. Social services personnel benefit from work centers because they can improve the quality of life for participants by helping them to become self-sufficient. Finally, the taxpayer benefits because increased participant employment results in the reduced expenditure of public funds. Given these benefits, it is somewhat surprising that work centers have not received heightened national attention following the passage of welfare reform legislation as an ideal program to promote self-sufficiency through employment and reduced welfare dependency.

Advocates point out that, in addition to benefiting participants, work centers affect all citizens because (1) increased participant employment results in decreased public assistance expenditures and lower taxes and (2) as rehabilitation facilities they can often sustain themselves financially without requiring large expenditures from taxpayer-supported public funds. Employing hard-to-place individuals is becoming increasingly important with welfare reforms that require work and set time limits on benefits. Many welfare recipients capable of working will have found employment by the time the first wave of time limits expires. Only those with significant barriers to employment will remain on the welfare rolls (Olson and Pavetti, 1996). These recipients can potentially benefit the most from work center services and support.

In addition to WorkCenter resources, human services clients (primarily CalWORKs or General Assistance [GA] recipients) have access to an additional array of services. In thirty-day intervals, human services case managers connect with clients after referral to the WorkCenter. If the participant is experiencing difficulties he or she is referred to income and employment service specialists (IESS) and/or staff in other county departments that specialize in health, mental health, substance abuse, and domestic violence issues. Often, personnel from these departments work together in a team. For example, the family self-sufficiency team combines professionals from substance abuse and mental health services to assist participants with barriers to employment.

If a CalWORKs recipient is not participating in the mandatory five-day job-search skills class, he or she will receive a home visit from a case manager to assess and help resolve the issues that interfere with attendance. Unlike their Aid to Families with Dependent Children (AFDC) predecessors, CalWORKs recipients do not work at the WorkCenter, but after the job-search skills class they receive ongoing assistance with finding employment. Recipients may receive federally mandated Temporary Assistance to Needy Families (TANF) sanctions if they do not comply with training, job search, or employment participation requirements. To prevent this from occurring, CalWORKs staff offer continuing services to facilitate participation and help clients progress in their goals.

Unlike the progressive nature of TANF sanctions, GA sanctions are immediate in that a client's case is closed if he or she is not participating in the job-search skills class followed by at least three days per week of job hunting. GA recipients that proceed to work at the WorkCenter, however, receive the same services as CalWORKs recipients when they are experiencing problems that interfere with employment. They, too, receive case manager home visits if, for example, they arrive at the WorkCenter intoxicated or they suddenly stop showing up for work. The family self-sufficiency team is frequently contacted to help GA recipients with undiagnosed mental health problems and/or substance dependence. The supports offered to human services clients by the county are as follows:

1. WorkCenter
   - Vocational rehabilitation services (VRS)
2. Support from human services
   - Home visits
   - Monthly meetings
3. Support from other county departments
   - Domestic violence services
   - Health services
   - Mental health services
   - Drug and alcohol services

This case study includes a brief literature review as a context for describing a unique public service work center operated by the Employment and Services Centers in San Mateo County, California. The description includes WorkCenter operations, staff, and services, followed by an in-depth look at the participants served. The case study concludes with a discussion of WorkCenter challenges and proposed solutions. In this case study the term *participants* is used to describe workers at the WorkCenter. Most participants are also county *clients* that may be *recipients* of public assistance (e.g., General Assistance or CalWORKs). *Staff* refers to county employees that supervise or counsel participants, and the term *customers* refers to businesses or agencies that hire the WorkCenter to complete job contracts.

BRIEF LITERATURE REVIEW

By providing employment experience, training, support, placement, and/or coaching, most work centers seek to fully integrate participants into the competitive workforce and the larger community (Visier, 1998). This goal can be traced back to the 1950s when a large number of work centers were established in the United States to serve people with psychiatric, physical, or developmental disabilities (Lamb, 1971). Prior to the 1950s, however, work centers functioned as the only alternative to mainstream employment for people with physical disabilities (Lamb, 1971).

Internationally, work centers vary in the way they view participants. From a survey sent to work center personnel in twenty-five countries, Visier

(1998) identified three types of work centers for participants who are (1) too disabled to be fully employed in the marketplace (Greece and Ireland), (2) considered trainees or clients en route to full-employee status (Australia and many European countries), and (3) considered full employees with job contracts and the right to organize (Sweden and Great Britain).

All of the work centers Visier surveyed varied on a continuum from entirely "therapeutic" to functioning as an entirely "normalized" work environment. Most work centers fall somewhere in the middle of this continuum. Visier's survey results revealed that participants are usually paid at the minimum wage, and their work typically involves packaging, assembly, or manufacturing.

On-site work centers are often combined with *supported employment,* or work that is done off site. This professional support can include on-the-job supervision and coaching, job adaptations and modifications, transportation, and assistance with social skills and money management (Rogan and Murphy, 1991). In most work center models, participants progress through a series of stages culminating in independent paid employment. These stages include preemployment training, adjustment to the workplace, time-limited employment services, and job placement (Parent, Hill, and Wehman, 1989).

One major challenge facing most work centers is finding the best balance between production and training (Rosen et al., 1993). If significant resources are devoted to the training of a large number of participants, then the work center may not have enough staff or participants for production and revenues will decline. On the other hand, future participant employability might be impeded if too few resources are devoted to training. Production will suffer if too many resources are devoted to therapeutic, medical, or social concerns and vice versa. It is difficult to find the most efficacious balance between production and rehabilitation (Visier, 1998).

In general, work centers that are more successful in training, supporting, and placing participants tend to have fewer participants available for production, which may lead to reduced revenues. In this respect, the business component of work centers competes with the rehabilitative component, resulting in the following critique primarily from within the field of vocational rehabilitation (Rosen et al., 1993):

1. The need to generate revenues may result in selecting participants who are the most productive (i.e., "creaming") in order to maximize revenues rather than serving the populations of more disabled, less productive individuals most in need of support (Rogan and Murphy, 1991).
2. The rehabilitative nature of work centers can justify the excessive *sheltering* of participants (protecting disabled participants from risk,

competition, frustration, and failure assumed to accompany independent employment). Critics believe that sheltering can isolate disabled individuals from the workforce and preclude community integration (Reker, Eikelmann, and Inhester, 1992; Rosen et al., 1993).
3. The rehabilitative nature of work centers can justify the absence of labor rights for participants, including the right to formally agree to a job contract and join a union (Visier, 1998).

Despite this critique, many authors (e.g., Rogan and Murphy, 1991; Rosen et al., 1993) discuss the potential of work centers to

- help social service and mental health clients find and maintain mainstream employment along with the material and psychological benefits of self-sufficiency;
- provide assessments of participants based on observed work performance (capability and productivity) that is not easy to obtain from participant interviews or testing;
- be located wherever a participant labor supply and organizations can provide work (Rosen et al., 1993); and
- serve people with more severe disabilities (health or mental health problems, lack of work skills or education, substance abuse, domestic violence issues, legal difficulties, or caretaker responsibilities) that are hard to place in the workforce (Rogan and Murphy, 1991; Rosen et al., 1993).

With these work center strengths and limitations in mind, it is now useful to look more closely at one of the few work centers in northern California. Participants at the WorkCenter are seen as job-search trainees that require varying amounts of rehabilitative services, but they are also viewed as productive and responsible members of the workforce. Rehabilitation staff at the WorkCenter, for example, will often support individual participants after they have found a job and help with job retention. Other times staff will assist whole work crews hired to complete off-site activities. Supervised, off-site jobs are often called *enclaves*.

THE EVOLUTION OF THE SAN MATEO COUNTY WORKCENTER

With a grant of approximately $200, the WorkCenter was established in 1967 to help welfare recipients find employment after assessing their work skills in a supervised setting. It was initially managed by a local priest and operated out of the basement of the county hospital, where participants, most of whom were women on AFDC, completed small jobs such as packaging surgical equipment and bandages. The San Mateo County Social Services Division (now the Human Services Agency) collaborated with the hospital and oversaw program operations.

By 1970 the county mental health division partnered with social services and rented a small, two-story building in San Carlos to house the WorkCenter. In addition to recipients of AFDC, the WorkCenter also began to employ people receiving ATD, or Aid to the Disabled (a precursor to SSI, or Supplemental Security Income). Welfare recipients worked on the bottom floor and ATD recipients, often mental health consumers, worked on the top floor. Staff at the WorkCenter consisted of four vocational rehabilitation counselors, one mental health clinician, a psychologist who completed weekly vocational testing, and a consulting psychiatrist.

In 1972 the San Mateo County Board of Supervisors approved a measure that would pay WorkCenter participants a wage. These wages would come from customer payments to the WorkCenter for completion of private-industry jobs (Anonymous, 1990). This legislation, the addition of mental health participants, and the relocation to a larger facility allowed for significant WorkCenter expansion.

A major WorkCenter activity in the early 1970s was electronics assembly. One of the larger job contracts was with Lenkert, a large electronics firm across the street from the WorkCenter. A Lenkert employee taught soldering, harnessing, and other electronic assembly skills to WorkCenter participants. Skills such as these enabled participants to earn a wage, complete WorkCenter jobs, and often find independent employment in the community. A large increase in the number of AFDC recipients at this time allowed for the continuing growth of the WorkCenter.

Along with an increase in AFDC recipients at the WorkCenter, General Assistance recipients were also referred to the WorkCenter in large numbers in the early 1970s. This followed a landmark case in which a GA applicant filed a lawsuit after being told he was employable and therefore not eligible for assistance. The lawsuit was successful, and the county began referring them to the WorkCenter.

In the early 1970s WorkCenter participants from mental health and social services began to work together as a team. A new director secured additional sources of revenue for the WorkCenter, and the number of vocational counselors grew from four to thirteen within a short period of time. Social and recreation programs were established for WorkCenter participants. Outreach programs were created to increase the number of referrals from board and care homes, psychiatric hospitals, and day treatment centers. Active efforts were also made to accommodate people with disabilities and other populations that could benefit from a supported work environment.

The WorkCenter again outgrew its facilities and relocated to Elmer Street in Belmont in 1975.

The Elmer Street location was much bigger and more staff were hired to oversee increasing numbers of job contracts. The GA Employment Program was developed at this time, whereby GA recipients earned their GA checks by working at the WorkCenter rather than paying back the cash assistance after finding employment. Throughout the late 1970s and early 1980s GA recipients could work toward completing their high school equivalency degree on site through collaboration with a local adult school that agreed to outstation a teacher.

The WorkCenter remained on Elmer Street for ten years before moving to its current Quarry Road address in San Carlos in 1985. Throughout the 1980s and early 1990s production revenues remained relatively high because of the availability of clients. Revenues have recently fallen, however, due to a shortage of participants during the strong economy of the 1990s.

To facilitate a more intimate understanding of the WorkCenter, the next section recounts the experiences of a single client. This is followed by a current description of the WorkCenter, its staff, the services they provide, and the participants that work and receive assistance.

THE EXPERIENCES OF A WORKCENTER CLIENT

At the age of thirty-seven Richard had recently been released from prison following a ten-month sentence based on domestic violence charges. When seen at the Department of Human Services it was determined that he was eligible for Food Stamps, bus passes, and a monthly GA payment of $265 based on an interest in looking for a job and participating in the WorkCenter. He lives in his brother's house in East Palo Alto and pays a monthly rent of $175. He said the following about his WorkCenter experience: "I needed help with food and paying rent, so I asked for assistance. Here they have a program which helps with government assistance and with Food Stamps, but you have to go to work before you receive anything. . . . A lot of different people come here, and it's a big help. We just need a chance to get back into society. I like to feel like I'm at least contributing something, so if I came here to at least give something while I am looking for a job.

"I work at the WorkCenter as part of the program. We are not here just to work at the WorkCenter—we are here to find employment. That's what this whole thing is about. I've put in so many applications since I've been here, and I'm getting calls. I have a couple of interviews next week. One is for Home Depot, and the other is working in sheet metal. That's what I do by trade. The sheet metal work you can make from nine to twenty-eight dollars an hour. I have two daughters, and that's why I am making an effort to find a job—so I can take care of my responsibilities toward them. As soon as I start working I'll move out of my brother's house. I'll probably move to Menlo Park. That's where I was before this altercation with my wife happened. I'm on probation now. Every Thursday I go to my domestic violence group, and I see my probation officer once a month. I have to pay a total of about one thousand dollars in fines.

"I go to the Network Center three days a week, when I am not at the WorkCenter. Everyone is asked to bring in three or four job leads. Sometimes they pan out and sometimes they don't. They teach you how to use the newspaper, how to fill out an application correctly, and how to use the phone. They even have posted the correct way to use the phone as far as using the person's name, not to say 'yeah' and all that on the phone, but to say 'yes.' They help you with a résumé and the do's and don'ts of interviews—even how to sit and hold your hands and throw in some light talk so the interview won't be all serious. We did a couple of mock interviews, where they videotaped us. We are our own critics as far as what we did wrong and what we did right. And then our job coach, Jerry, he told us our weak points and our strengths. We also got help using the computer. They will give you individual help if you need it and extra help in general. They even have maps to give locations of where to go and what buses to catch to jobs and interviews. It really works when they help you send out your résumé and use the phone. It's so much better than running up and down the street looking for some work.

"There are only two of us left from the group of eight that I came in with. Everybody is really taking the initiative to get out of there and look for work. I know one wanted to be a waitress and she became one, and one found work at the airport in customer service. There are a lot of jobs out there. I should have a job by next week. I feel that if you come here, put in the time, and ask people for a job, you'll find it. And if you don't, in my opinion, you're not even looking. You can tell when someone's not looking for a job, especially if the job offered won't pay the bills."

CURRENT WORKCENTER OPERATIONS

With over 45,000 square feet of floor space, the current facility has the modern equipment necessary to remain competitive in securing contracts with a wide variety of private industries in the greater San Francisco Bay Area and the Silicon Valley. The equipment includes shrink-wrap machines, forklifts, two delivery trucks, and electric conveyor-driven assembly lines. There are six sections of the production floor, each with a production supervisor and a participant lead client-worker. Two production managers oversee the entire floor, and a quality control manager ensures that jobs are completed according to customer specifications. A marketing director identifies and recruits customers, and an operations manager provides executive leadership.

WorkCenter participants complete a wide variety of jobs. The major on-site activity is called *fulfillment,* or the packaging and shipping of different products. Participants ship an average of 300 packages per day, learning job skills such as forklift operation and shipping and receiving. The WorkCenter serves about thirty different companies per month, with about five jobs in operation at any one time. Companies are charged between eighteen dollars and twenty-one dollars per hour to cover participant wages, overhead, equipment, shipping, and receiving. In addition, companies frequently send engineers to train and supervise participants in electronics assembly. For example, participants are currently building Internet video cameras for Vista Imaging. In the past, other types of on-site work activity have included bicycle repair, microfilming, and the refurbishing of office equipment. The WorkCenter is accredited by the Commission on Accreditation of Rehabilitation Facilities (CARF).

The WorkCenter off-site activities are also highly varied and include a food service catering operation, a recycling service, and a janitorial program. All three serve private industry and public organizations. The food service program, for example, caters to Cañada College and many other customers in addition to serving as a cafeteria for county employees. Other off-site jobs include staff-assisted participant placement in, for example, the medical or social service records department of hospitals or county departments.

From the perspective of the customer that contracts with the WorkCenter, the WorkCenter offers competitive pricing, quick job completion, and quality that competes favorably with private industry. For example, the local United Airlines Maintenance Center contracted with the WorkCenter for the mentally disabled to sort and inspect hundreds of pounds of nuts, bolts, and clamps which were generated from tearing down a jet engine (Anonymous, 1990).

Although most WorkCenter participants are paid the minimum wage, some off-site work can pay from eight dollars to ten dollars per hour. Lead workers, for example, often find higher-paying work after obtaining supervisory experience in one of the six sections of the WorkCenter production floor. Mental health clients are paid according to a productivity assessment that is determined in their first two weeks of work and reviewed every six months thereafter. They receive half the minimum wage, for example, if their work is half as productive as the work of a nondisabled individual.

GA recipients receive the minimum wage from GA county funds. In essence, these recipients work off their benefits and do not receive wages that exceed them. All participants are evaluated regularly.

WORKCENTER SERVICES

The WorkCenter is a part of several larger organizational structures, including Vocational Rehabilitation Services. VRS is itself a small component of one of three regional (the Central Region) Employment and Services Centers in San Mateo County that include various programs from the county human services agency. Participants are supported by a variety of VRS staff while they receive work assessment, training, and experience. If needed, transportation, child care, and interview clothes are provided throughout the job-search process.

At intake, screening, and assessment specialists determine eligibility and assess work skills through vocational testing and interviewing. To be eligible, participants must be U.S. citizens that reside in the county, and they must be willing to work. In addition, they should be receiving mental health services if deemed appropriate by a treating professional, or be referred from the State Department of Rehabilitation or another sponsoring agency.

The screening is followed by participation in a weeklong class on job-seeking skills in which interests are explored and résumés developed. The class is part of the Network Center. The center is equipped with computers, telephones, job listings, phone books, and other resources that assist in seeking employment, and it is staffed by job-search and placement specialists. A participant flowchart of the WorkCenter intake process is included in Figure 7.1. The curriculum encourages self-sufficiency and teaches job-search and retention skills. Like the earlier GA Employment Program, participation in this class is mandatory for GA and CalWORKs recipients unless they are exempted from work requirements. Recipients are usually exempted because they have a disability or they are caring for someone that has a disability.

After the job-search class, a ten-day WorkCenter participant assessment begins with the identification of significant barriers to employment. In the

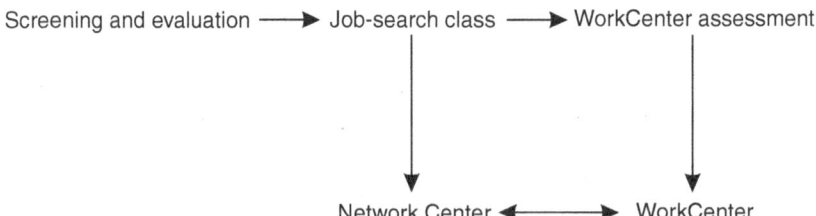

FIGURE 7.1. Flowchart of the WorkCenter Intake Processes

assessment, the participant is evaluated for work performance and stamina, as well as the ability to follow instructions, learn, get along with co-workers, and arrive at work on time. Information from the assessment is used to remove barriers to the client's employability. Participants continue to work at the WorkCenter and look for a job at the Network Center until employment is found.

A CLOSER LOOK AT WORKCENTER PARTICIPANTS

Recipients of GA and CalWORKs work together on a daily basis with a variety of other populations, providing an integrated and transitional employment experience. Although most participants are referred by county departments of mental health or human services, smaller numbers come from a prison work-furlough program, substance abuse programs, rehabilitation programs, and the family court for nonpayment of ordered child support. Mental health clients are also referred from the State Department of Rehabilitation. According to one senior employee, the biggest changes at the WorkCenter over the course of its history have been the addition of these new populations of participants.

Approximately 100 people work at the WorkCenter on a typical day, and about 2,500 people are served each year, based on the goal of a high turnover rate. Most WorkCenter positions are vacated more than twenty times per year. An estimated 25 percent of participants find competitive employment, while the remainder drop out of the program, periodically reenter, or continue as WorkCenter participants. Many of the remaining participants have chronic mental health disabilities and stay in the program for longer periods of time. Due to shortages in the labor market, WorkCenter participants are occasionally employed by a community organization in order to complete contracts in a timely manner.

The proportions of participants from these different populations have changed over time. In the 1980s and early 1990s about two-thirds of the participants were human services (GA or TANF/AFDC) recipients and about one-third were mental health clients. However, these percentages have recently reversed themselves. Now, about two-thirds of the participants are mental health clients and only one-third are human service clients. As a result of low unemployment in the county and welfare reform, there has been a dramatic decrease in public assistance recipients at the WorkCenter. For example, a few years ago there were about 285 GA recipients at the WorkCenter each day, whereas there are now only about sixty-five per day. This 77 percent decrease in GA recipients at the WorkCenter is caused by (1) a strong economy, (2) a very low (2 percent) local unemployment rate, with most GA clients finding competitive employment within a short period of time, and (3) a high cost of living in the county resulting in poor people moving to more affordable communities.

Largely due to a strong economy in the late 1990s, the WorkCenter completed fewer job contracts along with dramatically reduced revenues and the need for county subsidy. In 2000 the WorkCenter generated approximately $900,000, representing roughly 27 percent of total revenues. About 42 percent of total revenues are from the county human services agency, and the remainder (31 percent) is from the State Department of Rehabilitation and the county Mental Health Unit.

WORKCENTER CHALLENGES

In addition to a reduced supply of labor and revenue shortfalls, the WorkCenter faces several other challenges.

Participant Challenges

- A significant percentage of participants, especially the most disabled, are hard to place in the competitive workforce. Many of them have a fear of independent employment that further complicates the more apparent physical and psychiatric barriers to self-sufficiency. Flexible and creative approaches are often taken in placing these participants, yet new approaches still need to be developed and implemented.
- A significant percentage of participants, especially from human services, have difficulty retaining jobs once they are placed as a result of substance abuse, undiagnosed mental health problems, legal issues, or family problems. Although job coaching assists participants in keeping jobs, many return to VRS and the WorkCenter after varying periods of time.
- Conflicts sometimes arise among participants working together in an integrated work environment. GA recipients, for example, sometimes state they feel uncomfortable working with mental health clients. Other times the inappropriate behavior of some participants interferes with WorkCenter production. Problems such as these are handled at the WorkCenter by assessment and behavior modification techniques, followed by individual and group counseling if needed.

Administrative Challenges

- It is often difficult to obtain the types of customer jobs that Work-Center participants are able to complete. Participants can complete

packaging and assembly jobs within customer time limits, but other jobs are more complex and are more quickly completed by private industry. Competing with private industry, therefore, is an ongoing struggle.
- As a result of rapid changes due to welfare reform and the recent creation of the Employment Services Center for the central region of the county at VRS, many staff positions are changing quickly. For example, employees (IESS) that had primarily engaged in screening and eligibility now have many case management responsibilities, resulting in some role confusion.
- The majority of participants today are mental health clients with cognitive difficulties related to lack of concentration or attention skills that can lead to lower productivity.

To address the major challenge of reduced production revenues due to labor shortages, plans are being prepared to assist CalWORKs recipients to the WorkCenter when their two-year TANF time limit expires. This would enable them to fulfill their work requirements and continue their job search while providing needed WorkCenter labor. Another idea under consideration is to provide broader and more assertive outreach to underserved low-income or disabled populations.The future success of the WorkCenter is dependent on strategies that increase its capacity to involve a sufficient number of participants to meet the demands of new contracts.

The rehabilitative success of the WorkCenter, however, has remained constant for over thirty years. What started as a $200 operation out of a hospital basement has grown into an organization recognized nationally as a model for successful vocational rehabilitation services. In counseling, supervising, or helping with job search and retention, WorkCenter staff have viewed low-income and disabled individuals as capable and productive yet in need of temporary assistance. More importantly, staff members have helped people to overcome personal obstacles and find employment. Services that achieve this objective will be increasingly needed as greater numbers of people are encouraged to find work and exit public welfare and disability rolls.

In helping welfare recipients achieve self-sufficiency, the county human services agency offers a great deal of support to WorkCenter participants, including ongoing contact with a case manager, home visits, and referrals to a continuum of county professionals. In addition, welfare recipients receive services that are available to all participants, including (1) a job-search skills class; (2) access to a variety of rehabilitation staff; (3) assistance with transportation, child care, and clothes for interviews; (4) WorkCenter assessments and job experience; and (5) access to the Network Center and help with finding and retaining employment.

WorkCenter staff members have learned valuable lessons in delivering these services. First, it is important to keep an eye on the balance between productivity and employability. Although employing participants is the primary WorkCenter objective, success in achieving this objective will result in lower production revenues and increased public subsidy. In this respect the need for increased state and county funding is an indication of the rehabilitative success of the WorkCenter.

Staff members have also learned to change the way they view WorkCenter participants because they are no longer exclusively mental health clients or GA recipients. Participants have recently become much more diverse. Rather than qualifying for services because they are disabled or poor (deficit-based eligibility), participants now qualify for assistance because they have the desire to learn new skills and transition to higher-level employment (strength-based eligibility). As a result, staff roles have changed dramatically as the WorkCenter has opened its doors to the larger community.

REFERENCES

Anonymous (1990). People, work and pride: San Mateo County's Vocational Rehabilitation Services celebrates 33 years of service. *Special Supplement to the Peninsula Times Tribune,* September 12, p. F1.

Lamb, H.R. (1971). *Rehabilitation in community mental health.* San Francisco: Jossey Bass.

Olson, K. and Pavetti, L. (1996). Personal and family challenges to the successful transition from welfare to work. The Urban Institute.

Parent, W.S., Hill, M.L., and Wehman, P. (1989). From sheltered to supported employment outcomes: Challenges for rehabilitation facilities. *Journal of Rehabilitation,* 55 (October-December) 51-57.

Reker, T., Eikelmann, B., and Inhester, M.L. (1992). Pathways into sheltered employment. *Social Psychiatry and Psychiatric Epidemiology, 27,* 220-225.

Rogan, P. and Murphy, S. (1991). Supported employment and vocational rehabilitation: Merger or misadventure? *Journal of Rehabilitation,* 55(April-June), 39-45.

Rosen, M., Bussone, A., Dakunchak, P., and Cramp, J. (1993). Sheltered employment and the second generation workshop. *Journal of Rehabilitation,* 60(January-March), 30-34.

Visier, L. (1998). Sheltered employment for persons with disabilities. *International Labour Review, 137*(3), 347.

Chapter 8

The Family Loan Program as a Public-Private Partnership

Susan E. Doyle
Michael J. Austin

Recent federal welfare reform legislation has transformed the way counties approach serving their low-income populations. San Mateo County has responded to these changes with a series of programs designed to address the changing needs of clients. This case study highlights one such innovative effort, the Family Loan Program, which was established in January 1998 and is operated by the Family Service Agency of San Mateo County. This program is a replication of a family loan program developed by the McKnight Foundation in Minnesota in 1984. It reflects a public-private partnership to serve clients in three critical ways: (1) alleviating hardship and facilitating the parents' ability to work, (2) providing education and training in real-life skills, and (3) contributing to the family's asset-building ability. This case study covers the first eighteen months of program implementation (January 1998-July 1999). The case study includes the following sections: a review of the literature; the development and implementation in San Mateo County; a description of program operation; a discussion of lessons learned; and the identification of future areas for expansion.

REVIEW OF THE LITERATURE

Federal welfare reform has focused on getting welfare recipients into employment as soon as possible. However, the jobs former welfare recipients can expect to find are primarily entry-level, service-sector positions without many benefits or job security (Jones and Wattenberg, 1991). Therefore, the working poor seeking to become self-sufficient are still often vulnerable to large, unexpected expenses (such as car repairs) due to a lack of savings (Jones and Wattenberg, 1991; Raschick, 1997; Berde and Mueller, 1996). Low-interest loan programs are one way of addressing this issue.

Access to reliable and flexible transportation, in particular, has emerged as a vital component of a family's ability to attain and maintain employment or education. Transportation difficulties result, in part, from a persistent spatial mismatch between job seekers concentrated in inner cities and employment growth which is primarily in the suburbs. Irregular shifts, dropping children off at child care, and weekend work hours further exacerbate the situation (Reichert, 1997; Berde and Mueller, 1996; Lambert, 1998). Initiatives aimed at resolving the transportation crisis of the working poor include both asset-building activities, which promote automobile ownership, and direct transfers, such as bus and gas vouchers (Reichert, 1997). Low-interest loan programs focus on helping low-income populations build assets, which have been shown to contribute to improved life satisfaction and self-efficacy, the development of human çapital, increased community involvement, and the enhanced welfare of children (Finn, 1994; Page-Adams and Vosler, 1995; Page-Adams and Yadama, 1997).

ORIGINS OF THE PROGRAM

The original Family Loan Program was established in Minneapolis in 1984 by the McKnight Foundation, a private foundation committed to enhancing the abilities and productivity of the poor and disenfranchised. The idea started simply with a dinner party hosted by the McKnight Foundation and attended by ten low-income families from Minneapolis. The parents were asked what would most help them manage their lives better and increase their ability to be self-sufficient. Overwhelmingly, these parents expressed a need for financial assistance to address large, one-time expenses that were keeping them from being able to get better jobs or pursue educational opportunities. These unexpected expenses (related to car repair, child care, or car purchase) often result in lost jobs and family deprivation. In addition, these parents wanted assistance in the form of a loan, not a grant, because they wanted the self-respect that goes with being self-sufficient and honoring one's obligations.

The mission and philosophy of the new program were based on the views expressed by the low-income parents. What emerged was a public and private partnership that blended banking and social services to enable clients to build assets and repair damaged credit histories by learning real-world skills related to borrowing and budgeting. The following core values reflect the philosophy of the family loan program (Alliance for Children and Families, 1999):

- Recognizing that small amounts of money at the right moment can make a real difference in moving working low-income families along the path to self-sufficiency and away from welfare and dependency
- Welcoming and supporting applicants who exhibit a potential for success in work or school even though they may have had limited success with past credit experience
- Assuming the best about loan applicants, treating them with dignity and respect, and supporting them in living up to their highest aspirations
- Recognizing that creating a climate of mutual support and responsibility within informal local communities can provide built-in incentives for borrowers to repay loans from a revolving loan fund that serves others within that community

The original Minnesota program was called the Single Parent Loan Program when they handed out their first loans in 1984. The program expanded to include two-parent families in 1991 and the name was changed to the Family Loan Program. The program grew dramatically, and twelve expansion sites within the state of Minnesota were proposed and implemented by 1994. Beginning in 1995, the McKnight Foundation initiated their collaboration with the Alliance for Children and Families (formerly known separately as Family Service America, Inc., and the National Association of Homes and Services for Children) to help coordinate the national replication of the program.

The McKnight Foundation provides local sites with a matching grant and the Alliance offers technical support for the program's implementation. The matching grants are designed to cover $150,000 of the approximately $500,000 needed to start a loan program and operate it for three years. The remainder of the funding comes from a variety of local sources, including private foundations, the banking community, and the public sector. Nationally, a significant amount of local funding has come from the public sector, namely the Community Development Block Grant (CDBG) and similar welfare-to-work initiatives. State and local governments in such states as Virginia, New York, and Colorado have recognized the value of a low-interest loan program in removing barriers to employment and have dedicated some of their welfare reform money to these programs. However, one of the appealing features of this program is the involvement of the private sector. The program in San Mateo County operates solely with private funding.

At the time the original national expansion grants were made available, it was projected that five sites would be established in the first five years of the effort. In reality, local agencies had little difficulty raising the matching funds and those five sites were established in the first year. As a result, the Alliance approved the addition of more sites, and the McKnight Foundation committed the funds to provide additional matching grants. The program's name has gone through another change as well and is now known nationally as Ways to Work: A Family Loan Program.

IMPLEMENTATION AND DEVELOPMENT IN SAN MATEO COUNTY

In the fall of 1997, the director of the human service agency in San Mateo County heard about the Minnesota Family Loan Program. The Peninsula Community Foundation was asked to investigate the program and the possibility of bringing it to California. The foundation quickly discovered the availability of the matching grants being offered by the McKnight Foundation and applied to become one of the national replication sites. Within a few weeks, the Peninsula Community Foundation, along with the David and Lucile Packard Foundation, was able to raise the additional funding needed for the program from a variety of private sources.

Once the funding was secured, the human service agency approached the Family Service Agency (FSA) of San Mateo County to administer the program. The Family Service Agency is a private, nonprofit organization which provides comprehensive and ongoing services to the families of San Mateo County (counseling program, senior service program, child care, a visitation center, and child abuse treatment). The Family Loan Program represents a new direction for an agency focused mainly on counseling and support services.

Once the Family Service Agency was committed to the project and the funding was in place, the next step was to recruit a director for the new program. In keeping with the program's history of blending business and social services, the director was recruited from the private sector. The program's first and only director brought with him a background in finance and a business-oriented approach to the provision of social services, which he describes as

> very business-oriented, kind of like "tough love." This is not a warm and fuzzy program. We provide a service that educates clients on how things work in the real world. Some clients are used to a lot of hand-holding. With this program, clients need sufficient motivation and follow-through. The more work they do, the more likely they will succeed.

One additional part-time support staff position was provided and the program was fully staffed.

The final piece to the puzzle was to bring the local banks into the equation. The Family Service Agency approached local banks in November 1997 and asked them to administer the loan funds for clients of the Family Loan Program. A partnership was established quickly with three local banks (Bay Area Bank, Borel Bank and Trust, and Liberty Bank) and within three months, the first loan had been handed out. As a representative of the Peninsula Community Foundation noted, "This was philanthropy at the speed of light."

PROGRAM DESCRIPTION

The Family Loan Program in San Mateo County officially began on January 7, 1998, and the first loan was given out in February. The program offers loans of up to $3,000, at a low interest rate of 4 percent, for up to a maximum of twenty-four months, to help low-income families attain or maintain economic self-sufficiency. The applicant must show the loan committee how the loan will enable him or her to start or keep a job or further education goals. The most common uses of the loan money are for car purchases, car repairs, tools and uniforms for work or trade, help with housing costs, and child care. In addition to the loan money, the program also provides assistance with establishing and maintaining a realistic budget.

According to the program guidelines, clients must meet the following requirements to apply for a loan:

- employed or enrolled in vocational training at least twenty hours a week and been at their present employment or vocational training three months or longer;
- pursuing post–high school education (at least nine credits per semester);
- other loan sources exhausted and unable to qualify for conventional financing;
- sufficient disposable income (no less than eighty dollars per month);
- must be resident of San Mateo County (for at least three months);
- families must demonstrate the ability to make monthly payments;
- custodial parent of child(ren) under seventeen years of age, living in household (or eighteen if child is in high school);
- loans must be related to helping parents make employment or education a success; and
- loans are available to qualifying families regardless of race, sex, or religious affiliation.

Loan Process

As reflected in Figure 8.1, referrals in the first three months of the program were accepted only from the human service agency (HSA). The HSA sent information about the program to all of their CalWORKs clients each month (approximately 3,500/month). Starting on April 1, 1998, applications were made available to all residents of San Mateo County. Starting in January 1999, the HSA also began mailing information about the program

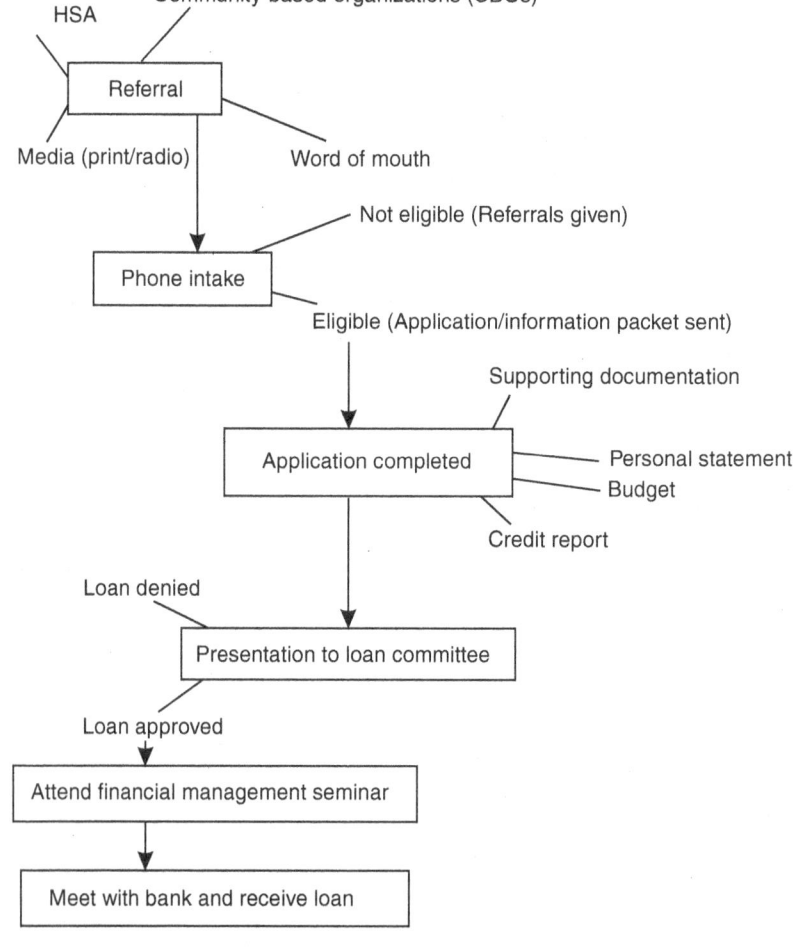

FIGURE 8.1. The Loan Process

to their Medi-Cal clients (approximately 1,100/month). County residents generally learn about the program through the HSA and other CBOs, print and radio media, and word of mouth. When potential loan applicants call the program, they go through an initial phone intake to determine if they meet the eligibility requirements for the program. Eligible applicants are then sent an application packet with various forms to complete. If, after the initial phone conversation, the program cannot serve the client, he or she is given information on what to do to become eligible or is referred to other county resources. When the application has been returned with all the appropriate supporting documentation (pay stubs, tax forms, residency verification, etc.), the file is turned over to the director for review and presentation to the loan committee.

The program director reviews each case thoroughly, paying particular attention to the budgets provided by the client. Several follow-up calls are usually needed to complete a file for presentation to the loan committee. For example, if the client's budget is not realistic, budget counseling is provided to make the application stronger and determine if they truly have the disposable income to support the loan repayment plan. Clients are also encouraged to include in their budgets a savings plan in addition to the repayment amount. At this point in the process, one of the program's employees commented:

> The very last thing I do with a case is pull the credit history. I know there will be problems on it and I don't want to prejudice myself against them before I look at the other pieces. When banks make loans, they look at the credit report to measure character; in this program, character is based on how well the clients communicate their needs and plans.

The next step is the confidential presentation of the file to the loan committee, which meets twice each month. After the director presents the relevant facts of each file, the merits are discussed among members and the loan is either approved or denied. The loan committee consists of a diverse group of three to six individuals and includes banking professionals, counselors, community volunteers, and social workers. The goal in forming each committee was to involve the community as much as possible. In the first year and a half of program operation it has taken an average of fifteen days from receipt of the application to review by the loan committee.

If a loan is approved, clients then attend a mandatory one-and-a-half-hour financial management workshop covering a variety of money-management topics with the following curriculum:

1. Developing a budget
   - Calculating income
   - Current expenses
   - Projected expenses, including savings and loan repayment
2. Where do you spend your money?
   - Bill-paying system
   - Adjusting your budget
   - Having fun
3. Money-saving tips

After attending the workshop, clients bring to the Family Loan Program proof, such as an invoice, for how the funds will be used. The entire file is then sent to the bank located closest to the client's residence for processing and the client becomes a bank customer. The bank services the loan in the same way as any other personal loan, except that the loan check is made out to the client's vendor. The client then receives monthly loan payment slips to send with payment to the bank.

CLIENT POPULATION

A typical loan recipient is a single mother with two children who needs a car, or serious car repairs, so that she can get her family back and forth between work, school, and day care. Based on demographic information collected by the program, the typical loan recipient is a thirty-five to fifty-four-year-old, Caucasian woman with an annual income of less than $25,000. The demographics of the client population, however, do not provide a complete picture of the families served by the program; the following are two illustrations:

Alicia, a forty-three-year-old mother of five, cares on her own for her two youngest sons, Pedro, ten, and Francisco, two. (The three older children have all graduated from high school.) Alicia worked two jobs to care for her family until she fell ill and was forced to rely on public assistance for a time. Last September, she got off welfare and secured a job as a bank teller. Though it took her two buses and forty-five minutes to get to work, she knew she was on her way back to self-sufficiency. Then a co-worker offered to sell her a car. It seemed like the perfect solution to her transportation issues, especially since an older daughter with asthma often needs emergency medical care.

Alicia came to the Family Loan Program in February buried under the weight of $500 monthly payments to her co-worker. She received a loan of $3,000 to pay off the car and to pay for six months of auto insurance. After signing her loan documents at Liberty Bank, she grinned and sighed with relief. "I feel like a million bucks," she said, knowing that now her family would be able to make ends meet.

Anne is a thirty-four-year-old mother whose priority is caring for her five-year-old son, Robert. Until recently a recipient of public assistance, Anne now works two jobs to make ends meet. Anne came to the Family Loan Program after a roommate left her stuck with a bill for back rent and her car needed expensive repairs. The Family Loan Program approved Ann for just over $1,500 to settle her obligations. She is now pursuing the possibility of a move to a better neighborhood for her son.

LESSONS LEARNED

Since 1984, the approval and repayment rates of the national Family Loan Program have all increased significantly, from 46 percent to 70 percent (Berde and Mueller, 1996; Jones and Wattenberg, 1991; Raschick, 1997). The San Mateo County program has benefited greatly from the experience of the national model, demonstrating similar successes as follows:

- Of the 203 applications received, eighty-nine (44 percent) were approved.
- 71 percent of approved loans were for car purchase. The remaining funds were used for housing-related expenses and child care.
- Average application processing time was fifteen days.
- 97 percent of those receiving loans are women.
- Average loan size was $2,594.
- Repayment rate is 91 percent (compared to the national rate of 70 to 75 percent).
- Clients report a 89.9 percent decrease in work time missed; a 92.61 percent reduction in travel time to work; and a 25.9 percent increase in attendance in job-related educational activities.

In addition, clients continue to state that the program was the "booster" they needed to overcome unexpected expenses. The primary strengths of the program include (1) the quality of the relationship formed between the program and the client; (2) the careful and fair judgment of the loan committee; (3) the development of community partnerships; and (4) the continuous program assessment and evaluation. Based on these strengths, four major lessons have been learned.

1. *A trusting relationship between the program and clients needs to be established in order to promote successful participation and high repayment rates.* The quality of the interactions between the program and the client has been shown to be critical to the successful repayment of loans (Berde and

Mueller, 1996). In San Mateo County, the program-client relationship develops from the very first phone call and involves a balance between being supportive and demanding accountability. The program reports a 91 percent repayment rate on its loans, which is significantly higher than the national average (approximately 70 percent). If a client runs into a problem with loan payment, the program-client relationship appears to be strong enough to discuss any difficulties. In return, the program treats each client with dignity and considers each recipient on an individual basis. If a payment is missed, the bank will contact the client in an attempt to collect the money. If, after sixty days, the bank is unable to recover the loan payment, the Family Service Agency buys the loan back from the bank and starts collection procedures themselves. In the first eighteen months of operation (January 1998 through June 1999), only three out of eighty-nine loans granted (3.4 percent) have been charged off. The bank was repaid from the loan pool and the program was unable to recover the money from the client or is pursuing recovery through small claims.

2. *Loan committee members need to be carefully selected because the program relies heavily on their judgment of client risk related to repayment.* One unique feature of this program is the autonomy given to the loan committee in approving and denying loan applications. The task of assessing risk in these applications is difficult and relies heavily on the committee's experience and knowledge of the issues facing low-income populations. Some of the factors that might cause an application to be denied are recent credit problems (within the previous six months); insufficient proof of need; loan seemingly unrelated to employment or education; insufficient disposable income; and inconsistencies in the application. In a regular loan process, banks judge an applicant by the "4 Cs": collateral, credit, cash flow, and character. With the Family Loan Program, demonstration of character is the largest part of the decision to approve or deny an application, as described by one loan committee member:

> I'm not only looking for a hard-luck story because everyone has one. The three things I look for are (1) the client's goals and goal-oriented activity, (2) how the loan will help the individual like nothing else can, and (3) an indication of being a responsible person.

The committee's overall goal is to encourage clients to focus on positive outcomes as they struggle to attain self-sufficiency. When a loan application is not strong enough for immediate approval, the committee often approves it on a provisional basis. If clients are able to meet the additional conditions set by the committee, they will receive their loan. In this way, the client is given some control over the process.

3. *Strong working partnerships need to be established with local banks and businesses.* The Family Loan Program relies greatly on the partnerships it has developed with public and private agencies for each step of its operation. As a referral source, local agencies are indispensable for getting the word out about the program. The banking partnerships provide the vehicle for dispensing loan funds and an opportunity for clients to learn real-world skills. Community collaborations are also essential to making the loan experience a positive one for clients by linking them with additional resources in their community. One of the program's employees noted that "no Family Loan Program can operate as a stand alone CBO. Community involvement and support is necessary for it to fulfill its mission. There are two types of partners: banking partners and community partners."

- *Banking partners.* Participation in the Family Loan Program is attractive to financial institutions for several reasons. It does not create a heavy burden for the banks, it represents a sign of good will to the community, and it qualifies the bank for federal funding under the Community Reinvestment Act (CRA).

  The San Mateo County program could be developed and implemented quickly because the banks are able to treat Family Loan Program clients like any other bank customer. Participation in the program does not require the hiring of new bank staff or developing new products or procedures. It should be noted, however, that it does require a significant commitment of bank resources and personnel time. A loan officer at each bank volunteers his or her time to serve on the loan committee as well as service the loans for clients once they are approved. The banks do not charge the program for servicing the loans, although each installment loan, regardless of size or interest rate, incurs a minimum cost (excluding staff time) to the bank. These costs are not covered by the client's interest payments, but financial institutions are willing to incur them as a way to give back to the community.

  Participation in the Family Loan Program also qualifies banks to receive low-interest federal funding under the requirements of the Community Reinvestment Act. Under the CRA, banks receiving these funds must use a percentage of them for "qualified investments" in "community development" within the bank's assessment area. Qualified investments are defined as having the primary purpose of fostering community development by supporting community services targeted to low- or moderate-income individuals. The banks receive "positive consideration" by those who administer the Community Reinvestment Act as a result of their participation in the Family Loan Program. The positive considerations include (1) contributing to the program's loan pool; (2) contributions to fund the program's administration; (3) providing low-interest loans to the program to expand the loan pool once the original pool is funded from other sources; and (4) servicing loans for clients of the Family Loan Program.

- *Community partnerships.* The collaboration between the Family Loan Program and the Human Investment Project (HIP) is one example of fostering new partnerships to serve low-income populations. Since 1972 HIP has operated a nonprofit organization that develops permanent housing options for low-income residents of San Mateo County. In 1998, they wanted to designate funds to be made available as loans to their clients for emergency expenses that were interfering with self-sufficiency, but could not find one that was willing to administer such a small amount of money. With the arrival of the Family Loan Program, HIP was able to take advantage of their banking relationships based on sharing a similar mission and philosophy.

4. *Continuous assessment and program evaluation needs to be built into the program model. This means that the program is accountable to itself, its public and private sector partners, and the clients that it serves.* Program assessment has been built into the national model for the Family Loan Program from the beginning. The San Mateo County program produces demographic and outcome data every six months as a way to measure its progress. Not only does the program know who they are serving but also who they are not serving. From this information, the program operation can be fine-tuned and new products and services can be developed.

Program assessment has led to the exploration of new ways to expand the Family Loan Program in the future by focusing on reaching the clients that currently cannot be served. As noted in the following list, there are a variety of reasons why a potential applicant might not be eligible for a loan.

Reasons for ineligibility*	Percent of inquiries	
Work/school requirement not met	40	percent
Requested use of loan not appropriate	12	percent
No children or none in custodial care	11	percent
Resident requirement not met	9	percent
Currently receiving disability and/or unemployment insurance	7	percent
Request for information only	6	percent
Emergency need requesting twenty-four-hour turnaround	5	percent
Insufficient income	3	percent

*Random sample of 100 of the 505 ineligible inquiries.

In response to these factors, the program plans to develop new loan products that might be more helpful.
Several new products are currently being explored:

- *Higher-risk loans or emergency loans.* Clients would be able to get small loans at a higher interest rate. Positive repayment history would allow them to "graduate" to lower-interest loan products.
- *Individual development accounts.* A savings account for low-income individuals that matches the amount that they deposit.
- *Loan rebates.* Offer clients a rebate for a positive repayment history.
- *Additional locations.* Establish low-interest loan programs in different locations such as vocational schools and workplaces with high numbers of low-wage workers.
- *Public funding.* Increase the level of public-private partnership through increased use of public funding.

These products are an indication of the program's potential for future development, not a mandated path that the program must take. It is a priority of the current program director to pace the expansion according to a realistic time frame and not grow too quickly.

CONCLUSION

Low-income families face many challenges to self-sufficiency. Most notably, they find that large expenses, such as car repairs and child care, can hinder their ability to maintain employment or pursue further education. In response to this reality, low-interest loan programs across the country have been helping these families make ends meet since 1984. The Family Loan Program operated by the Family Service Agency of San Mateo County has been offering this service to low-income county residents since January 1998. In addition to providing financial assistance that would not otherwise be available to this population, this program offers clients an opportunity to expand their skills by providing training and support around budgeting and borrowing issues.

The undeniable success of this program can be attributed primarily to its ability to establish and maintain strong relationships with clients and community partners, to whom the program holds itself accountable. The high repayment rate reported in the first eighteen months of operation (91 percent) is one indicator of the strength of the program-client relationship. In addition, the dedication and expertise of the loan committee members, banking partners, and community agencies further enables clients to attain their goals and fulfill their obligations. Given this proven track record, the Family Loan Program of San Mateo County can expect to continue to support its client families as well as expand and improve its countywide services.

REFERENCES

Alliance for Children and Families (1999). *Ways to Work: A Family Loan Program.* Milwaukee, WI: Author.

Berde, C. and Mueller, M. (1996). Minnesota's family loan program: Small interest-free loans can help low-income families stay on the job or in school. *Public Welfare,* 54(2), 32-42.

Finn, C.M. (1994). Empowerment in Habitat for Humanity housing: Individual and organizational dynamics. Doctoral dissertation, Case Western Reserve University, Cleveland, OH.

Jones, L. and Wattenberg, E. (1991). Working, still poor: A loan program's role in the lives of low-income single parents. *Social Work,* 36(2), 146-153.

Lambert, T. (1998). The poor and transportation: A comment on Marlene Kim's "The Working Poor: Lousy Jobs or Lousy Workers?" *Journal of Economic Issues,* 32(4), 1140-1142.

Page-Adam, D. and Vosler, N. (1995). Effects of home ownership on well-being among blue-collar workers. Paper presented at the Seventh International Conference of the Society for the Advancement of Socio-Economics, Washington, DC.

Page-Adam, D. and Yadama, M. (1997). Asset building as a community revitalization strategy. *Social Work,* 42(5), 423-434.

Raschick, M. (1997). Helping working poor families with low-interest loans. *Families in Society,* 78(1), 26-36.

Reichert, D. (1997). On the road to self-sufficiency. *State Legislature,* 23(10), 32-33.

Chapter 9

The Adopt-A-Family Program: Building Networks of Support

Susan E. Doyle
Michael J. Austin

It is a common phenomenon that donations of time and money are higher during the holidays, even though the needs of low-income families are year-round. The San Mateo County Adopt-A-Family program, established in November 1997 by Al Teglia, legislative aide to San Mateo County Supervisor Mary Griffin, seeks to expand on the popular holiday programs run each year to ease the hardships of low-income families on a more continuous basis. The focus of the year-round Adopt-A-Family program is to provide for the physical needs of these families as well as build a supportive relationship between "godparents" and their adopted families. In the course of its development, it has also emerged as a valuable countywide network able to link available resources with those in need.

This case study explores the development of the program over the first eighteen months of operation. It is divided into the following sections: (1) a brief review of similar programs, (2) the development of the San Mateo County program, (3) a program description of the impact on its key players (referring agencies, godparents, and client families), and (4) a discussion of program outcomes and lessons learned.

REVIEW OF SIMILAR PROGRAMS

The underlying concept of the Adopt-A-Family program is not new or unique to San Mateo County. Holiday programs that link families in need with individual or group sponsors can be found in many communities across the country. Although they are often operated in conjunction with county social services, they mostly function as a component of private organizations. Organizations that currently operate local holiday programs include the United Way, Kiwanis clubs, universities, trade unions, and public service employees. The bulk of programs operate exclusively during the annual winter holiday season (primarily Thanksgiving and Christmas) and do not include an expectation of an ongoing relationship between the family and their sponsor. In several instances, the family and their sponsor will never meet and the program acts as a clearinghouse for the collection and distribution of donations. Typically, these programs serve anywhere from a handful of families to several hundred each season.

The primary assistance offered through the typical adopt-a-family programs is material. The most frequently donated items include food, gifts, children's toys and clothes, furniture and household items, money, and gift certificates. A small minority of the programs, including the subject of this case study, encourage the development of a relationship between the family and their sponsor. These relationships offer emotional support to families under stress. Activities may include coming together with the family for holiday and birthday parties or helping school-age children with their schoolwork. One program, the Dial-a-Granny program, is exclusively based on offering emotional support to families at risk for child abuse. In this program, surrogate grandparents adopt an at-risk family and share their parenting experience with them. It is designed to be a preventive measure to alleviate the stress of the often isolated and overburdened parents (Barbour, 1983).

Social isolation is becoming an increasing concern in communities across the nation. The stress of modern, everyday life in this complex society takes a heavy toll on families with few resources and support. It is often those in the poorest neighborhoods who have the least interaction with members of the larger community, although they may be located near more affluent areas (Wilson, 1996). As one of the Adopt-A-Family's participating godparents noted, "We all know that there are poor people out there, but we don't realize they live that close to us."

In the era of welfare reform, programs that facilitate greater community support for low-income and at-risk families are becoming increasingly more important. As part of rebuilding neighborhood support systems, these programs help to foster an increase in social interaction between members of the community. Through these interactions a sense of community is built and problem-solving skills are developed (Morrison et al., 1997).

PROGRAM DEVELOPMENT

The popular programs that provide food and gifts to needy families during the holidays inspired the San Mateo County Adopt-A-Family program.

It was conceived as an expansion of these programs, in which low-income families would be supported throughout the year in their struggle for self-sufficiency. The driving force behind the creation of the program is Al Teglia, who started matching families with godparents in November 1997.

The idea for the program did not develop overnight and was based on a growing recognition of the social isolation of low-income families within the county. Teglia felt that untapped resources existed within the county and that they could easily be mobilized to help build a stronger sense of community. Many of the families served by this program are in need of the most basic household items, such as diapers and laundry detergent, as well as items that many people probably have stored in their basements or attics, such as children's clothing and furniture. In addition to the need for material support, Teglia recognized the importance of fostering personal relationships that could benefit both families.

To establish the program, Teglia drew on the knowledge, experience, and connections he had developed during his long career of public service in Daly City. He has been a champion of the needs of families in San Mateo County, most notably during his four terms as mayor of Daly City. His current position with the San Mateo County Board of Supervisors was also instrumental in the successful beginning of the Adopt-A-Family program. With the full support of Supervisor Mary Griffin, Teglia is able to spend approximately 25 percent of his time working on the Adopt-A-Family program. The reputation and resources offered by the supervisor's office have contributed to the success and rapid growth of the program.

The philosophy of the Adopt-A-Family program is to use grassroots networking to connect existing and available county resources with struggling families. The program is becoming a vital link in the county network of resources based on its commitment to minimizing bureaucratic red tape. Once the program has linked families with godparents it assumes a minimal role. The program does not define client needs or godparent resources. Material support provided by godparents goes directly to the family in need. The relationship that develops is determined solely by the family and their godparent.

The program was launched with a presentation to potential client families at a human service workshop conducted at a local SUCCESS Center of the San Mateo County Human Service Agency. In keeping with the informal nature of the program, the site was chosen because a group of clients was available to hear Teglia's announcement of the new program. Once the first family was identified, Teglia approached local businesses to become the first "godparent." The Daly City branch of the Bank of America was the first to agree, and the first "adoption" took place soon after. In the first two years of operation, approximately 100 families have been matched with middle-class families and businesses throughout San Mateo County. The program is constantly evolving as either new needs are recognized or new opportunities or resources become available.

PROGRAM DESCRIPTION

The Adopt-A-Family program is essentially a network of resources which depends on information, both access to information about godparent resources and sharing information about the program with low-income families. The program's success is based on two initiatives: (1) identifying the families who are in need of help and (2) reaching out to community members to get them involved.

Client families are identified by caseworkers in various social service agencies throughout the county. In order to be referred to the Adopt-A-Family program, the client families need to be prescreened by the referring agency and have a recognized need. To increase the chance of a successful match, the agency caseworker must be willing to help facilitate the match and provide some follow-up throughout the relationship.

Introducing the program to potential godparents is accomplished by spreading the word about the opportunity to give back to the community through the use of the following methods:

- *Community presentations:* Teglia takes advantage of any opportunity to introduce the program at the meetings of various community groups such as Rotary clubs, Kiwanis, and chambers of commerce.
- *Publicity:* A partnership has been formed with local newspaper journalists. Articles describing the program successes and ways to become involved appear on a semiregular basis. A flyer is currently being developed for the program, and information on the program is listed on the Web site for the local Children's Fund.
- *Word of mouth:* Contact with many of the referring agencies has developed informally, and each match that is made opens up new networking possibilities for new godparents.

The process of matching a family with a godparent begins with a phone call. The call can come from a caseworker making a client referral or from an individual or business interested in adopting. Once Teglia receives the information, he reaches into the resource network to make the match. Matches are made at monthly Adopt-A-Family program committee meetings that include Teglia, representatives from the human service agency of San Mateo County, representatives of referring agencies, and a newly integrated public relations person who schedules community presentations. In addition to formalizing the matches, these meetings provide an opportunity for program updates, for feedback on how to improve the structure and operation of the program, and discussion of possibilities for program expansion.

When a family is referred, they are asked to develop a wish list of items needed to help them become self-sufficient. Once this is done, it is forwarded to Teglia and eventually to the individual or business sponsoring that family. The first meeting between the family and their godparent is set up and facilitated by Teglia and the referring caseworker. After the initial meeting, the relationship that develops is entirely up to the family and their godparent. Follow-up is provided by the referring caseworker and is based on his or her continued service contact with the client family. The amount of follow-up done varies greatly based on the involvement of the referring agency and the individual caseworker.

There are no formalized entry criteria within the Adopt-A-Family program for screening the participants or making the matches. Client families are prescreened by the referring agency. The program expectations are explained to potential godparents when they inquire. If they are willing to make the one-year commitment to support the family in whatever way they can, they are deemed appropriate for the program. From interviews with the key players in the program, the following informal guidelines for matching the families seem to be in operation:

- *Geography:* Families are matched with godparents who are usually in the same city.
- *Family characteristics:* The size of the family, ethnicity, language, and the ages of the children may determine the type of match that will be most appropriate for that family.
- *Level of need:* Different families have different levels of need. Those with greater need are primarily matched with godparents who feel they have the necessary resources.

There is no funding for the Adopt-A-Family program since there are no employee salaries or administrative costs. The program is operated through donations of staff time, resources, and goods. Each participant in the network donates a portion of his or her time and energy to making and maintaining the matches. The costs of the program other than staff time (primarily phone calls, mailings, and meeting space) are incurred jointly by the human service agency and the office of Supervisor Mary Griffin. No cash donations are accepted by the program, and at this point only a small number of material donations are accepted due to the lack of storage space for such items. Cash donations would increase the overhead costs and create more bureaucracy than is desired. Even the godparents are not encouraged to spend money on their families. If they choose to do so, the items are given directly to the family without the program becoming the middleman.

Referring Agencies

Numerous agencies throughout the county refer clients to the Adopt-A-Family program, and any human service agency in the county is eligible to make referrals. Caseworkers find it quite easy to include the Adopt-A-Family program in the resources that they offer to their clients. As one caseworker noted, "I can easily fit the program into my regular duties. The only hard part is finding time in everyone's schedule for the initial meeting to match the family with the godparent."

The caseworker will introduce the program to a family he or she thinks would be interested in participating and would benefit from it. The family then creates their wish list. Caseworkers emphasize that there is no guarantee the families will receive all the items on the wish list. Many caseworkers also help their clients to finalize their wish list by making sure that it is realistic and includes the basic necessities. The typical wish list might include the following:

- Clothing (especially for the children)
- Food
- Diapers
- Basic household items (detergent, soap)
- Children's books and toys
- Furniture and bedding (especially cribs)

Once the wish list is finalized, it is forwarded on to Teglia so that the program committee can match the family with an appropriate godparent. After a godparent is found, Teglia or his human service agency counterpart, Judy Bardales, arranges the initial meeting that includes the family, the godparents, and the caseworker. The length of time between referral and adoption varies from a few days to a few weeks.

Each caseworker utilizes different criteria, in addition to need, in determining which families to recruit into the program. Most, however, look for a certain level of openness to accepting and welcoming newcomers into their lives. They have found that the relationship works better when the family is looking to get more from the program than the material items on their wish list. Many find that the social support offered by the program can be even more important than the material support. One caseworker noted, "The most important part is building relationships between families and their communities. Some families are really surprised at how much people care."

After the initial meeting between godparent and family, the role of the program and the caseworker is minimal. Although no paperwork is involved in follow-up, it is important for caseworkers to stay in touch with their families in order to monitor their experience with the Adopt-A-Family program. The primary goal of doing follow-up work is to facilitate the development of an independent relationship between the godparents and the adopted family. Ideally, the clients will learn to call their godparent first when they are in need of assistance instead of contacting the agency. One of the indirect benefits of the program is the opportunity to teach clients how to access and utilize community resources directly and become more independent.

There are no set guidelines for the development of the relationship between the godparents and their families. Some godparents wish to maintain anonymity and fulfill the wish list without meeting with the family more than once. Others want more of a relationship with the family and invite them to holiday and birthday parties. One company even gave one of the family members a job. Although some families meet with their godparents only once, most will meet four or more times over the course of a year.

Godparent Experience

One godparent heard about the Adopt-A-Family program from a friend and got involved with the support of her co-workers, friends, and family. She was matched up with a Latino family with three children, one of whom had a learning disability and needed special schooling. The godparent met with the family and the caseworker, who acted as translator, because the parents spoke limited English. At the start of the relationship, the godparent noted,

> I didn't really have a lot of expectations going in, just to help the family out with their basic necessities. After the first meeting, though, I took a real interest in them. The parents were so devoted to their kids; I could tell that right away. I was impressed with how resourceful they were with what they had. One of the children has a learning disability and was in a special school that involved a one and one-half hour commute each way every day. On her own, the mom found him a different program that was only fifteen minutes away. It was inspiring to see such loving and concerned parents.

This godparent worked closely with the family's caseworker and Teglia to tap into resources for the family. Most significantly, they applied for and received a grant from the Gift of Love program, another program founded by Teglia, which is run by the Italian Catholic Federation. The grant enabled the family to buy a specialized computer to help their son overcome his learning disability. To fill the family's wish list, this godparent enlisted the help of her family, friends, and co-workers to donate time, money, and information on available resources. She describes her efforts in the following way:

> Some of my co-workers helped out by giving me hand-me-downs from their kids, or small monthly donations that I used to buy things at garage sales. All my friends knew about my family and were always giving me suggestions about where to find things for them. There's an annual sale at St. Anne's in San Francisco and a great book sale every summer in Palo Alto. And if you're there at the end of the day, you can get some great bargains. They are practically giving things away. I even ended up pinning a copy of the wish list in my car so it would be handy if I happened to pass a garage sale. It was fun, kind of like a scavenger hunt.

In addition to providing the family with material items, this godparent was interested in overcoming the language and cultural barriers and developing a relationship with them. Throughout the year, she was in close contact with the family, meeting with them at least once a month, but usually more often than that.

> It wasn't always easy to communicate, but the family was willing and the caseworker was great about translating for us. The kids were fluent and the dad spoke some English, so we were able to make do. After a few visits, I wouldn't just drop things off for them and leave. One time, we brought over a bed for one of the children. We put it together with the family and then stayed and had coffee with them. This family had a great attitude.

Her year commitment with the family was officially over in June, but she is planning one more meeting to say good-bye and give them a final box of goods that she has collected for them. She is planning to adopt another family in the near future and looks forward to repeating the positive experience. When asked to reflect on her experience with the Adopt-A-Family program, she replied:

> Al and the caseworker were great, very attentive to my attempts to find resources for the family. But what I really liked was how hands-on the program was. You could set your own boundaries with the family, wherever you were comfortable. It's not as rewarding to just contribute money and not even know where it all goes. With this program, you get to see the impact you have on the family.

There is very little I would change about my experience. It was inspiring and gratifying to get to meet a family that I would not have otherwise met. In retrospect, there is one thing that I would do differently. I think with my next family, I'll try to show them where the resources are so they can keep using them when our year together is over. If I can, I'll take them with me to the annual garage sales that I find.

The Experiences of Adopted Families

Client families also report having a positive experience with the program. One family, adopted by a local business, admitted to having low expectations at the start of the program because they were not sure what type of support they would receive. Once the relationship began, however, this same family described being overwhelmed by the amount of material assistance and emotional support they received. In addition to providing the items on the family's wish list, the company invited the family to all of their picnics and holiday celebrations. Over the course of the year, this family met with their godparents more than ten times. When asked about the specific support her family received from their godparents, the mother replied,

We received clothes, pots and pans, and things for the children. Most of it was used, but that didn't matter because it was in really good shape. Everything they gave us was so helpful, but what I wanted most was for my children's wishes to be fulfilled, and they were.

As with many adoptions, there was a language barrier between the Spanish-speaking client family and the English-speaking godparents. The caseworker involved with this match was central to the development of this relationship because she was willing to take an active role as translator. The only regret this family had regarding their participation in the program was that the language barrier prevented them from being able to express their gratitude as well as they would have liked. However, they describe their overall experience in the following manner: "Everyone was so nice, friendly, and supportive. I am really grateful for everything the program did for me and my family, and I hope that it continues to help other families in the future."

LESSONS LEARNED AND FUTURE CHALLENGES

In its first two years of operation, the Adopt-A-Family program in San Mateo County has already demonstrated its effectiveness in linking existing needs with available resources. There have been over 100 adoptions countywide. There are three major lessons learned to date and three challenges which will impact its future.

1. *Build a strong resource network.* The commitment and experience of the founder, Al Teglia, significantly aided the establishment of this program. With over forty-eight years of public service experience in San Mateo County, his knowledge about the needs of the county's families and the potential resources available was extremely valuable in the implementation of the program. Despite the unique experiences of Al Teglia, this program can be replicated elsewhere. Special attention needs to be given to establishing a network of agency and business representatives which focuses on two main areas: cultivating relationships with social service agencies who can refer clients and wide dissemination of program information throughout the community to reach potential godparents.
2. *Minimize bureaucratic procedures and costs.* Unlike most programs for low-income populations, this one is not interested in getting more funding. In fact, the success of its implementation and expansion is, in part, because it is based exclusively on donations of time and materials. Outside of the staff time needed to establish and develop a program like this, the overhead costs are minimal. The program continues to refuse to accept cash donations because it would create too much red tape. Any money that does change hands goes directly from the godparent to the family, without incurring administrative costs.
3. *Make it easy to participate.* The network-based approach and the minimal bureaucracy make it easy for the key players (referring agencies, godparents, and client families) to participate. This program places only a small burden on the staff time and resources of referring agencies. The only requirement placed on clients is that they be pre-screened by a social service agency in the county. Godparents need to commit to helping their family in whatever way they can for a period of one year. Beyond this, the program places no requirements on participants.

With these lessons in mind, this innovative program also faces several challenges, including the following:

1. *Need for increased public awareness of the program:* Continued public exposure of the program is critical for its future, especially keeping the program uppermost in the minds of referring caseworkers to encourage appropriate families to participate. It is also crucial to maintain a sufficient number of godparents who want to adopt these fami-

lies through the use of flyers, Web sites, and volunteers who give presentations to local community groups, which is the program's primary method of recruiting godparents.
2. *Need for additional services:* The flexibility of the Adopt-A-Family program makes it possible to expand the types of goods and services it can offer to client families. As new resources come to the attention of the program's manager, they should be incorporated into the program, given the changing needs of client families.
3. *Need for program self-sufficiency:* This represents the greatest challenge to the future development of the program. The program is currently dependent on the personality and reputation of its founder, Al Teglia. The human service agency of San Mateo County has recently created a community liaison position to provide support to the Adopt-A-Family program in addition to numerous other community outreach projects. The newly hired community liaison is helping to develop the program's operating protocol, advertising materials, and job description for when she becomes the main contact of the resource network. As the transition develops, the community liaison will be more and more responsible for keeping track of potential godparents and client families, making the matches, and arranging the meetings between godparents and families. While Teglia continues to coordinate the program, the partnership with the community liaison at the human service agency will ensure that the program continues to flourish.

CONCLUSION

The strength of this program can be found in its simplicity. It seeks to mobilize existing resources to fill existing needs, without bureaucracy. From inspiration to implementation, the program has stayed true to this founding principle and is emerging as a vital link in the countywide network of resources. The potential for future expansion of the Adopt-A-Family program is limited only by the amount of time, energy, and resources which can be mobilized without burdening it with too much red tape.

REFERENCES

Barbour, P. (1983). Dial-a-Granny. *Child Abuse and Neglect,* 7(4): 477-478.
Morrison, J., Howard, J., Johnson, C., and Navarro, F. (1997). Strengthening neighborhoods by developing community networks. *Social Work,* 42(5): 527-534.
Wilson, W. (1996). *When work disappears: The world of the new urban poor.* New York: Alfred A. Knopf.

Chapter 10

Utilizing Hotline Services to Sustain Employment

Christine M. Schmidt
Michael J. Austin

With the passage of 1996's Personal Responsibility and Work Opportunity Reconciliation Act, the welfare system in the United States shifted from one focused on eligibility and economic assistance to one focused on propelling welfare recipients into the workforce. The new Temporary Assistance for Needy Families (TANF) applied lifetime limits to assistance and required states to devise and implement welfare-to-work plans that address barriers to employment and move welfare recipients into sustainable jobs in the workforce. Under the California program (CalWORKs), adult recipients of aid who do not meet exemption criteria are required to meet work requirements by participating in welfare-to-work activities in order to maintain their cash assistance.

In an effort to remove these barriers to employment, California counties, including Santa Clara, have developed and implemented a series of support services for CalWORKs participants. One such service is the JobKeeper Hotline, which provides round-the-clock counseling, crisis intervention, and information and referral services. The hotline is considered a preventive measure, designed to help employees retain their jobs and help the unemployed gain access to needed resources that may help them find a job. This is a case study of how Santa Clara County Social Services Agency (SSA), along with community partners, developed and implemented a telephone hotline to address the complexities of obtaining and maintaining long-term employment for CalWORKs recipients.

BRIEF LITERATURE REVIEW

In terms of welfare-to-work strategies, it is noteworthy that there is little or no published evidence of programs such as JobKeeper which provide information and referral services specifically geared toward job retention through a hotline for welfare recipients. Although hotlines have been in existence for decades, until recently they have generally been geared toward crisis intervention in fields such as domestic violence, child abuse, rape, suicide, and health-related issues. In an early study of their use, Rosenbaum and Calhoun (1977) cite several reasons why hotlines came to be regarded as accepted, successful methods of disseminating information and referrals to the public:

1. Callers have more control over the situation
2. Callers can remain anonymous if they so choose
3. Hotlines can break geographic barriers
4. Operators can also remain anonymous

Practitioners in health, mental health, and social service agencies have utilized hotlines (or helplines, as they are sometimes called) to provide information and referral to callers since the 1960s. Typically, agency-based hotlines provide an opportunity for caregivers to intervene in the lives of those who would seek only anonymous help. Hotline callers are usually in the midst of a crisis and are not sure where to go for necessary services (Loring and Wimberley, 1993).

Hotlines have been developed to address a diversity of social and health problems and issues. Researchers have explored hotline use in assault and rape (Renner and Wackett, 1987), learning problems (Adelman and Taylor, 1984), suicidal ideation (Glatt, 1987; Glatt, Sherwood, and Amisson, 1986; Green and Wilson, 1988; Rustici, 1988), parenting stress (Elmer and Maloni, 1988), child abuse (Fandetti and Ohsberg, 1987), and eating disorders (Burket and Hodgin, 1989), to name a few. Similarly, the use of the telephone has been particularly effective in connecting elderly persons with resources. Providing community referral has been found to be an important service component, as the problems facing older adults tend to involve less situational crises and more long-term problems with life management and independence (Winogrond and Mirassou, 1983). Many are afraid to seek services due to feelings of shame, suspicion, or fear of losing control of one's life, such as forced institutionalization. Calling in to a hotline offers the advantage of help while protecting the elderly from having to self-identify (Loring, Smith, and Thomas, 1994).

In addition to seeking information and/or referral, more callers are utilizing hotlines and helplines as a means of social support. Helplines have become an established part of many community social services, and Goud (1985) states that their popularity stems from accessibility, increased willingness of people to seek help in times of stress, declining opportunities for intimate relationships, or a preference for a quick fix. Ouchi and Johnson (1978) attribute the increase in helplines to the weakening or lack of traditional forms of social support such as the family, church, and community.

Several studies suggest that callers to helplines are seeking, first and foremost, social support, which can be defined as "the degree to which the person's basic social needs are gratified through interaction with others" (Thoits, 1982, p. 147). According to Thoits, basic needs include affection, esteem or approval, belonging, identity, and security, to which others would add instrumental, informational, and emotional support (Himle, Jayaratne, and Thyness, 1989; Kauffman and Beehr, 1989). It is often the case that callers to social service hotlines do not have an emergent problem but rather a need for someone to engage in active listening.

Although telephone hotlines and helplines are available in many communities, it is an ongoing challenge for agencies to evaluate their effectiveness for the people who use them. First, many hotlines and helplines are anonymous, with no contact information given for follow-up, so outcome assessment is impossible. Although some hotlines are able to ask callers about satisfaction with services, client satisfaction alone is a weak indicator of success, as clients of social services often report satisfaction at rates in excess of 90 percent (Gingerich, Gurney, and Wirtz, 1988). Measuring effectiveness through outcomes can also be difficult, as it is not always clear which outcome to measure. There is no universal definition of effectiveness, and different programs operate with different outcomes in mind.

SANTA CLARA VALLEY EMPLOYMENT SUPPORT INITIATIVE

In February 1996, County Supervisor James T. Beall Jr. and the social service agency's executive team initiated a local planning effort to address the anticipated welfare reform legislation. Local businesses, community groups, public and private agencies, and public assistance recipients were invited to participate in a series of community forums to address welfare reform as a community issue. The goal of these discussions was to find ways "to strengthen low-income parents' access to the resources they need to care for their children through employment and related service" (Employment Support Initiative [ESI], 1996, p. 4).

To facilitate this process, an oversight team was created, chaired by Supervisor Beall, the SSA director of income maintenance, another elected county supervisor, a county executive, and an expanding group of community leaders. This group, in turn, initiated a variety of specialized work teams that focused on specific issues such as child and youth services, immigrant issues, housing, and job-retention services. In subsequent months, these work groups gathered information, refined ideas, and made recommendations that eventually led to the development of a concept paper titled "The Santa Clara Valley Employment Support Initiative: An Agenda for Children and Their Families." The JobKeeper Hotline was one of the recommendations.

Planning for the JobKeeper Hotline began in October 1997, and it opened in July 1998. It is a hotline to help CalWORKs participants find ways to deal with crises on the job as well as gain support for locating employment. JobKeeper was developed through the collective efforts of the Career Retention Employment Support Team (CREST), one of the initial work groups of the ESI, whose goal was to assist customers in obtaining long-term, sustainable employment. Currently, the team is represented by over twenty organizations that provide education, training, and support services for CalWORKs participants throughout Santa Clara County. The purpose of the collaboration was to develop and coordinate employment and retention services countywide and provide feedback to the CalWORKs Employment Services Retention and Advancement Units in the Santa Clara County Social Services Agency (Employment Support Initiative, 1999).

Although CREST team members provided most of the services utilized by CalWORKs participants, many of the participants were either unaware of available services or did not know how to access them. To address the information gap, CREST envisioned a hotline which customers could call anytime of the day or night for resource information and referral. Although the primary goal of the JobKeeper Hotline is to maximize job retention through immediate assistance in addressing barriers to employment, it was agreed that callers would also be able to get help with non-employment-related issues.

CONTACT CARES, INC.

Contact Cares, or simply Contact, is a nonprofit organization (accredited by Contact USA and affiliated with Lifeline International and the United Way of Santa Clara County) that provides a twenty-four-hour per day, seven-day per week hotline service to Santa Clara County. The agency is staffed by trained volunteers and operates seventeen other hotlines in addition to JobKeeper. The services include telephone listening and support, crisis intervention, information and referral, and answering services. Specially trained personnel are on hand at all times to lend support and assistance to volunteers. Using an extensive computer library, Contact is able to access a network of community resources and links to human service agencies. The agency is funded by individuals, corporations, foundations, religious organizations, service clubs, and the United Way.

Contact training includes a paraprofessional thirteen-week, fifty-hour course consisting of listening skills, strategies for helping those in need or under stress, and basic understanding of human personality and needs. Although Contact training is open to anyone, teens and college students with interests in psychology, counseling, or human services are encouraged to gain experience through volunteering. Both experiential and didactic training are used through lectures, readings, and facilitated group work. Although Contact training is available to those who wish to volunteer (for one dollar per hour of training), sessions are also open at a higher fee to professionals and community members seeking to enhance their skills.

To recruit volunteers for the agency, Contact sends out public service announcements to a variety of media sources and makes personal recruiting presentations at locations such as churches, schools, community colleges, job fairs, and corporations. In addition, Santa Clara SSA publishes an all-staff memo prior to each biannual training session in an effort to recruit agency staff members to serve as volunteers. There is no age limit (young or old) to volunteer in the program, but youth under the age of eighteen must be accompanied by a parent and often take a more limited number of calls. Volunteers generally work four-hour shifts, although some of the late-night volunteers have opted recently to work a full eight hours while phone lines are less hectic.

Trainees are given assistance and practice with communications skills and are trained to refer callers to mental health and community resources. Twelve hours of apprenticeship with experienced Contact volunteers is included, and volunteers are asked to make a minimum commitment of eight hours of service per month for a period of one year. Training topics include the following (Contact of Santa Clara County, 1999):

- Orientation
- Communications I and II
- Crisis intervention
- Family relationships
- Adolescence/young adult issues
- Mental illness
- Human sexuality
- Parenting/parental stress
- Domestic violence/child abuse
- Death and dying
- Depression/suicide

- Substance abuse
- Reality therapy
- Caring confrontation
- Community resources
- Job retention

The thirteen weekly training sessions last three hours per night, with an initial orientation session at the outset and a Saturday workshop to complete the training. At the final Saturday workshop, Contact staff members explain policies and procedures with the potential volunteers and conduct a final interview to determine the applicant's suitability. The final steps are taken when new volunteers sign an agency confidentiality agreement and have their pictures taken and displayed at the agency for security reasons.

The Santa Clara County Social Services Agency assists Contact in recruiting volunteers to work the hotline and also provides meeting space for many of the volunteer training sessions in addition to the sessions reserved specifically for JobKeeper training. The following is a description of the JobKeeper hotline service along with information and statistics on the first year of operation.

JOBKEEPER

When contacting JobKeeper, callers reach trained, volunteer phone counselors who can provide support, information or assistance, crisis intervention, or active listening. Some counselors speak Spanish or Vietnamese, and all counselors have access to translation services. Each JobKeeper volunteer is familiar with and actively uses the Santa Clara County Job Support Resource Directory.

Produced by the Employment Support Initiative in conjunction with CREST, the directory is a comprehensive source of information and referral related to child care, employment services, education and training programs, legal and mediation services, and transportation. These topics were selected based on the most commonly requested subjects from callers during the first year of operation. Each listing in the various sections contains agency name, address, phone and fax numbers, eligibility and fee requirements, transportation options, physical accessibility, languages spoken, and listings of any other available services. Sections of the directory are color coded according to topic so that volunteers can quickly refer to the appropriate section to provide the caller with resources.

In its first year (July 1998 through June 1999), JobKeeper received a total of 770 calls, and 68 percent of the callers were female. The types of requested information included child care, skills or education, transportation, job search/résumé, and legal services. The job search requests accounted for nearly one-third of all calls. The language spoken was primarily English (87 percent), and 80 percent of the calls came from the city of San Jose, where 77 percent of all CalWORKs participants reside. Half of those who called in were currently employed.

At present, JobKeeper receives between forty-five and sixty-five calls per month, reflecting a continuous rate of increase despite limited advertising. When calls come in, callers are asked how they heard about the program. Although most referrals come from community providers, an increasing number of callers are referred by a friend or a relative, or are self-referred based on seeing a flyer. With the growing success of the program, staff members are exploring ways to reach a larger population.

SUCCESSES

One of the ways which JobKeeper has continued to improve its services is through the development of a seamless system of service. For example, individuals who call during business hours with child care questions are now transferred to the Community Coordinated Child Development Council for immediate response by a professional. Likewise, callers seeking employment information are now transferred directly to a professional counselor at the Employment Connection. Because of the many calls related to child care and employment, it has proven beneficial to have a professional in these fields available during peak calling times to provide immediate assistance and free volunteers to assist other callers.

Given the unusually low rate of unemployment in Santa Clara County in the late 1990s, many people were able to move off cash assistance and retain support services for a period of up to one year. This is an important time for participants to utilize JobKeeper in an effort to sustain long-term employment and self-sufficiency. In addition, although JobKeeper was designed to assist CalWORKs participants in finding and maintaining jobs, persons who are no longer eligible for CalWORKs may still utilize JobKeeper for information and referral to non-CalWORKs services.

To further improve services, JobKeeper is updating their technology to include a faster and more efficient phone system to allow volunteers to be available to answer additional calls. The CREST committee continues to meet on a quarterly basis in order to monitor operations and identify opportunities for improving the service.

CHALLENGES

In implementing any new pilot program, there will be challenges related to establishing and marketing the service. For example, in an effort to expedite start-up, the county neglected to utilize an 800 number, rather than a local area number, requiring some callers to make a long-distance call to access the service. This was corrected immediately and incurred additional expenses to change printed flyers and marketing tools (key chains and magnets) that advertised the local number.

Another ongoing challenge is to maintain a sufficient pool of trained volunteers. Given the extensive array of community resources, JobKeeper volunteers must be able to absorb a large quantity of information, quickly learn to use the available technology, and apply the policies and procedures that govern their work.

In the context of a strong economy and low unemployment rate, maintaining employment has become more of an issue than obtaining a job. In the past, employment services were geared primarily toward finding jobs and helping people remove the barriers to gaining employment. Now, the challenge is to make it possible for participants to obtain the skill upgrades needed to sustain long-term employment. Competition for good jobs is an issue in Silicon Valley, and earning a living wage is a continuing challenge when prices for food, housing, and services continue to rise. It is only through increased skills that persons moving off cash assistance will be able to compete for living-wage jobs.

Finally, program evaluation is also a continuing challenge. Although volunteers are expected to record information from each call, the crisis nature of the calls does not always lend itself to answering service evaluation questions. Also, because the service is confidential (no name or number), there appears to be no easy way to evaluate through follow-up whether the service has been of use to the caller. Although the numbers of people utilizing JobKeeper has increased, it seems equally important to assess the impact of the hotline service on the callers.

LESSONS LEARNED

In looking back on its past two years of services, those involved with the planning and implementation of the JobKeeper Hotline identified the following lessons related to program development, staff training, and evaluation:

1. When launching a pilot program, it is important to develop a marketing plan. It is helpful to seek out the opinions of the people who will be served when deciding how to best reach that target audience.
2. It is necessary to provide initial and ongoing training for program volunteers. When orienting volunteers to the new program and whenever introducing them to additional technology or program responsibilities, it is important to conduct informational sessions utilizing skilled trainers.
3. A system needs to be in place to update program data. It is necessary to keep updated information by identifying someone to work exclusively on this task, or to make it a job duty for all volunteers.
4. It is necessary to incorporate evaluation into every program. It is important to have information that can help clarify how a program is being utilized, as well as identify areas for improvement.
5. It is sometimes necessary to provide for the confidentiality of program staff as well as for program customers. The location of the JobKeeper program is kept a secret, except to those who administer or volunteer for the program. Due to the sensitive nature of information exchanged and safety concerns of volunteers who work through the night, the location of the JobKeeper program is not advertised.

REFERENCES

Adelman, H.S. and Taylor, L. (1984). A helpline for learning problems. *Journal of Learning Disabilities,* 17, 237-239.

Burket, R.C. and Hodgin, J.D. (1989). An eating disorders hotline: Organization, implementation, and initial experience. *Journal of American College Health,* 37, 183-186.

Contact of Santa Clara County (1999). Listening and caring: Orientation, training, and registration form. Available at <http://www.contactcares.org>. Santa Clara County, CA.

Elmer, E. and Maloni, J.A. (1988). Parent support through telephone consultation. *Maternal Child Nursing Journal,* 17, 13-23.

Employment Support Initiative (1996). *The Santa Clara Valley Employment Support Initiative: An agenda for children and their families.* Santa Clara County, CA: Author.

Employment Support Initiative (1999). *The Safety Net Project: Update, October 1999.* Santa Clara County, CA: Author.

Fandetti, K.M. and Ohsberg, L.A. (1987). Rhode Island's child protective service system. *Child Welfare,* 66, 529-538.

Gingerich, W.J., Gurney, R.J., and Wirtz, T.S. (1988). How helpful are helplines? A survey of callers. *Social Casework: The Journal of Contemporary Social Work,* 69:10, 634-639.

Glatt, K.M. (1987). Helpline: Suicidal prevention at a suicide site. *Suicide and Life Threatening Behavior,* 17, 299-309.

Glatt, K.M., Sherwood, D.W., and Amisson, T.J. (1986). Telephone helplines at a suicide site. *Hospital and Community Psychiatry,* 37, 178-180.

Goud, N. (1985). Dial-a-need hotlines. *Journal of Humanistic Education and Development,* 24:2, 76-80.

Green, L.W. and Wilson, C.R. (1988). Guidelines for non-professionals who receive suicidal phone calls. *Hospital and Community Psychiatry,* 39, 310-311.

Himle, D.P., Jayaratne, S., and Thyness, P.A. (1989). The buffering effects of four types of supervisory support on work stress. *Administration in Social Work,* 13:1, 19-34.

Kauffman, G.M. and Beehr, T.A. (1989). Occupational stressors, individual strains and social supports among police officers. *Human Relations,* 42:2, 185-197.

Loring, M.T., Smith, R.W., and Thomas, T. (1994). Utilization of a time-limited holiday hotline by older adults. *The Gerontologist,* 34:4, 557-560.

Loring, M.T. and Wimberley, E.T. (1993). The time-limited hotline. *Social Work,* 38:3, 344-346.

Ouchi, W.G. and Johnson, J.B. (1978). Types of organizational control and their relationship to emotional well-being. *Administrative Science Quarterly,* 23:2, 293-317.

Renner, K.E. and Wackett, C. (1987). Sexual assault: Social and stranger rape. Canadian Journal of Community Mental Health, 6, 49-56.

Rosenbaum, A. and Calhoun, J.F. (1977). The use of the telephone hotline in crisis intervention: A review. *Journal of Community Psychology,* 5, 328.

Rustici, C.J. (1988). Teenline: A CMHC-based adolescent suicide prevention and intervention program. *Journal of Mental Health Administration,* 15, 15-20.

Thoits, P.A. (1982). Life stress, social support, and psychological vulnerability: Epidemiological considerations. *Journal of Community Psychology,* 10:3, 144-154.

Winogrond, I.R. and Mirassou, M.M. (1983). A crisis intervention service: Comparison of younger and older adult clients. *The Gerontologist,* 23, 370-376.

Chapter 11

Hiring TANF Participants to Work in a County Human Services Agency

Kirsten A. Deichert
Michael J. Austin

HISTORY

Although the San Mateo County Human Services Agency has a history of hiring clients for temporary assignments, the agency's most recent effort to hire clients into full-time, permanent positions occurred with the implementation of welfare reform. The primary goal was to address the agency's staffing needs by providing meaningful employment for former welfare recipients as well as set an example for the larger community. In 1997, the San Mateo County Human Services Agency developed a new service delivery model called SUCCESS (Shared Undertaking to Change the Community to Enable Self-Sufficiency) which included restructuring the benefit analysts positions into new case-management roles. The transfer of employees from one unit to another left many vacant positions, especially in the Medi-Cal benefits unit which has the largest caseload. In their effort to fill these positions, the human services agency began hiring their own clients and this case study describes that process.

While the Medi-Cal eligibility unit deliberately hires current and former clients to fill open positions, other areas in the agency also do the same. With the implementation of the SUCCESS model in 1997, welfare recipients were hired in all three of the agency's regional SUCCESS Centers, as well as elsewhere in the agency. Outside the agency, but still within county government, the family support division in the district attorney's office obtained a grant to hire seven to eight TANF recipients to perform child-support collections duties. These former TANF recipients were eligible to compete for full-time positions in the family support division in March 2000 when the grant expired.

Earlier efforts to hire clients date back to 1989 when the agency created internships for welfare clients who needed work experience that would qualify them for a greater number of employment opportunities. A number of the interns later went on to become valued, permanent employees of the agency. One such employee has worked for the agency for several years and now holds a supervisory position. Another intern went on to earn permanent employment at the central county government office. Throughout the agency's efforts to hire its own clients, the goal has been to set an example for the larger community to hire welfare recipients.

REVIEW OF RELEVANT LITERATURE

On August 22, 1996, the Personal Responsibility and Work Opportunity Reconciliation Act (PRWORA) established lifetime restrictions on the amount of time individuals could receive public assistance funds, while also establishing a "work-first" expectation that welfare recipients obtain any employment as soon as possible. One-stop centers provide a single point of entry for employment-related services to welfare recipients. In San Mateo County, these one-stop career centers are located in its three regional SUCCESS Centers or Work First Centers. Recruitment of welfare recipients for human services agency positions is conducted through the SUCCESS employment centers. While PRWORA challenges public assistance recipients to obtain employment, it also challenges employers to hire them.

On March 8, 1997, President Clinton issued a memorandum to the heads of executive departments and agencies, directing the federal government, as the nation's largest employer, to hire people off the welfare rolls into government jobs (The White House, 1997a). To assist in these hiring efforts, the president created the Worker Trainee Program to allow federal agencies to bypass the complex federal personnel hiring rules and procedures to hire entry-level persons for up to three years. Seven months later, in October 1997, Vice President Gore announced that the federal government had already hired nearly 2,000 welfare recipients and was well on its way to achieving the president's goal: to hire 10,000 people by year 2000 (The White House, 1997b). By giving welfare recipients the opportunity to work for the federal government, they set "a powerful example for the private sector," said the Vice President (The White House, 1997b).

Recognizing that the government could not bear the entire burden of putting all welfare recipients to work, and in response to President Clinton's encouragement of the private sector to hire people on public assistance, five major corporations formed the Welfare to Work Partnership. The CEOs of United Airlines, Burger King, Sprint, Monsanto, and UPS formed the national, independent, nonpartisan organization to help the business community hire and retain welfare recipients, without displacing existing employees. For instance, in less than two years UPS hired 10,000 welfare recipients, estimating that about 70 percent were retained (Jacoby, 1998). Providing information, technical assistance, and support for all businesses, the Welfare to Work Partnership involves business leaders and government officials in achieving the common goal of putting welfare recipients to work.

In a follow-up survey of the impact of their efforts, the Welfare to Work Partnership (Carroll, 1999) found that

- child care and transportation are the primary obstacles among working welfare recipients;
- creating a welfare-to-work program does not cost a company extra money (16 percent report they saved money by creating a program);
- 82 percent who have hired former welfare recipients describe them as "good, productive employees";
- 27 percent hire welfare recipients into salaried positions; and
- 77 percent hire welfare recipients into promotional track positions.

A common thread running through each of these findings is that job-retention strategies must address the needs of both employers and employees. Employers identified the following major obstacles facing their newly hired former welfare clients: child care, transportation, technical skills, motivation/attitude, education/training, job-readiness skills, and the need for mentors/positive reinforcement (The Welfare to Work Partnership, 2000).

The need for welfare recipients to acquire "soft skills" (e.g., motivation, understand appropriate behavior in a work setting, manage family and work responsibilities, reliability, time management) is considered more important than their technical or training needs (National Governor's Association, 1999). As noted in Jacoby (1998), "You cannot push someone out there who has never done this before and expect them to succeed (without help)." For example, Candleworks, Inc., an Iowa City company, offers weekly "life counseling" to its employees, approximately half of whom are welfare recipients, on topics including nutrition, drug abuse, and financial planning (Jacoby, 1998).

Specific strategies for employers to utilize in helping welfare recipients retain their jobs include the following (Jacoby, 1998):

- *Providing ongoing case management:* Case managers could help employees cope with the workplace, the public service system, household difficulties, and the social service network through counseling, advice, support, and assistance in accessing services and resources.
- *Developing effective mentoring programs:* Mentors could be volunteers from the community, current employees of the agency, or peer

mentors who are former recipients and can assist new employees with such issues as managing time and stress, balancing work and home demands, managing finances, adjusting to new responsibilities, developing appropriate work habits, and understanding office relationships.

- *Improving access to support services:* Employers could ensure that former welfare recipients know about and understand the application processes for accessing state-sponsored Transitional Child Care and Transitional Medicaid, in addition to other local resources for the provision of child care and medical attention available to low-income workers. Employers could also make sure employees understand their eligibility for the federal earned income tax credit (EITC), as well as its advance payment option that allows a portion of the credit to be added to each paycheck. Even though 80 to 86 percent of eligible families receive the credit, less than 1 percent utilize the advance payment option.
- *Providing opportunities for career advancement within the organization:* When welfare recipients obtain entry-level jobs, they experience the high cost of working, which can include new or additional child care, transportation and clothing costs, reductions in case assistance and Food Stamps, and even higher rent for those living in subsidized housing. Therefore, career advancement and promotions are critical in moving welfare recipients from just any employment to long-term self-sufficiency.

In addition to the San Mateo Human Services Agency, other public agencies throughout the nation are making efforts to fill vacant positions with TANF recipients. Hennepin County, Minnesota, piloted a Community Workforce Partnership to train and hire twenty TANF recipients for permanent positions in county departments experiencing labor shortages (American Federation of State, County, and Municipal Employees [AFSCME], 1999). Throughout the training period, participants are paid a rate equivalent to 90 percent of the entry-level salary for the position in which they will be eventually hired. Philadelphia, Pennsylvania, has implemented a transitional work program using funding obtained from donations and funds previously earmarked for TANF benefits (Cohen, 1999). The program provides six-month positions in public and nonprofit agencies for 3,000 TANF recipients over a three-year period. Working twenty-five hours per week and receiving ten hours of training per week, participants learn skills, receive the workplace support of mentors, and receive the minimum wage and a bonus of up to $800 upon obtaining a permanent job. In Kansas City, Missouri, Mayor Emanuel Cleaver earmarked more than 150 city jobs for TANF recipients (Kniss, Mathews, and Thurmaier, 1998).

HIRING FORMER CLIENTS AT THE SAN MATEO HUMAN SERVICES AGENCY

Although welfare reform legislation added new pressures to welfare recipients to obtain employment, these expectations have also given employers a new pool of potential applicants from which to draw. Since the federal government began its recruitment of welfare recipients and set an example for private and public agencies to follow, welfare recipients continue to find jobs with employers eager to hire them. However, both TANF recipients and their employers acknowledge the extra support they require to retain these jobs.

The San Mateo Human Services Agency's first efforts to hire clients predate welfare reform with the internships they offered during the GAIN program. The internship was designed to provide participants with enough current work experience to augment their job applications and résumés. One former intern has worked for the agency for over four years and is the supervisor of the human services agency records center. After receiving public assistance for three years and having not worked for almost ten years, she reported that she was surprised at how much she had missed the opportunity to work. Believing that, "no one's going to hire me" and that the "odds were against" her, she began a two-month, unpaid internship at the agency. These two months, she said, gave her time to gain basic computer skills and learn how to use current office machinery. The two months of work experience gave her confidence and a transition period for "getting in the routine" of working. It was the agency's willingness to "take a chance on her" that gave her the opportunity to believe in her own abilities and continue advancing her career in the agency.

The agency has hired clients to fill a variety of positions during the past decade; some went on to obtain permanent employment and supervisory positions within the agency. One of its most extensive efforts to hire TANF recipients, however, has been in filling vacant Benefits Analysts I positions. This case study describes the strategies used in hiring, training, and recruiting clients to fill this position, along with the lessons learned.

Job Description and Hiring Practices

A detailed description of the Medi-Cal Benefits Analyst I position, including minimum qualifications, is included in Box 11.1. Because eligibility requirements of public assistance programs are complex and ever-changing, benefits analysts need to retain a significant amount of information, make quick and accurate mathematical computations, and organize a considerable amount of paperwork. The agency makes a concerted effort to staff the Medi-Cal Benefits Analyst I positions with either agency clients or

> **BOX 11.1. Benefits Analyst—Extra Help Job Description**
>
> *The Position*
>
> The trainee-level position in the Benefits Analyst series in the Human Service Agency. Benefits analysts receive intensive training to perform a variety of duties including interviewing applicants for public assistance, applying regulations and procedures for eligibility determination, maintaining accurate records, and providing referrals to community resource agencies.
>
> *Minimum Qualifications*
>
> California driver's license
>
> *Experience and Education*
>
> Any combination of education and experience that would likely provide the required knowledge, skills, and abilities is qualifying. A typical way to qualify is equivalent to two years of clerical or public contact work which involves responsibility for interviewing and record keeping or two years of college course work.
>
> *Knowledge and Education*
>
> - Principles of eligibility determination
> - Public assistance laws and regulations
> - Basic interviewing techniques
> - Basic office procedures and record keeping
>
> *Skills Required*
>
> - Organize and maintain a heavy workload within deadlines
> - Make arithmetic computations quickly and accurately
> - Utilize data-processing systems
> - Communicate effectively, orally and in writing, with people from a wide variety of socioeconomic backgrounds
> - Prepare, maintain, and interpret records and reports
> - Interview effectively and secure cooperation of applications in obtaining pertinent personal information
> - Interpret and apply laws, rules, and regulations
> - Work under pressure with frequent interruptions

current clerical staff. This policy gives public assistance clients a better chance of becoming county employees than applicants from the general public.

Initially, the position is open to clients under the status of "extra help," a trainee-level position without medical or vacation benefits or job guarantees. Periodically, permanent positions become available within the agency and the extra help employees are encouraged to pursue the civil service testing process to secure permanent employment with the agency.

Recruiting

To recruit for the Medi-Cal eligibility positions, the Medi-Cal program training specialist sends flyers advertising the positions to SUCCESS Centers, the income and employment services specialists (case managers), the agency's clerical staff, and the lead instructor of the human services certificate program at the San Mateo community colleges. At the SUCCESS Centers, all job leads are shared with all participants and it is left to individual participants to decide whether to apply for agency positions. According to management staff, the positive attitudes, personal experiences, and enthusiasm for the work make former clients ideal employees. Although the positions for which clients were recruited were identified as new and additional positions, with no displacement of current employees, management staff needed to reassure current employees and their unions that they would not be displaced.

During the first few years, recruiting qualified applicants from SUCCESS Centers for positions in the human services agency was a relatively easy task. Recently, however, the applications received from clients have begun to reflect those individuals on aid who lack many basic skills and relevant work experience and face significant barriers to employment (e.g., alcohol and other drug abuse, mental illness). As a result, it has become increasingly difficult to find already-qualified employees among the ranks of public assistance clients.

Training and Hiring

To train applicants for these positions, four cycles of training were completed (July 1998, January 1999, May 1999, and August 1999). Each training cycle included approximately ten to twelve participants. Approximately six trainees were offered positions at the end of each training session. Trainees are not retained in the event that their absences during training are too high, scores on tests given during training are too low, they voluntarily decide not to continue, or they have not admitted criminal history revealed in background checks.

The training for Medi-Cal Benefits Analyst I positions involves a seven-week program. The first four weeks include academic/classroom instruction, followed by two weeks of on-the-job training, and one week of both academic and computer training. On-the-job training is provided by a lead worker who is selected by a district office manager. Program-specific information and interpersonal relations issues are presented and discussed in training. Trainees are tested each of the six weeks on cumulative material and must score 80 percent or better in order to be hired. A total of eight extra help staff have been hired from the client population and three have become permanent employees in the Medi-Cal Benefits Unit. Unfortunately, six to ten clients hired from the SUCCESS Centers to fill extra help positions have been terminated because they did not pass the civil service testing process.

A significant challenge for many former clients during training (and throughout their employment) is related to being absent. Missing even one day of training due to illness or lack of child care can result in not only a loss of pay, but also a loss of a significant amount of information, making it difficult to pass the training tests. All of this is compounded by the fact that the training experience is fast paced and covers a lot of information in a short period of time.

Impact

Agency employees support hiring clients, especially since it sets an example for other county agencies and the larger community to hire public assistance recipients. Hiring clients also promotes increased diversity among the agency's employees, since the cultural, language, and income backgrounds of clients are often quite different from those of the agency's other staff.

Administrators and program managers have been pleasantly surprised by the high quality of employees who had been clients. The former clients are described as highly motivated, eager, committed, and very bright. For example, one agency employee who was impressed by the former clients' passion for work noted, "We can teach anyone the tasks of the job, but we can't teach people to have a positive attitude about the work they do." In the case of former clients working in the SUCCESS Centers, one manager attributes the success of the centers to the very nature of having ex-clients as employees.

The opportunity to become permanent county employees is a significant accomplishment for individuals receiving public assistance. The welfare reform time limits have placed new pressures on public assistance clients to obtain both employment and long-term self-sufficiency. In the event that an individual hired as extra help does not pass the civil service testing process, he or she will leave the agency with a new set of transferable skills, including time management and interpersonal communications.

Although obtaining employment has the reward of income, it also involves new expenses such as transportation, child care, medical care, and work clothes. Although extra help staff do not have employer-provided health coverage, former CalWORKs recipients are eligible to receive transitional Medi-Cal at zero share of cost for two years following their receipt of public assistance.

Another difficulty for former clients is that many are likely to have insufficient support networks in their personal lives. This not only intensifies their problems with child care, but also makes them less likely to have the resources needed to cope with some of the aspects of their new jobs (e.g., stress, feeling overwhelmed, interpersonal conflicts). In addition, former clients may not have the experience to handle such workplace issues as interpersonal tension/conflict with co-workers and managers, time management, or organizing the flow of work. Although these capabilities are required of any successful employee, this group of employees has had fewer work-related opportunities to acquire them.

The chief obstacle in hiring clients as permanent employees is the civil service application process. Although there are obvious benefits to becoming a permanent employee (e.g., health care, sick leave, job guarantee, wage increase), most clients hired as extra help do not successfully pass the civil service testing process. Many former clients perform their jobs successfully for a year or more, but they are not able to pass the civil service application process due to the broad nature of the questions and the lack of preparation for the panel interviews.

LESSONS LEARNED

The San Mateo Human Services Agency supports hiring former clients and reports positively on their job performance and attitudes. However, as the welfare rolls decline, the pool of qualified applicants shrinks. Future staffing needs and caseload sizes, coupled with the ability to find qualified individuals among those on public assistance, will impact the agency's future efforts to hire former welfare recipients. Interviews with administrators, staff trainers, and former clients employed by the agency revealed that the following lessons have been learned in hiring TANF recipients to work in the agency:

1. It is crucial to find ways to address the obstacle of the civil service exam. One approach is to support supervisors in helping prepare extra help staff for the civil service exam and interviews. It remains to be seen if coaching from supervisors will be sufficient to help prepare former clients for successfully passing the exam.

    The second, and more radical, recommendation is to develop a policy which exempts former clients from the civil service hiring process and grant permanent status to extra help employees who have demonstrated on-the-job proficiency. In this way, advancement to permanent positions could be based solely on performance and the support of the employee's supervisor (e.g., letters of reference). However, this approach would need to be negotiated with the unions.

2. Job advancement requires new ways to address the need for support networks and soft skills. With regard to learning soft skills and constructing a support network, a mentoring relationship with a coworker or supervisor during the first year of employment could be established to assist former clients with a more successful transition into the work world. The demanding nature of the job coupled with the lack of work experience can lead to the need for more support than may be the case for other employees. Mentoring relationships could focus on preparation for the civil service testing process, as well as provide former clients with a resource to acquire skills needed to deal with workplace issues and conflicts.

Another way to equip former recipients with soft skills is to expand internship opportunities for the client population. The internships can lead to the hiring of the best interns as extra help. An internship program would give former welfare recipients more time to gain on-the-job experience and the skills needed for successful employment and advancement. The benefits of internships have been illustrated in the success stories of former clients who participated in internships during the GAIN program. The extra support and transitional time significantly contributed to their retention and to the attainment of permanent employment with the agency.

REFERENCES

American Federation of State, County, and Municipal Employers (AFSCME) (1999). We do it best! Flexible workforce and good labor-management relations. Available at <http://www.afscme.org/pol-leg/nobod05.htm>.

Carroll, R. (1999). Welfare reform: Assessing the progress of work-related provisions. Congressional testimony to the House Committee on Education and the Workforce, 106th Congress. Available at <http://edworkforce.house.gov/hearings/106th/pet/welfare9999/carroll.htm>.

Cohen, M. (1999). Work experience and publicly-funded jobs for TANF recipients. The Welfare Information Network. Available at <http://www.financeprojectinfo.org/Publications/newwork.htm>.

Jacoby, N. (1998). From welfare to work. <http://money.cnn.com/1998/08/14/smbusiness/welfare>.

Kniss, C., Mathews, K., and Thurmaier, K. (1998). Implementing welfare reform in Kansas: A study of 4 communities. Available at <http://www.huhttp.cc.ukans.edu/~kupa/projects/837s98exex.html>.

National Governor's Association (1999). Helping welfare recipients stay employed. Available at <http://www.nga.org/center/divisions/1,1188,C_ISSUE_BRIEF^D_1854,00.html>.

The Welfare to Work Partnership (2000). Member survey: Taking the next step. Available at <http://www.welfaretowork.org/publications/wirthlin/2000.pdf>.

The White House (1997a). Presidential memorandum for the heads of executive departments and agencies: Government employment for welfare recipients. Office of the Press Secretary. Available at <http://www.opm.gov/wtw/htm/welfarem.htm>.

The White House (1997b). Press release: Nearly 2,000 former welfare recipients hired by government. Office of the Vice President. Available at <http://govinfo.library.unt.edu/npr/library/news/welfare.html>.

Chapter 12

Promoting Self-Sufficiency Through Individual Development Accounts (IDAs)

Judie Svihula
Michael J. Austin

Many Americans are asset poor. The average American family holds only $3,700 in net financial assets, and nearly one-third of American households operate with zero or negative net financial assets (Oliver and Shapiro, 1995). Half of all Americans have less than $1,000 of assets to invest. Thus, absent any safety nets, the typical family is only about three monthly paychecks away from financial ruin. The low asset levels are not surprising considering the low savings rate (5 percent) of U.S. households and the lack of government support for asset building among the low- and middle-income population.

Although the federal government subsidizes $200 billion annually for asset acquisition in the forms of home mortgage deductions, preferential capital gains, and pension fund exclusions, many Americans lack the resources to take advantage of these subsidies. Federal welfare policy historically has denied eligibility to public assistance recipients who exceeded the $1,000 asset limit. In addition, asset poverty is increasing. Based on the level of net worth needed to meet the poverty threshold for three months, the asset poverty rate increased from 22.4 percent in 1983 to 25.5 percent percent in 1998 (Haverman and Wolff, 2001).

Welfare reform legislation calls for millions of families to become self-sufficient, yet those with the highest rates of asset poverty are those who have been on welfare, including female heads of households with children (64 percent) and heads of households less than twenty-five years of age (75 percent). To enable struggling families to build assets and achieve economic well-being, a new program has emerged called the individual development account (IDA). IDAs are special savings accounts designed to help people build assets to reach life goals and to achieve long-term security (IDANetwork, 2001b). Account holders receive matching funds as they

165

save for purposes such as buying a first home, attending job training, going to college, or financing a small business. Funding for IDAs can come from public and/or private sources.

The emergence of IDAs following the implementation of welfare reform provided an opportunity to implement a community partnership utilizing public and private resources (Sherraden, 2000). This case study describes the implementation of an IDA pilot program by the San Mateo County Human Services Agency (HSA). Following a brief history and description of IDAs at the national, state, and regional level, the case study elaborates on the implementation of IDAs as a pilot program in a one-stop service center. It concludes with a discussion of lessons learned and future challenges.

HISTORY

Asset building as an antipoverty strategy emerged in the 1980s and 1990s as a result of several publications: *The Safety Net As Ladder* (Friedman, 1988), *Assets and the Poor* (Sherraden, 1991), and *Black Wealth/White Wealth* (Oliver and Shapiro, 1995). IDAs as an asset-based policy and program evolved over several years out of discussions between Michael Sherraden (2000) and academic colleagues, social workers, and welfare recipients. He suggested that savings and asset accumulation are more related to providing structures and incentives than the result of personal preferences. In addition to deferred consumption, he also noted that assets may have a wide range of positive psychological, social, and economic impacts (Sherraden, 1988, 1991).

The first policy reports on IDAs were published in 1989 and 1990 by the Corporation for Enterprise Development (CFED) and the Progressive Policy Institute (PPI), creating a policy discussion that has expanded over the past decade (Sherraden, 2000). As a result of the discussions, there has been a change in the federal policy restrictions on asset holding for those who receive means-tested benefits, namely, more flexibility and increased possibilities to build assets. IDA proposals typically receive bipartisan support because they do not fit a "liberal" or "conservative" mold.

The first IDAs were initiated by community-based organizations in the early 1990s. By 2001, more than 400 community-based IDA programs were in various stages of development across the country. Nonprofit organizations in at least forty-seven states are implementing or planning IDA programs, with or without state support. The first large-scale national demonstration of IDAs is the American Dream Demonstration (ADD), which was launched by the Corporation for Enterprise Development in September 1997 (Center for Social Development, 2000).

The ADD involves thirteen host organizations to design, implement, and administer IDA initiatives in their local communities. These programs have established more than 2,000 IDAs in low-income communities across the country. The following preliminary ADD results indicate that IDAs encourage the poor to save and accumulate assets: (1) the IDA-matched funding is attracting participants, (2) each hour up to twelve hours of financial education is associated with higher average monthly net deposits, and (3) higher match rates encourage participant retention and maintenance of account balances (Center for Social Development, 2001a).

REVIEW OF NATIONAL AND STATE IDA INITIATIVES

Numerous policy initiatives at the federal, state, and local levels have contributed to a rapid expansion of IDAs in recent years (IDANetwork, 2001b). Three major federal laws provide funding and support for individual development accounts: (1) the Personal Responsibility and Work Opportunity Reconciliation Act of 1996 (PRWORA), (2) the Assets for Independence Act of 1998 (AFIA), and (3) the 1977 Community Reinvestment Act (CRA) that has encouraged community investments (IDANetwork, 2001a). The latest legislative proposal, titled Savings for Working Families Act (SWFA), would provide additional incentives for investment in IDAs and could foster the creation of millions of new accounts (Charity, Aid, Recovery, and Empowerment Act [CARE], 2003).

1. *Personal Responsibility and Work Opportunity Reconciliation Act:* Under PRWORA, states are permitted to include IDAs in welfare reform plans or welfare-to-work grants and are allowed to fund IDA initiatives under the block granted to the Temporary Assistance to Needy Families (TANF) program. TANF-funded IDAs may be used for postsecondary education, first home purchase, or business start-up. As of 1999, TANF-funded IDA benefits are
   - excluded from the definition of "assistance,"
   - exempt from impacting a recipient's five-year time limit,
   - separate from and do not jeopardize the receipt of other welfare benefits, and
   - exempted from impacting eligibility for many federal means-tested programs.
2. *Assets for Independence Act:* The 1998 AFIA authorized the U.S. Department of Health and Human Services to establish and administer a five-year, $125 million demonstration of IDAs. This is the first federal program established to test the efficacy of IDAs as a poverty-reduction strategy for low-income Americans. The demonstration received

$10 million in fiscal years (FY) 1999 and 2000 that enabled forty nonprofits to establish IDA programs. It is estimated by the Corporation for Enterprise Development that this demonstration will fund between 27,000 and 33,000 IDAs with the full $25 million it received in FY 2001. Moreover, recent amendments have expanded eligibility for IDAs.

3. *Community Reinvestment Act:* The CRA is intended to encourage financial institutions to help meet the credit needs of the communities in which they operate. IDAs can satisfy a number of different CRA criteria, depending on the type and extent of services and products that banks provide. For example, financial institutions may become involved in IDA programs by

- providing matching funds for account holders or operating support for community organizations running an IDA program,
- offering accounts which may be structured as traditional savings accounts,
- helping design and implement IDA programs, including developing and teaching financial literacy courses,
- enhancing accounts by offering special account benefits, including higher interest rates, ATM services, or waived minimum balance requirements, and
- making loans to account holders once they have achieved their savings goals.

4. *Savings for Working Families Act:* The SWFA is a legislative proposal that would provide additional incentives for IDA investment and potentially create millions of new accounts. Current legislation would provide a 100 percent tax credit to financial institutions to provide one to one matches up to $500 per qualified individual saving in an IDA. The SWFA was nearly passed in 2000. In 2001, language mirroring the SWFA was included in the House and Senate Charitable Giving Package. In addition, President Bush included a version of SWFA in his FY 2002 budget.

As of December 2000, thirty-two states, including California, planned to use TANF funds for IDAs (Center for Social Development, 2001b). About half of these states were already using TANF funds for IDAs. Twenty-nine states had passed IDA legislation for TANF recipients and/or low-income citizens. Eight states had created pilot programs for IDAs by administrative rule. IDAs were included in California's welfare reform of 1997 as part of the California Savings and Asset Project. The implementation of this provision was dependent on federal appropriations, other than TANF block grant funds, specified for the purpose of establishing IDAs. The state's own welfare reform program, the California Work Pays Demonstration Project, allows $5,000 of unmatched savings to be accumulated and disregarded as income for the uses of home ownership, small business development, or educational expenses.

There is currently no state legislation on IDA in California (Center for Social Development Washington University, 2001). Two unsuccessful IDA bills were introduced in the 1997-1998 legislative session. AB 692 was introduced in 2001 by Assembly Member Dion Aroner, requesting state general funds to create the California Savings and Asset Project, based on the PRWORA and the AFIA.

Supported by foundations and financial institutions, over forty IDA programs are either in operation or under development in California. The following regional IDA coalitions have emerged in California: the San Francisco Asset Building Initiative, the Assets for All Alliance in San Jose, Assets CAN: the California Action Network, IDA coalitions in Southern California, and youth IDA programs. California participates in the national demonstration program (ADD) at the East Bay Asian Local Development Corporation site in Oakland.

THE IDA IN SAN MATEO COUNTY

The San Mateo County Human Services Agency, as part of the Peninsula Partnership for Children and Families since 1995, had been working with the Peninsula Community Foundation (PCF) to reduce family and child poverty in San Mateo County. PCF is part of a regional coalition that provided support for an IDA pilot with one of the HSA's contractors, The Samaritan House. The Samaritan House pilot served a small number of low-income working families and was having difficulty recruiting. The following sections describe the regional IDA coalition and the HSA's implementation of an IDA pilot at a one-stop service center.

The Regional IDA Coalition

The Center for Venture Philanthropy (CVP) and Lenders for Community Development (LCD) partnered with the Peninsula Community Foundation to form a regional IDA coalition called Assets for All Alliance (Alliance). CVP, based in Menlo Park, is a forum for community donors to collaborate and catalyze societal change, which creates avenues for investors from Silicon Valley to engage in new philanthropy. LCD, based in San Jose, is a consortium of twenty-three banks that provide fixed-rate term loans of up to $50,000 for qualifying microloan programs designed for women and minority-owned businesses as well as businesses located in low-income communities. PCF, based in San Mateo, has total assets over $400 million and provides funding and expertise to support an array of community programs to assist local donors in meeting their philanthropic goals (Peninsula Community Foundation, 2000).

The Alliance supports low-income families as they save money for purchasing a home, going to college, starting a business, or retiring with financial security (Assets for All Alliance, 2001a). The IDAs are held in savings accounts at local banks. CVP and LCD work with seven community-based nonprofit agencies that serve low-income families in order to identify, recruit, and support qualified IDA program participants among their existing clients. Financial trainers, provided through the Alliance, focus their classes on expanding the abilities of participants to save. As noted in Box 12.1, there are three types of support for the IDA program: community partners, investors, and managing partners (Assets for All Alliance, 2001b). IDA community partners include LCD, Catholic Charities of Santa Clara, North Central College Institute of Samaritan House in San Mateo, Lifetime, PeninsulaWorks-Daly City, De Anza College, and Family Support Center of the Mid-Peninsula. CVP and LCD serve as managing partners of the Alliance. The Alliance investors include San Mateo Human Services Agency, the Peninsula Community Foundation donor advisors, The David and Lucile Packard Foundation, Community Foundation Silicon Valley, the Candelaria Foundation, Citibank, and Bank of America. The relationship between the investors (HSA and foundations), the managing partners (financial and philanthropic institutions), and the community partners (service organizations) is illustrated in Figure 12.1. In September 1999, the Alliance began a six-year plan that will offer IDAs to 840 Silicon Valley participants (Assets for All Alliance, 2001c).

Implementation of the IDA Pilot

When the HSA received its CalWORKs incentive money, the HSA director initiated a discussion with the regional IDA coalition about partnering with the HSA on the IDA initiative. The HSA had access to families who were in transition from welfare to work as well as the PeninsulaWorks one-stop employment centers. To the HSA director, the IDA initiative seemed like a wonderful opportunity to bolster the earnings of low-income workers and increase their financial skills, as well as expand their awareness of educational and training programs at PeninsulaWorks. In so doing, the HSA director also hoped to increase numbers of well-trained workers San Mateo desperately needs in its job market. The IDA could be instrumental in lifting families out of poverty, engaging them in lifelong learning and education, and helping the community relieve its shortage of workers. The HSA chose PeninsulaWorks-Daly City as its first IDA pilot site.

> **BOX 12.1. The Merging Partnership of the Assets for All Alliance: Division of Responsibilities**
>
> **IDA Investment Council (Problem-Solving Quarterly Meetings)**
>
> - Shares expertise
> - Monitors results and holds partners accountable
>
> **Managing Partners**
>
> *Lenders for Community Development (LCD)*
>
> - Leads planning process for Alliance
> - Oversees partners with depository and financial training roles
> - Monitors participant account activity and allocation of matched funds
> - Reports and analyzes progress toward program milestones and savings targets
> - Oversees community partners in day-to-day operations
>
> *Center for Venture Philanthropy (CVP)*
>
> - Raises fund pledges from investors
> - Recruits and supports Investment Advisory Council
> - Develops and tracks Memorandum of Understanding (MOU) signed by all partners (Includes targets, key process outcomes, and commitments)
>
> *LCD and CVP Joint Responsibilities*
>
> - Determine eligibility requirements for participants
> - Select partner community organizations
> - Implement MOU accountability-results process from the venture capital world
> - Track learning and innovation generated at community partner level
> - Coordinate reports to the community

The HSA would have two roles; it would be an investor and a community partner. As an investor, the HSA would commit $100,000 of TANF funds to the asset development fund and participate as a coinvesting partner with the Alliance. As a community partner HSA would

- identify potential participants;
- support participation by helping participants with forms, sending meeting notifications, and making arrangements for meetings to ensure families attain their savings goals and increase their self-sufficiency;

- review monthly savings statements and follow up with clients as needed;
- attend an orientation to IDA principles and other meetings as necessary; and
- promote regular communication with the Alliance.

The Alliance would provide IDA trainers and offer the program to families identified by the HSA based on the following eligibility criteria:

- residence in San Mateo County and association with PeninsulaWorks-Daly City,
- half of the families would have a household income less than 185 percent of the federal poverty level and half would have a household income less than 80 percent of the median income in San Mateo County,
- possession of household net worth of less than $10,000 excluding one primary residence and one car,
- status of head of household and at least eighteen years of age,
- completion by the head of household of the WorkFirst curriculum including a comprehensive course in employment and life skills,
- receipt of income from gainful employment,
- indication of stable lives,
- development of asset goals that are compatible with the pilot project, and
- positive response to the opportunity to participate in the program.

Potential participants would be identified by PeninsulaWorks staff, attend an Alliance orientation, participate in an assessment conducted by PeninsulaWorks staff, and sign an IDA program agreement. The LCD staff would evaluate the application and admit or reject the applicant. If the applicant seemed promising but did not meet the eligibility criteria, the LCD staff could provide written indication of what factors the applicant would need to change in order to participate. With all the procedures in place, the pilot program was launched in September 2000.

HSA/PENINSULAWORKS-DALY CITY IDA PROGRAM

Start-Up

When the IDA pilot began in November 2000, ten PeninsulaWorks staff members were selected to oversee the program as part of their regular work responsibilities. They would manage the projected fifty participants over the three pilot years. One was selected to lead the project; all were experi-

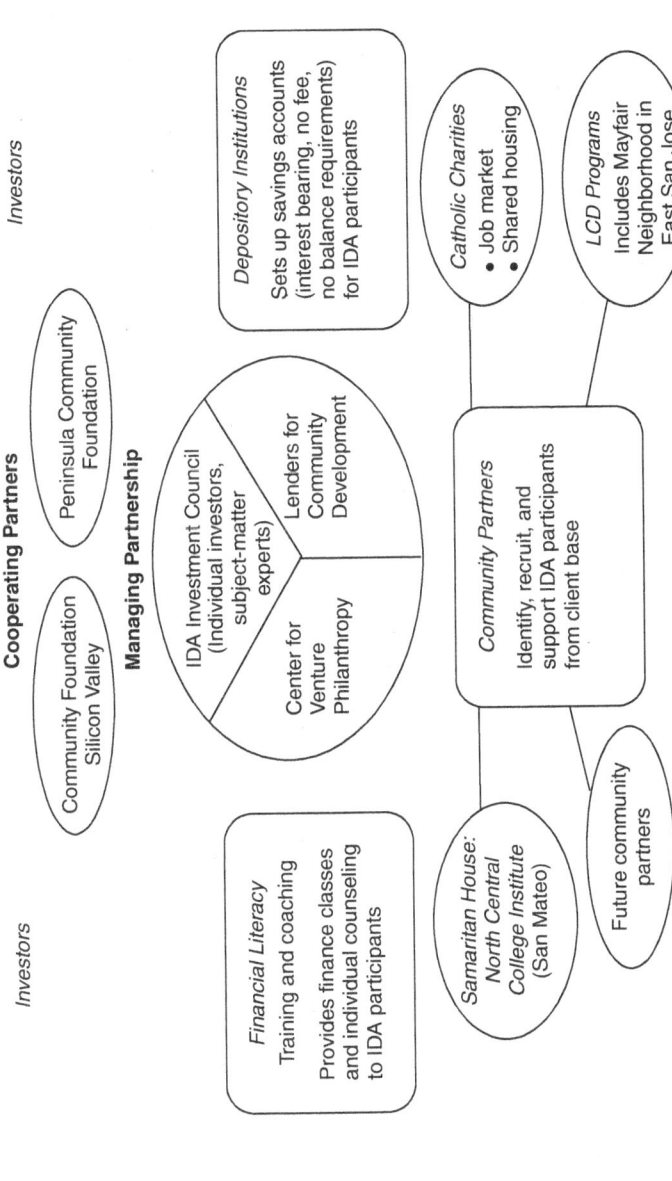

FIGURE 12.1. The Assets for All Alliance Individual Development Accounts (IDAs): A Savings Program for the Working Poor

enced case managers. The staff members began their search by selecting participants who had stable employment, successfully completed a San Mateo County job-search program, and demonstrated commitment toward self-sufficiency. To enroll the target of fifty participants, four sets of money-management classes would be scheduled over the first program year. With much optimism, the staff members put in extra effort and hours to get the program started.

As a recruitment strategy, staff members reviewed their past caseload and contacted individuals who might be qualified and interested in the IDA program. Follow-up mailings and reminder phone calls were made to ensure the highest possible attendance at the orientation. The leader posted a sign-up board outside her office to keep track of the invitations and provided weekly updates to staff and management on the program's progress.

The forty people who showed up for the first IDA orientation were welcomed with food and child care. The staff members were introduced and participants were given the opportunity to share their employment success stories. Thirty-two of the forty attendees signed up for the program at the first orientation. After the first set of money-management classes, the staff leader videotaped the first group of IDA participants for a presentation by the HSA director to the San Mateo County Board of Supervisors. Twenty-three individuals were invited to the second orientation and nine attended, with seven qualifying for the program.

As of March 2001, PeninsulaWorks had enrolled forty-seven participants and was beginning its third set of financial management classes. These forty-seven participants were all women; most were single (52 percent) or divorced (32 percent) and raising one or more children. The median income of participants was $26,400. Over half of the participants lived in households with more than one adult. All participants had a high school diploma or GED; some had attended college (49 percent), and almost a quarter had a four-year college degree. Most participants were working full-time (72 percent), while the rest were either working part-time (14 percent) or more than full-time (14 percent). A majority (55 percent) earned over $2,000 per month; 41.8 percent earned between $1,000 to $2,000. Over half (55 percent) of the participants had health insurance.

The Program

The IDA program has three major components: a five-week money-management class, one goal-specific seminar, and six meetings of the investor club annually. Figure 12.2 is an IDA client flowchart. Following the orientation

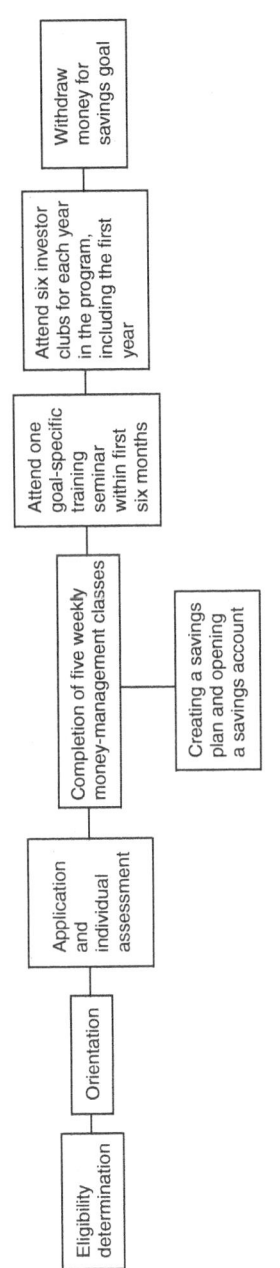

FIGURE 12.2. IDA Client Flowchart

and signed agreement, participants are required to successfully complete the five-week money-management class titled "Master Your Money." The five course topics and materials focus on the following issues:

1. Getting organized and budgeting
   - Introduction to the IDA program
   - Getting organized (e.g., course overview such as setting financial goals, tracking daily expenses)
   - Education on the distribution of wealth
   - Budgeting basics
   - The money pie (e.g., visualization of target amounts for participant expenses such as housing, transportation, debt, and savings)
   - Food for thought on how secure you feel about money (a quiz for participants to understand how they feel about money so they might balance their financial lives)
2. Goal setting and financial health
   - Assessing your financial values (a quiz for participants to determine what items are essential in their financial planning)
   - Goal setting (e.g., helps participants realize importance of establishing short- and long-term goals)
   - Asset-building action plan (helps participants begin to think about their savings plan)
   - Your money life (questions that help participants determine their financial status)
   - Ten steps to financial health
3. Money in your pocket and credit basics
   - Increase your income and reduce your expenses
   - Building your savings
   - Money down the drain
   - 101 ways to save money
   - Shopping the seasons
   - Credit IQ (a quiz for matching credit terms with definitions)
   - Cost of credit (a table providing interest based on annual percentage rates)
   - Credit basics (provides definitions for credit terms such as secured and unsecured credit, and two-tier billing cycle, as well as explaining various credit topics such as efficient dept repayment, credit and marriage, and the Fair Debt Collections Practices Act)
4. Credit! Credit! Credit! Credit!
   - Your credit report
   - Establishing and reestablishing credit
   - Cleaning up that credit report

- Obtaining a credit report
- Identify theft (provides guidelines on what to do if victimized by theft of credit cards, checks, etc.)

5. The spending plan
   - Savings agreement (stipulates conditions for participation such as being involved for at least two years, using the savings for their specified goal by December 15, 2005, missed deposits)
   - Spending plan (outline of monthly expenses and income)
   - Evaluation (ratings of workshops and presentations, best times and days for scheduling seminars, what topics are of interest for investor clubs)

During the fifth class, participants open their bank account with $10.00 and choose one of the following savings goals: (1) business start-up or expansion, (2) postsecondary education or job skills training for themselves or their children, (3) home purchase or improvements, or (4) retirement. The purpose of the classes is to assist participants with setting realistic, yet challenging, financial goals. Participants are able to adapt their savings goals between $20 and $84 per month and are allowed to miss two deposits per year. Family savings are matched at $2.00 for each $1.00 that the participant saves, up to a match of $4,000 or a combined total of $6,000.

Shortly after the five classes, participants attend a meeting to review and implement their budget to ensure they are able to achieve their goal. In addition, participants are required to attend one training class on the savings goal they have chosen and six investor clubs for each year they are in the program. The goal-specific training class provides in-depth information on the participant's selected savings goal (e.g., home ownership, education, retirement, or business start-up). The investor clubs are designed to provide additional financial education (e.g., tenant rights, income taxes, insurance), as well as ongoing individual and group support.

The structure and content of the classes appeared to be appropriate for the participants, using clearly stated concepts. Although many participants found the money-management classes to be a review, they frequently learned something new and helpful. Participants reported that the credit management and budgeting classes were particularly useful and motivated them to change their financial situation. The credit report was a reality check for most. The budgets demonstrated the feasibility of reaching their goals.

Overall, the classes proved to be a confirmation of good habits and provided self-confidence for improvement. One participant stated the IDA seminars helped to modify her self-perception from "poor" to "money-saver." Another participant said the course helped her to avoid becoming overdrawn at the end of the month. In addition, participants felt the course materials were an excellent information resource and source of strategies for saving money (e.g., packing lunch, riding BART, and taking children to story time at libraries, to parks, and to free museums). A few participants required occasional Spanish translation provided by bilingual trainers. Participants eagerly looked forward to the investor clubs to gain additional knowledge about money management.

The trainers created a comfortable learning environment that included food and child care arrangements. Participants described the trainers as "friendly," "nice," "considerate," "understanding," "hopeful," "having a sense of humor," and "self-disclosing." One trainer, described as a "grandmother type," brought her husband to help them read credit reports and give advice on balancing needs with wants. For example, if automobile maintenance costs are low then a new car is not needed, or making fewer trips can help reduce gas and auto repairs. One participant made frequent trips to visit her family in San Jose, Scotts Valley, and Santa Maria and now visits primarily when the family gathers together in one place. In addition, participants reported great appreciation of the provision of food and child care.

PROGRAM STRENGTHS, CHALLENGES, AND STRATEGIES

This section includes a sample of the strengths, challenges, and strategies for change that were identified by the trainers, program staff, and participants.

Strengths

Participation

- Personal contact, especially face to face, with a trusted PeninsulaWorks staff member had the highest recruitment results. Building on their prior worker-client relationships, participants appreciated being recruited into the program.
- The recruitment procedures that involved personal contact, mailings, and reminder calls before orientation were the most successful.
- The dinners and child care are helpful to the participants and were appreciated.

Program

- The trainers were friendly, knowledgeable, helpful, and understanding.
- The credit report and budgeting classes are perceived by participants as motivational and valuable course content.

- The binder is a wonderful resource for participants to achieve their goals.
- The financial changes led to better family relationships and healthier lifestyles. The class content reinforces good habits and provides motivation to change bad habits. Moreover, children are learning to save through their parents' example.

Challenges

Participation

- Participants need to be convinced that the 2:1 money match is real.
- Participants may have work hours that conflict with or make it difficult to attend meetings. Moreover, the lack of transportation made it difficult for some participants to attend the seminars, especially in the evening when public transportation is limited and travel can be dangerous. In addition, it is difficult for participants to arrive at class on time when they have little time to pick up their children between work and class.
- Participants with extremely low incomes may not be able to commit to a monthly savings program.
- To be eligible, participants must be current or former PeninsulaWorks program participants. This population may be limited because the community may not be aware of the services that PeninsulaWorks offers or its extended evening hours.

Staff

- It is difficult for other PeninsulaWorks staff to remember to disseminate IDA program information when teaching other classes.
- It is difficult for staff members to give the IDA program the attention it deserves when they have other work priorities and unclear expectations of what efforts are required for success. Moreover, it is difficult to maintain enthusiasm for the program when staff members must wait years to see the results of their efforts.
- Depending on the size and needs of the class, more trainers or staff members are needed to review the budgets and credit reports of each participant.

Program

- The money-management concepts are basic and need to be more closely matched to the needs of the participants. Sometimes it is hard

for participants to remain focused in the evening after work when the material is too simplistic. In addition, the class presentations were repetitious of the binder materials, giving little incentive for participants to read the materials in advance. Also, there is a need for greater clarity on what topics are to be covered in the investor clubs that differ from the goal-specific seminars.
- Sometimes the children are distracting. Moreover, participants and/or trainers who arrive late cause disruption or delays.
- Some participants initially felt pressured to save more than the minimum amount. Participants require patience and empathy, especially during the budget review and credit processes. This may be the first time they have allowed someone to see their financial information.

Strategies

Participation

- Utilize the original successful recruitment procedures.
- Greater participation may be attained for the five money-management classes through (1) arranging a more flexible schedule, (2) providing participants with choices regarding the scheduling of days and hours, and (3) providing classes at locations that may be more accessible to participants.
- Increase contacts with the community and HSA personnel to share program information (e.g., presentations to all line staff and outside agencies, publicity releases, a monthly newsletter, and a supply of IDA materials for staff to distribute).
- A greater number of low-income families would benefit if the IDA program was cosponsored with other community organizations.
- Continue to provide food and child care.
- Bring back successful graduates to share their successes and advice.

Staff

- Explore the possibility of hiring one highly interested, full-time staff member to oversee the program when resources become available.
- Ensure program coverage by bringing in extra staff when needed.
- Keep staff morale high by reporting outcomes and giving staff recognition through newsletters as well as publicity releases.
- Provide clear guidelines as well as incentives for staff participation.

Program

- Provide an outline of the topics to be covered in the money-management classes, goal-specific seminars, and investor clubs during orientation.
- Experiment with the program structure. Some participants expressed an interest in a lecture/homework structure with questions and answers during class.

PARTICIPANT FEEDBACK

Most of the participants learned of the IDA program through their contact with PeninsulaWorks, such as through a former or current employment specialist. Some heard through relatives or fellow employees, and one learned about it through her work at the Peninsula Community Foundation. They gave various reasons for participating. Most said they wanted to save money for their goals (e.g., child's education, home purchase). Others wanted to improve their self-sufficiency or learn how to manage their money or invest wisely.

Personal financial changes led to other positive lifestyle changes as well. Participants repeatedly stated that they were becoming more involved with their families. Discussing and planning financial goals together helped their family work together as a team. Their children were learning the value of saving and enjoying it. Some had allowances and piggy banks. At times, the adults had to borrow from their children! One mother relayed the following poignant story:

> One time during the Christmas season I told my son I felt like a "bad mommy" because I could not buy him the things he wanted. He had been asking for everything he had seen on television. His reply was "Oh no, you're a good mommy! Kids are supposed to want everything and not get them. Otherwise, they'll be spoiled."

Participants said that by saving together their family spends more quality time together and lives healthier lives. One participant quit smoking to reduce her expenses. As a result she is able to spend longer periods of time with her daughter, whose asthma had been irritated by her smoking. Others have stated they eat more healthily by spending less on fast foods and cooking at home, as well as packing lunches.

Participants share the following advice with their peers:

- Be assured that you have much to gain and nothing to lose. These seminars are designed for low-income, single parents—they are designed for you!
- Plan ahead on the day before class to make sure that you will have everything ready and arrive on time.
- Be sure to attend all the classes. They change the way you think about things. Even if you don't like it, you will learn.
- The program requires a lot of commitment and incentive. It is important to identify your goals and values so that you will be motivated to budget and save. Continually reevaluate yourself and maintain focus on your dreams.

LESSONS LEARNED

Capturing the key lessons from implementing the IDA program can assist with future program changes as well as alert others contemplating the start-up of a similar program. This case study offers lessons in the following four areas: (1) resources, (2) flexibility, (3) program development, and (4) personal transformation.

1. *Resources:* Building on current resources was critical to success. The resources included the leadership of the HSA and community partners. CalWORKs funding, in conjunction with enterprising staff, was also key to initial successes. The personal relationships between the workers and their clients were central to the recruitment efforts. Moreover, the IDA built on the strengths and resources of each participant.

   When the population of former PeninsulaWorks-Daly City participants had been reached for recruitment, new strategies began to emerge. Suggestions were made for information dissemination through HSA line staff, community agencies, and the media. Expansion of the target population beyond former PeninsulaWorks participants was explored.

2. *Flexibility:* Flexibility is an important factor for the IDA to reach its full potential in recruitment, retention, and programming. For example, after the second set of money-management classes, the program content was reorganized. Instead of setting up bank accounts and reviewing budgets in the first money-management class, these tasks were placed in the fifth class. As a result, trainers have time to establish a relationship with the participants and participants have time to plan realistic savings strategies.

   Flexibility based on participant characteristics and feedback will be vital to the program. Despite their desire to participate, many individuals have work schedules, modes of transportation, and family obligations that may affect attendance. Flexible schedules and additional locations will make the IDA program accessible to more families. In addition, greater program flexibility with regard to minimum monthly deposits and/or extended periods of time may benefit participants with extremely low incomes and encourage them to participate.

3. *Program development:* In implementing successful strategies, it is important to identify program strengths and weaknesses. The second and third recruitment efforts were not as successful as the first one. Staff members examined strategies and agreed that personal contact, with follow-up mailings and telephone reminders worked best. Moreover, oversight has been given to staff who demonstrated a high interest in the program. These IDA staff will receive additional pay for the extra time and effort the program requires. The Alliance trainers as well as PeninsulaWorks case managers recognized the need for additional assistance during the budget reviews and have provided more staff based on the size and needs of the class.

Based on participant feedback, the Alliance has added new content and materials to their lectures and binders, such as frequently asked questions and an outline of program requirements. Moreover, in April 2001, they published the first issue of *The Investor Gazette,* a quarterly newsletter that reports program outcomes, upcoming investor clubs and events, participant success stories, and other interesting news and facts. This is helpful in reminding participants about investor club meetings, providing staff and participant recognition through success stories, and disseminating information to the IDA community.

4. *Personal transformation:* The money-management seminars, presented in a family-like environment by friendly professionals, have led to other outcomes beyond financial gains. Participants reported improvements in their family relationships, healthier lifestyles, and high motivation and self-confidence about improving their futures. Moreover, the children were learning from role models provided by their parents. In addition, participants have expressed appreciation and gratitude for the community support. Several have declared their intention to help others similar to themselves.

CONCLUSION

Similar to many start-up programs, the implementation of the IDA pilot at PeninsulaWorks-Daly City has faced challenges on the road to success, yet forty-seven out of the goal of fifty participants were enrolled within the first six months. Initial feedback from participants has been positive, with reports of increased financial literacy, improved money-management capabilities, increased self-confidence and self-esteem, and new hope about the future. Early results indicate the PenninsulaWorks-Daly City IDA program is helping low-income participants establish savings habits and accumulate assets. As of May 2001, participants had saved $9,396 with a match of $18,792, totaling $28,188. Ninety-two percent of the participants had demonstrated a regular pattern of savings, exceeding both the program performance goals and the national average. Eighty-four percent had met their monthly savings goal. Based on these initial successes, the HSA is extending the program throughout the county with an additional investment of $300,000 for seventy-five new low-income welfare participants who are below 200 percent of the federal poverty line. There are plans to provide additional matching funds from other investment partners for forty more low-income participants who are at or below 80 percent of the median income in San Mateo County.

The next steps include continued monitoring and evaluation to assess the abilities of participants to establish regular savings patterns and attain their investment goals. The community partners gather and report data to LCD, which then analyzes and reports their progress toward IDA project milestones and participant savings targets. The Alliance reports the outcomes and knowledge gained from the project to relevant policy, funding, and private sector audiences. The goal for the future is to reach new populations and encourage greater community investment. A key to reaching this goal is advocacy for appropriations to implement state bill AB 692, which will provide additional resources for IDA programs throughout California.

REFERENCES

Assets for All Alliance (2001a). *IDA factsheet.* San Jose, CA: Center for Venture Philanthropy, a division of Peninsula Community Foundation.
Assets for All Alliance (2001b). Quick facts. *The Investor Gazette,* 1 (Winter), 3.
Assets for All Alliance (2001c). *Year two MOU: September 2000-September 2001 target summary report.* San Jose, CA: Center for Venture Philanthropy, a division of Peninsula Community Foundation.
Center for Social Development (2000). *Saving patterns in IDA programs: Downpayments on the American Dream Policy Demonstration, a national demonstration of individual development accounts.* St. Louis, MO: Washington University.
Center for Social Development (2001a). *Savings and asset accumulation in individual development accounts: Downpayments on the American Dream Policy Demonstration, a national demonstration of individual development accounts.* St. Louis, MO: Washington University.

Center for Social Development (2001b). *State IDA policy profiles*. St. Louis, MO: Ford Foundation and Washington University.
Center for Social Development Washington University (2001). *California IDA policy profile*. St. Louis, MO: Ford Foundation.
Charity, Aid, Recovery, and Empowerment Act (CARE) (2003). S. 476, 108th Congress, 1st Session (incorporated the Savings Opportunity and Charitable Giving Act, S. 592, 107th Congress, 1st Session, 2001).
Friedman, R. (1988). *The safety net as a ladder: Transfer payments and economic development*. Washington, DC: Council of State Policy and Planning Agencies.
Haverman, R. and Wolff, E. (2001). Who are the asset poor?: Trends in asset poverty, 1983-1998. *Assets*, Winter, 6-7.
IDANetwork (2001a). *Exchanging information on individual development accounts: Laws*. The Corporation for Enterprise Development. Available at <http: www.cfed.org>.
IDANetwork (2001b). *Exchanging information on individual development accounts: Overview*. The Corporation for Enterprise Development. Available at <http:www.cfed.org>.
Oliver, M. and Shapiro, T. (1995). *Black wealth/white wealth: A new perspective on racial inequality*. New York: Routledge.
Peninsula Community Foundation (2000). *Peninsula Community Foundation: Program and application guidelines*. San Mateo, CA: Author.
Sherraden, M. (1988). Rethinking social welfare: Toward assets. *Social Policy*, 18(3), 37-43.
Sherraden, M. (1991). *Assets and the poor*. New York: M.E. Sharpe.
Sherraden, M. (2000). From research to policy: Lessons from individual development accounts. *Journal of Consumer Affairs*, 34(2), 159-181.

SECTION III: ENHANCING COMMUNITY PARTNERSHIPS

NEIGHBORHOOD PARTNERSHIPS

Chapter 13

Fostering Neighborhood Involvement in Workforce Development: The Alameda County Neighborhood Jobs Pilot Initiative

Judie Svihula
Michael J. Austin

Many counties and communities have designed creative approaches to integrating multiple funding streams through an array of federal and state programs to promote workforce development. This case study tells the story of three neighborhoods in Alameda County that implemented a neighborhood jobs pilot initiative (NJPI) with public and private funding support. Following a brief history and a literature review, the case study describes how the neighborhoods implemented the NJPI, as well as their strengths and challenges and the lessons they learned from the NJPI experience.

HISTORY OF THE NEIGHBORHOOD JOBS PILOT INITIATIVE

The Neighborhood Jobs Pilot Initiative (NJPI) is public-private sponsored, neighborhood-based workforce development system.[1] The NJPI be-

---

This chapter originally appeared in *Journal of Community Practice* 9(3): 55-72. Copyright 2001 The Haworth Press, Inc.

gan with a partnership between Alameda County Social Services Agency (SSA) and the Rockefeller Foundation. In 1995, the Alameda County Private Industry Council (PIC) director was approached by the Equal Employment Program director of the Rockefeller Foundation to explore the possibility expanding its Jobs Intiatives[2] to Alameda County. In 1996, the SSA director, assistant agency director of workforce and resource development, and the Alameda County Private Industry Council director were invited to a Rockefeller Foundation-sponsored conference on the NJPI to discuss the possibility of Alameda County's participation.

In addition to economic and workforce development, the Rockefeller Foundation intended for the NJPI to support community-based organizations (CBOs) that would develop strong networks with their residents to address issues such as housing, family support, and resident leadership as well as access resources and assistance from national and local partners. The Rockefeller Foundation envisioned that the SSA would participate actively in funding these community collaboratives in order to build the neighborhood infrastructures as well as the employment pilots. A final concept paper was accepted by the Rockefeller Foundation in November 1997.

Subsequently, a committee composed of SSA program staff, community-based employment and training providers, and community building organizations met over several months to develop a plan for implementing an alternative employment service system. The planning process was funded by the Rockefeller Foundation with in-kind contributions from the SSA staff. The implementation plan was to include a budget proposal to leverage federal, state, and county welfare funds as well as foundation and corporation grants. A target date was set for June 1998.

The Interagency Children's Policy Council (ICPC)[3] helped the planning committee identify three target neighborhoods from the twenty-two communities included in the United Way Alameda: Community Assessment 1997. Three neighborhoods were selected based on their high rates of poverty, infant mortality, at-risk children, and their well-established SB620 Healthy Start pilots, as well as their history of community activism: South Hayward, Prescott, and, at a later date, Lower San Antonio/Fruitvale (LSAF). The NJPI became part of the ICPC mission to improve outcomes for children and families while promoting institutional changes at the county level. ICPC is responsible for coordinating the planning activities between two of the community collaboratives and the SSA, as well as administering the Rockefeller Foundation planning grant. Technical assistance and planning grants were awarded to ICPC for the initial implementation of the NJPI in South Hayward and Prescott, and to the East Bay Asian Local Development Corporation (EBALDC) for LSAF.

Utilizing Rockefeller Foundation grant funds as seed money, the NJPI provided the framework for workforce development and cultivated community access to employment and training resources, community-based economic development, and job retention and lifelong learning activities. Funds were used to develop one-stop employment resource centers in all three communities: The Institute for Success in South Hayward, the Prescott Resource Center in Prescott, and the Unity Council in Lower San Antonio/Fruitvale. The employment resource centers link the communities to current job-related labor market information and provide job-training opportunities. The goal is for each employment resource center to be independent of Rockefeller Foundation funding after two years and to be self-supporting. The anticipated types of self-support include membership dues, community volunteering, public and private job services contracts, temporary agency contracts with corporations, and space rental from local colleges for job skills and basic education classes. The goal of the NJPI is that the employment resource centers will become valuable community-owned resources for building long-term self-sufficiency.

BRIEF LITERATURE REVIEW

In some states the staff of welfare agencies provide job-search assistance and employment services; in other states programs are integrated into one-stop career centers that might include employment services, education, and other services (Martinson, 1999). It is important to understand the Department of Labor welfare-to-work (DOL-WtW) grant programs which provide supplemental funds and services to help welfare recipients, especially those with the most serious employment problems, gain and maintain employment. This grant program provides the foundation for neighborhood-based workforce development services.

Welfare-to-work grant programs operate under the authority of the Department of Labor and private industry councils and are designed to support Temporary Assistance to Needy Families (TANF)[4] services and focus on improving the job skills of participants (Nightingale, Trutko, and Barnow, 1999). DOL-WtW usually focuses on immediate job entry, known as WorkFirst (Trutko et al., 1999). With assistance, TANF recipients are expected to explore the labor market to see if they can find jobs. DOL-WtW staff assist clients with job-readiness training, counseling, job-search workshops, job clubs, and/or job leads. If individuals are not successful in their initial efforts to secure regular employment, TANF programs then engage the unemployed in other activities such as training or community service job assignments.

In an Urban Institute study, Trutko and colleagues (1999) found that the first eleven states to receive DOL-WtW funds were utilizing the resources to collaborate with other agencies and programs to expand the range and availability of support services (e.g., transportation, child care, housing, substance abuse services, and domestic violence services). There were indications that postemployment and career-advancement services (e.g., customized training at employer sites, workplace-based computer learning centers, workplace mentors, and extended case-management services) were being expanded along with longer follow-up periods. Some promising program features included targeting of individuals with multiple barriers to employment, mandating services to noncustodial parents, allowing open-ended periods during which job retention and postemployment services may be provided, and coordinating the welfare and workforce development systems at state and local levels.

Under the DOL-WtW program, states are required to match every $2 of federal DOL-WtW funds expended with $1 of state or local in-kind or cash expenditures (Trutko et al., 1999). Up to 50 percent of the state match can be in-kind rather than cash and may be provided entirely with state funds or a match through a combination of state and local funds. In Alameda County, the NJPI combines private foundation support with county and local resources in a comprehensive workforce development system which extends funding from the California Work Opportunity and Responsibility to Kids (CalWORKs) program, California's version of TANF.

A study by Holcomb and colleagues (1993) of one-stop service centers found considerable variation according to the target population, type of agencies and programs, and array of services and activities. The variation in target populations included all job seekers, disadvantaged workers, dislocated workers, unemployment insurance claimants, welfare recipients, youth, homeless, and ex-offenders. The variety of programs and agencies at the state and local level included employment services, cash assistance programs, secondary and postsecondary academic education, vocational education, economic development, and vocational rehabilitation. The spectrum of services or activities related to coordination or service integration included client services such as intake and eligibility determination, assessment and case management, and delivery of employment and training services. In addition, coordination may occur around activities involving agency operations such as planning, training, and information exchange, integrated management information systems (MIS), and colocation of facilities.

Following the national trend, California's employment and training system has attempted to move toward an integrated, seamless delivery model that meets the needs of all low-income, disadvantaged job seekers. California's strong commitment to the development of a one-stop center system began in the mid-1990s when the state placed a high priority on developing a statewide system which provides universal access to services, promotes customer choice, provides integrated access to a full spectrum of workforce preparation programs, and is performance based. California's goal is to convert the partnerships at the state and local levels, as well as between the public and private sectors, into a one-stop career center system built on the objectives of integrated, comprehensive, customer-focused, and performance-based services (Employment Development Department, 1997). In January 1997 California received $8 million, the first of a three-year U.S. Department of Labor one-stop implementation grant. In July of the same year, Governor Pete Wilson awarded eighteen grants, totaling almost $5 million, to local one-stop partnerships throughout California. The state vision for one-stop career centers is that they will provide services and benefits for clients including service directories, job availability information, labor market data, assessments, and referrals to program and support services. Similar services and benefits are to be provided to employers including services directories, resource for placing job orders and obtaining referrals, labor market data, information and referral on training resources, and business assistance.

Studies on coordination efforts report that substantial benefits can potentially accrue to clients as well as programs (Holcomb et al., 1993; Trutko et al., 1991). Coordination frequently enables clients to access a wider range of services than would otherwise be available. Moreover, clients may experience a reduction in barriers to accessing services, primarily through simplified referral processes that reduce the associated cost and time. Agencies may be able to reduce service duplication through coordination and, as a result, might offer expanded or more intensive services that benefit their clientele. Agencies also might experience access to additional resources, greater flexibility in using funds, increased knowledge and communication among agency staff, enhanced ability to serve different target groups, and an improved image with clients, employers, and the communities served.

In summary, one-stop employment centers, despite their variation in population, structure, and service offerings, have been reported to provide clients with greater access to a wider range of services with little duplication of services among agencies. The NJPI coordination goals are similar to California's Employment Development Department in developing one-stop employment centers. In Alameda County, the SSA and the Rockefeller Foundation are building on existing community support networks to offer one-stop employment services as part of a continuum of services.

SOUTH HAYWARD NEIGHBORHOOD

Description

South Hayward is centrally located in Alameda County. It is framed on the west by the Nimitz Freeway; on the north by Harder Road, a major east-west thoroughfare; on the south by Industrial Parkway, a light industrial area bordered by five mobile home parks consisting primarily of retired senior citizens; and on the east by Mission Boulevard. Due to high rates of transiency, South Hayward is recognized as a gateway community by its residents and institutions. Immigration combined with the high percentage of rental housing (70 percent) versus home ownership and lack of employment opportunities cause instability in the neighborhood. South Hayward's largest ethnic groups are Latino, Asian, and African American. Fifty-six languages are spoken by students at local schools. As a social system, South Hayward is missing an essential ingredient to its successful functioning: employment opportunities. Most businesses on the outskirts of the community are grocery stores, fast-food outlets, auto repair shops, gas stations, or small family-operated businesses. In addition, access to jobs outside the community through public transportation is difficult.

South Hayward's population of 14,080 is mainly comprised of low-income, blue-collar residents. A community analysis indicates that over 1,300 families in South Hayward are dependent on public assistance. Welfare reform legislation will require many individuals in these families to find employment with minimal or no education, employment history, or job skills. Eighteen percent of the residents do not have a high school diploma. Fifteen percent of South Hayward's residents, and one-quarter of its children, live below the poverty level. Limited resources coupled with the commitment of residents to improving the quality of life in South Hayward have created an environment of cooperation between service providers, churches, and citizen volunteers. Community-based organizations in South Hayward provide a range of services and activities to the community.

Collaborative Efforts

The South Hayward Neighborhood Collaborative (SoHNC) emerged in 1973 when a neighborhood association, the Harder-Tennyson Community Organization, conducted a needs assessment. The neighborhood relied on community-based services and committed individuals to address its needs. The SoHNC is a cooperative venture of more than thirty members including public and private service providers, churches, community-based organizations (CBOs), the City of Hayward, and volunteer organizations to provide services and activities to address the needs of families in the communities. The major stakeholders are the Glad Tidings Church, Institute for Success, Shepard Family Resource Center, Healthy Start Elementary School, Tennyson Middle School Family Resource Center, La Familia, Family Support Network (FSN) Family Resource Center, the Eden Youth and Family Center, and the SSA.

Programs

In 1997, with the implementation of welfare reform, time limits were imposed through the WorkFirst program. SoHNC had been awarded the Rockefeller Foundation NJPI planning grant to develop community infrastructure and capacity for employment as well as economic development training and activities. Concurrently, Glad Tidings Church (GT) was hoping to establish on-site education and training services. The collaborative worked with GT to establish the Glad Tidings Community Campus (GTCC) which offers high school and college programs as well as business training for the working poor and welfare recipients. The GTCC houses a jobs placement center that provides employment placement, development, and postemployment support and soon will offer child care to provide a safe environment for children two and one-half to five years of age while their parents are enrolled in on-site programs.

In January 1999, GT created the Institute for Success (IFS), which is a thirty-day WorkFirst employment model that concentrates on job search activities, motivation, critical thinking skills, and retention. The facility has a training center and lab with twelve computers and a career library. Key components of the IFS program include personal plan development, weekly progress evaluation, a learning objectives workbook, self-esteem and personal development exercises, and interpersonal communication and job search strategies. Soft skills training as well as customized job search, career, and family planning services are provided through the IFS curriculum and staff. The Hayward Adult School provides on-site computer, GED, English as a second language (ESL), vocational ESL (VESL), vocational training (such as basic food preparation, carpentry, typist, and data entry), and certificate programs. Chabot College, a county assessment contractor, provides CalWORKs assessments. The IFS enhances the thirty-day job club program with support services to assist with the transition to work. Measures of success are based on numbers of participants enrolled, placed in jobs, and job retention at thirty, sixty, and ninety days.

The IFS combines successful traditional employment placement strategies with transferable skills and innovative learning techniques from the Les Brown and Associates Inc. model. The county has traditionally used the Dean Curtis job club model that includes one week of learning a variety of job search skills followed by a three-week job search component wherein they are supported by networking with other participants and meeting with employment counselors on a daily basis. South Hayward has added the Les Brown model which adds a motivational piece to the elements of the job club. The curriculum includes topics such as independent thinking and problem-solving skills, dealing with authority, motivation and positive work ethics, completing assigned tasks and activities, following directions and instructions, assessing strengths and weakness, and making good career decisions.

The IFS also serves as the hub for intake information. Although they are separate nonprofits, the partners of the collaborative share a universal intake form. The IFS enters client intake information from its partners into its on-site database. The collaborative partners are building a shared data system.

The SoHNC has accessed other resources to meet its community employment goals. For example, CalWORKs money was utilized to employ a retention counselor who links clients with the family support services through the IFS. In addition, SoHNC partnered with the Greater Bay Area Family Resource Network and with support from the Irvine Foundation created the Employment Journey project, which provides services such as job search, career development, and family advocacy through the family resource centers. GT is involved in neighborhood rental property development through its nonprofit, the Northern California Community Development Corporation (NCCD). Through money it receives from rental units, the NCCD provides assistance to individuals ineligible for county funds.

Employment support services are provided through La Familia and Eden Youth and Family Center. La Familia is the fiscal agent for the Family Support Network (FSN) which includes child care, mental health, and youth leadership services, family advocates who provide case management services, and a family resource center. Eden Youth and Family Center provides colocated services such as a pediatrics clinic, a dental clinic, day school, child care center, Head Start, and a respite care center. A multidisciplinary team meeting is conducted twice each month in which partners discuss client issues.

Clients

Clients learn about services mainly through flyers, brochures, advertisements in school class schedules, and word of mouth. Eligibility is determined by the county SSA which provides a list of individuals qualified for WorkFirst by zip code. CalWORKs clients are referred to the IFS through the collaborative partners as diagramed in Figure 13.1. Client assessment and enrollment occurs through the IFS. The IFS assesses the skill and education levels of the client and provides job-search workshops. During the

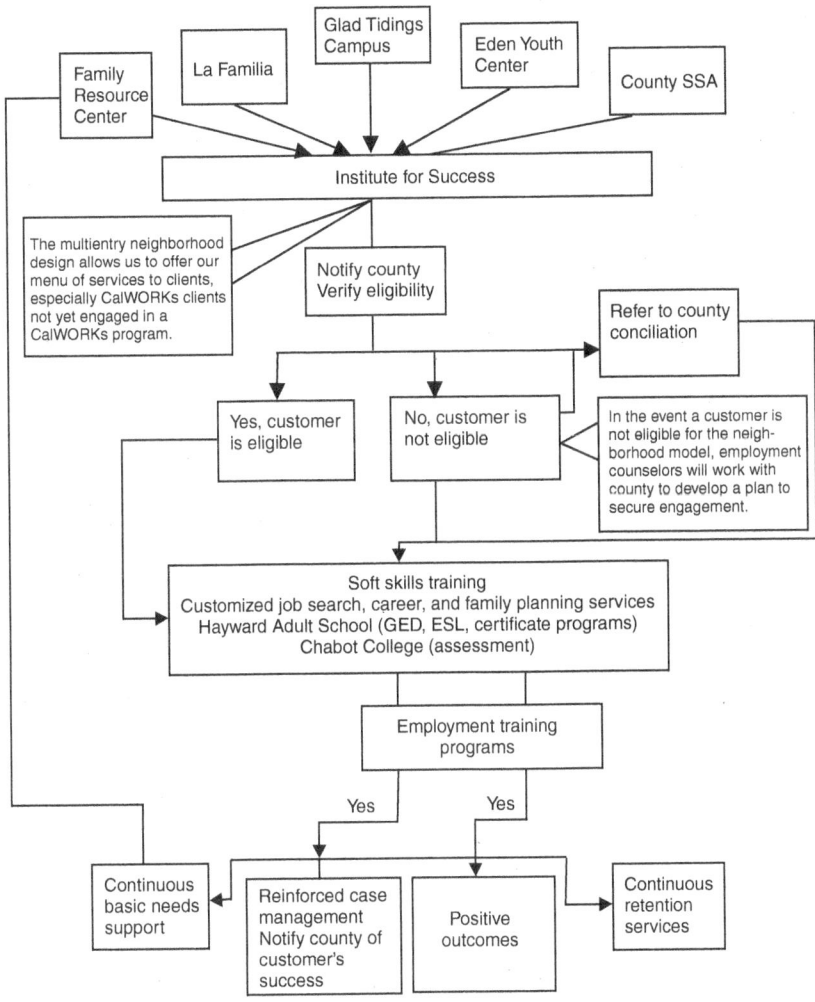

Note: Institute members / South Hayward Neighborhood Collaborative (SoHNC)

FIGURE 13.1. Institute for Success Client Flowchart

first two weeks, the client works with a job coach on a customized job-search plan and motivational skills. The coach accompanies the client to job club activities where they provide one-on-one assistance to the client in activities such as posting résumés and calling prospective employers. The coach continually seeks to strengthen the client's motivational skills. Glad Tidings and the FSN Family Resource Centers provide résumé assistance. Jobs are available through the IFS employment service job club. There is access to the Internet and job listings as well as employment postings. During fiscal year 1999, IFS exceeded its WorkFirst targets with 214 enrollments, ninety-six completions, twenty-three placements, thirty-two thirty-day retentions, thirty-five ninety-day retentions, and eleven 180-day retentions.

Strengths and Challenges

The following strengths were identified by SoHNC members:

- The ongoing tenacity, hard work, and dedication of the SoHNC partners who maintain a high level of communication and trust.
- Universal access to services. The one-stop philosophy of linkage and referrals is not only beneficial to clients, but also helps the organizations handle increased numbers of clients.
- Universal intake forms and a centralized database facilitate client referrals.
- The strength-based model builds on the assets of the poor who frequently rely on family, friends, and faith-based organizations for help.
- The NCCD provides assistance to individuals ineligible for county funds through money it receives from rental properties.

The following challenges were identified by SoHNC members:

- The collaborative process is not easy. The partners have a diversity of opinions and beliefs that need to be blended to move toward collaborative goals.
- Community resources are inadequate for CBOs and faith-based organizations to provide the amount of support services (such as child care and ESL classes) required by WorkFirst and CalWORKs clients. The SoHNC goals are to support low-income families, but only poor families and a portion of the support services are funded by CalWORKs.
- Outreach is difficult in a transient, multilingual community, especially when 44 percent speak a language other than English at home. It is also difficult to reach isolated clients, as well as those with substance abuse and mental health issues.

With SSA support, the IFS seeks to address the challenges with new services that include post-WorkFirst employment activities, on-the-job training programs, an employment training panel, a microenterprise project, enhanced postemployment retention services, complete CalWORKs asessments, in-home family assessments, and on-site drop-in child care. In addition, GT has entered into partnerships with Hayward Adult School for the development of adult education and entrepreneurial centers and with Chabot Community College for a CalWORKs assessment center to be housed at the GTCC. Moreover, GTCC hopes to offer a shuttle for transportation to and from the assessment and training centers to job interviews or job sites, and to the main campuses of community college and adult school. WorkFirst services will be provided to new immigrant and low-income families with an emphasis on those who are non-English speakers.

SoHNC has broadened the scope of CalWORKs activities, leveraged funding from multiple sources, and forged strong alliances with employers and training operators. New and innovative services are being offered to South Hayward residents so that they may become self-sufficient.

PRESCOTT/WEST OAKLAND NEIGHBORHOOD

Description

The Prescott neighborhood has a population of approximately 6,000 people. It is located in West Oakland and is bounded by West Grand in the north, Mandela Parkway in the east, Third Street in the south, and Southern Pacific Depot in the west. Prescott is an English-speaking, working-class community comprised primarily of people of color.

Before World War I, Prescott had a strong economy and a flourishing recreational and cultural life. Economic decline followed the closing of the ferry and railway services after World War II. The downturn in the economy resulted in inadequate adult education centers, a dearth of local support services, and the loss of recreational and cultural organizations. The deterioration of the residential neighborhood was exacerbated by major construction projects such as the BART station and tracks, the U.S. post office distribution facility, and the building of the Nimitz Freeway through the center of community. The final blow to the neighborhood came with the 1989 earthquake which destroyed the freeway as well as the neighborhood and left the community without an economic base or service infrastructure. The community economy was decimated by the closure of the army base in 1994. The recent development of industrial and commercial buildings continues to divide West Oakland and separate the Prescott neighborhood from downtown Oakland. The ongoing deterioration of the neighborhood is reinforced by banking practices of redlining and denying low-income families access to bank resources to promote home renovation. Poverty, domestic violence, homicide, lack of home ownership, and the need for more after-school programs have been identified as crucial community concerns.

Thirty-seven percent of Prescott's families live in poverty. The CalWORKs caseload is approximately 1,144, one of the highest in Alameda County. It is estimated that of the CalWORKs-eligible population 84 percent are women, 70 percent are African American, and 27 percent are of Asian, Latino, or Native American descent; over 50 percent do not have a high school diploma or equivalent. Over half of the CalWORKs population indicate they need assistance paying for transportation and locating and paying for child care. Most have limited transportation options. For example, 70 percent do not have a valid driver's license, 85 percent do not have access to a vehicle, and 40 percent indicate they need assistance finding transportation. More than 70 percent of Prescott's CalWORKs residents are neither working nor looking for work, perhaps due to the lack of local employment opportunities or the education and skills for available jobs. Preliminary results of a survey being conducted by the Women's Economic Agenda Project (WEAP) and the Prescott Resource Center indicate that the community is in favor of a redevelopment plan but would like to have a strong voice and influence in the planning and implementation processes.

Collaborative Efforts

The neighborhood's first collaborative, the Prescott Parent Collaborative, was established in 1995. Over its first few years the efforts of the collaborative to establish an employment resource center were stalled due to turnover in both lead and fiscal agencies,[5] as well as much staff turnover. ICPC which is responsible for coordinating Prescott's neighborhood planning activities and administering the Rockefeller Foundation planning grant had four consecutive directors and two different community liaisons. However, during the initial NJPI planning process in 1997-1998, ICPC formed the Prescott Community Collaborative (PCC) that included community residents, CBOs, and city and county representatives. The collaborative developed a community needs assessment that identified a range of issues such as food, clothing, housing, jobs, child care, and case management. A site was selected at 800 Pine for the Prescott Family Resource Center (PFRC).

In January 1999, the county released a request for a proposal to identify a new lead agency for the family resource center to coordinate a continuum of social services to neighborhood residents, economic development programs, technical assistance, and community outreach and capacity building.

In April the Women's Economic Agenda Project was chosen as the lead agency based on their eighteen-year history of advocacy for low-income, disenfranchised communities and individuals.

WEAP hired a director for PFRC and began to work with the collaborative, which included developing a governance structure and defining community goals and vision with local parents. WEAP and the PFRC, which was renamed the Prescott Resource Center (PRC) in 1999, collaborate with a variety of service providers in the Prescott community. The Prescott Community Parent Collaborative (PCPC) formed an interim governance structure with two parents as co-chairs in August 1999 and meets on a monthly basis to address various community issues.

The PCPC has created a forum in which the community members talk with elected officials about their concerns, such as safety, crime, and housing. Many of the basic services that the community identified in the original needs assessment are in place. WEAP and PCPC are designing an economic development model with the business community that will include job training and development along with entrepreneurial opportunities to assist residents in obtaining living-wage jobs as well as enhance the economic viability of the Prescott community.

The greatest potentials for employment growth in West Oakland are in the areas of transportation, communication, utilities, finance, insurance, and real estate. WEAP's employment focus is on training residents for jobs that pay a living wage, such as computer technology and information systems, and building construction. Combined with the PRC social services as well as community education and involvement, WEAP aims to (1) close the "digital divide," (2) transfer information and skills to community members in order to enhance their efficacy in resolving community needs, and (3) provide and coordinate social and health services. Existing employment resources in Prescott include

- training in the building trades (e.g., carpentry, cabinetmaking, computer-aided design and drafting related to manufacturing, and plumbing) provided by Asian Neighborhood Design,
- Goodwill Industries programs for residents with barriers to employment,
- job training and career counseling provided by Jubilee West, and
- job training and employment by the West Side Missionary Baptist Church at the Jack London Gateway Plaza.

Programs

The PRC, the only family resource center in Prescott, offers a one-stop program. The on-site Prescott Business Center (PBC) has several computers, a printer, a fax machine, and a photocopy machine that are accessible to the community. Staff members utilize the on-site business center to assist clients with résumé preparation, sending faxes, making copies, and calling prospective employers. The PRC has been added to the Alameda County Job Announcement mailing list that includes current job openings and promotions within Alameda County. The PRC has also established an on-site job announcement bulletin board and a job placement book. WEAP is upgrading the PRC in order to provide basic and intermediate computer training, job-readiness training, and job-placement services for area residents. Residents will have the option of enrolling in Cisco courses at WEAP's downtown office that will prepare them for positions as network administrators. An additional job-training component is the teen volunteers program. Teen volunteers arrive after school and receive a small stipend to help with various jobs at the PRC. By assisting the PRC staff they are able to learn about office work and procedures.

Informal support services available through the PRC include a food pantry, a clothing closet, emergency child care, basic literacy and parent training classes, family advocacy and peer support through case management, as well as child and family counseling. All residents have access to the parent drop-in room, a large room with comfortable furniture, videos, magazines, the daily paper and books, service provider listings, and other informational brochures. County on-site health and social services include eligibility determination, child welfare case management, maternal and child health outreach, and public health services. Collaborative partners participate in a biweekly seventeen-member multidisciplinary team meeting to help resolve client and community issues.

Clients

Clients learn about the PRC programs through outreach efforts, word of mouth, and referrals from the collaborative partners including the county SSA. Outreach efforts include block parties and neighborhood events attended by public figures as well as local musicians and CBOs. Community meetings, which frequently include speakers such as local politicians and experts in various fields, are well attended. Approximately 40 percent of the people who access the Prescott Resource Center's Business Services are seeking first-time jobs. Over 700 families have been served at the PRC.

Intakes and assessments are performed on-site by the community family advocate/case manager. The basic needs of clients are met through on-site programs such as the food pantry, emergency funds, or emergency respite child care. Clients are referred, based on their needs, to other on-site services such as the business center, the family literacy or parent training classes, or outside agencies.

Strengths and Challenges

The following strengths were identified by ICPC, PRC, and WEAP staff members:

- Prescott is a community of long-term residents committed to positive change based on strong family values.
- The PRC infuses trust and cooperation and a sense of pride into the community. Staff stability and understanding have gained the support of Prescott's residents. For example, residents from the community voluntarily help with setup and cleanup of all neighborhood events and block parties. Once, when a PRC coffee pot was stolen, it was returned the next morning by one of the residents. One building maintenance man stated that he no longer finds it necessary to carry a gun.
- Through the planning process, WEAP designed and implemented a systematic outreach strategy. Two local community outreach workers and one volunteer worker have been trained in community presentation skills and utilize outreach tools such as flyers, phone trees, and letters that WEAP has developed. The PRC brochure has been distributed to agencies, at meetings, and through the various program components (e.g., food basket, clothes closet).
- Employment opportunities are in close proximity to the neighborhood (e.g., Port of Oakland, U.S. post office, Emeryville, and San Francisco are accessible by public transportation).

The following challenges were identified by ICPC, PRC, and WEAP staff members:

- Although WEAP has a positive reputation among the Prescott residents, it had to overcome the negative perceptions of the predecessor agencies.
- It is difficult to offer comprehensive long-term support services based on categorical funding streams. Clients are unable to obtain and retain employment without long-term support services such as child care. In addition, higher levels of education and training are needed for participants to gain employment at a living wage.
- Reporting, which is based on the use of performance-based goals required by funding sources, has been difficult during the initial start-up period.

WEAP and PRC have linked with various resources to address some of these challenges. In addition to Rockefeller Foundation funding, the Prescott neighborhood has received support from the Hewlett Foundation for the implementation of economic development activities. The SSA has committed to support CalWORKs job-related activities. WEAP plans to reinitiate a neighborhood economic development collaborative by engaging area interests such as businesses, training facilities, schools, residents, and developers. Moreover, WEAP has partnered with the Port of Oakland, U.S. post office, Bay Area Economics, and the Alameda County Board of Supervisors in addition to other local businesses and area training programs to enhance neighborhood employment opportunities. Plans for future employment in West Oakland include the Seventh Street/McClymonds Corridor Neighborhood Improvement Initiative, which entails

- creating partnerships with businesses in the West Oakland First Hire Program,
- subsidizing training in building and construction maintenance programs at the Oakland Army Base with CalWORKs funding for welfare recipients,
- attracting computer assembly manufacturers to West Oakland,
- networking all classrooms to the Internet and assuring access and training to all households,
- developing on-the-job training and programs for high school students, and
- linking residents through transportation to job training and placement opportunities.

With the assistance of public and private funds, the PRC, PCPC, and WEAP are on their way to developing multiple strategies to promote neighborhood self-sufficiency.

LOWER SAN ANTONIO/FRUITVALE NEIGHBORHOOD

Description

The Lower San Antonio/Fruitvale neighborhood is located east of downtown Oakland. Its population represents 4.4 percent of the city of Oakland's population. LSAF is a predominantly immigrant neighborhood characterized by high unemployment, poverty, linguistic isolation, and low educational attainment rates. Fruitvale and Lower San Antonio are two very distinct communities despite similar socioeconomic circumstances and adjacent location. Lower San Antonio's population is mainly Asian; whereas Fruitvale's is mainly Latino. Of the total combined population of 21,367 people, about 23 percent receive public assistance and over 25 percent fall under the poverty level. Almost two-thirds of the 4,000 CalWORKs recipients, which comprise about 5 percent of the neighborhood population, are limited English speakers. CalWORKs recipients in the LSAF neighborhood represent 17 percent of the county CalWORKs caseload and 30 percent of the City of Oakland caseload. Thirty-six percent of the county's CalWORKs Spanish speakers and 47 percent of the Asian language speakers live in the LSAF neighborhood. SSA estimates approximately 14 percent of CalWORKs recipients in LSAF have been receiving aid for longer than thirty months.

Closures of big factories and warehouses over the past ten years have contributed to the loss of 4,857 jobs. The larger employers have been replaced by smaller businesses such as restaurants and nail salons which do not employ many people. Unemployment rates have remained at approximately 15 percent for the neighborhood, more than double the state rate (6.9 percent) and over triple the unemployment rate of the county (3.8 percent). Moreover, the disparity between unsubsidized earned wages ($11 to $14) per each public assistance dollar is approximately half that of the City of Oakland ($25) and about a fifth of California's rate ($61). Over 25 percent of LSAF residents fall beneath the poverty level, double the California rate and two and one-half times the county rate.

A large percentage of adults over eighteen years of age report low educational attainment. In both communities, 21 percent of residents over age eighteen have less than a ninth-grade education, while as many as 42 percent in the Fruitvale district do not have a high school diploma.

The county DOL-WtW service system is targeted almost exclusively to English-speaking clients. For example, the WorkFirst model places all clients in a four-week, self-paced job club from which very few limited-English proficiency (LEP) clients benefit. Clients had been handed English language job listings and expected to look for work on their own. To help resolve this dilemma, the SSA now allows LEP clients to waive job club requirements and move directly to postassessment programs. However, assessments and related written tests are currently offered only in English. Many clients in the LSAF neighborhood are not literate in their own language. It appears that, although they may have bilingual staff, current SSA and PIC systems as well as the community agencies with which they contract do not have the capacity to match language resources with client needs. None of the CalWORKs programs exclusively target LEP clients, and none of the federal competitive or governors 15 percent DOL-WtW grants funded in Oakland target this population. Recognizing that neither the SSA nor PICs have the capacity to develop an alternate service system for limited LEP clientele, the SSA awarded contracts to several CBOs to serve LEP clients.

Collaborative Efforts

As a result of the NJPI planning process, two neighborhoods joined together to address employment issues by forming the LSAF collaborative (LSAFC). In 1997, the East Bay Asian Local Development Corporation was approached by the SSA to develop an alternative to the DOL-WtW plan for the LSAF. The SSA and the Rockefeller Foundation provided a planning grant to build and implement a job-readiness program for LEP clients. The Unity Council,[6] located in Fruitvale, was asked to participate based on the model it used for its Spanish-speaking clientele. A thirty-five member partnership board, composed of local churches, community groups, ethnic associations, and service organizations, formed work groups to identify issues regarding welfare reform. In addition, focus groups of community residents were convened as part of the planning process. The planning committees came up with questions about client needs (ranging from child care to job transportation) which were incorporated in a questionnaire administered to clients in various agencies. In addition to identifying client needs, the focus groups gave the planning committee an opportunity to assess the number of clients the agencies were able to attract. Based on the focus group data, the SSA provided a CalWORKs grant to EBALDC to extend the planning process to job-readiness programs. The result was a comprehensive, integrated approach for restructuring the social service delivery system. Separate funding was provided for EBALDC to manage two pilot projects: WorkFirst, which is a job-readiness program, and a transportation contract to teach people how to use public transportation.

Programs

LSAFC has colocated their employment efforts at the Unity Council site and contracted with EBALDC for a project manager to oversee both programs. The employment program created as a result of the NJPI planning process, the Comprehensive Integrated Resources for CalWORKs Limited English Speakers (CIRCLES), focuses specifically on the needs of LEP welfare recipients in both neighborhoods. The CIRCLES program offers work experience, skills training, peer support, and job placement to participants while they improve their vocational English skills. Partnership agencies[7] provide on-site eligibility, assessment, case management, peer support, and ongoing retention services for CIRCLES participants. The CIRCLES team has linguistic and cultural experts that serve five groups: Cambodian, Laotian, Latino, Mein, and Vietnamese. Case managers provide up to one year of intensive job coaching and two years of peer support. The model offers intensive English as a second language and vocational English as a second language training, but ensures that a person is not simply learning English while other plans are put on hold. The VESL training integrates career path preparation and English language skills into a vocationally specific English language program. This component begins with basic ESL services (four to six months) and expands to on-site career path classes provided through community colleges that teach workplace appropriate language skills as well as technical skills.

CIRCLES has created a range of work experience opportunities within a supportive environment for participants. Temporary, subsidized positions that meet the WorkFirst requirements are available with private employers and community nonprofit organizations. EBALDC provides centralized job development and placement services for the different language groups, trains supervisors for the transitional work experience positions, and conducts extensive outreach to develop relationships with local employers. Goodwill Staffing Services of San Francisco (GSS), a nonprofit organization, and the Unity Council are two examples of placement opportunities. GSS serves as administrator of CalWORKs benefits and functions as employer of record to clients in positions such as retail and warehouse workers, drivers, and administrative support personnel. The Unity Council which has two divisions, the Economic Development Division and the Community and Family Asset Development Division, is able to place people in positions including early childhood education, security, administrative support, home care assistants for seniors, and janitorial.

An innovative structure called grant-based employment (GBE) administered by GSS converts a portion of county CalWORKs client grants to a wages rather than benefits. GBE clients perform community service work at local CBOs or public agencies and receive paychecks subsidized by competitive grant dollars to cover payroll taxes, workers compensation, and liability insurance. GBE payments allow recipients to be eligible for earned income tax credits which can have a substantial impact on increasing their annual income as well as providing the psychological benefits of paid employment.

In addition, the educational specialist links clients with resources for supportive services such as transportation, child care, and mental health services. Child care/transportation advocates help clients identify child care and transportation alternatives and provide training to enable clients to plan their trips to work. Two mental health care organizations, La Clinica de la Raza and Asian Community Mental Health Services, provide ongoing support as needed.

Clients

Clients are referred through the county WorkFirst program, but mostly through outreach efforts as diagramed in Figure 13.2. The eligibility process is handled by the SSA. Intake at the Unity Council is comprehensive and is based on clients' employment interests. When a person enters the program, he or she is matched with the services required, such as routine time

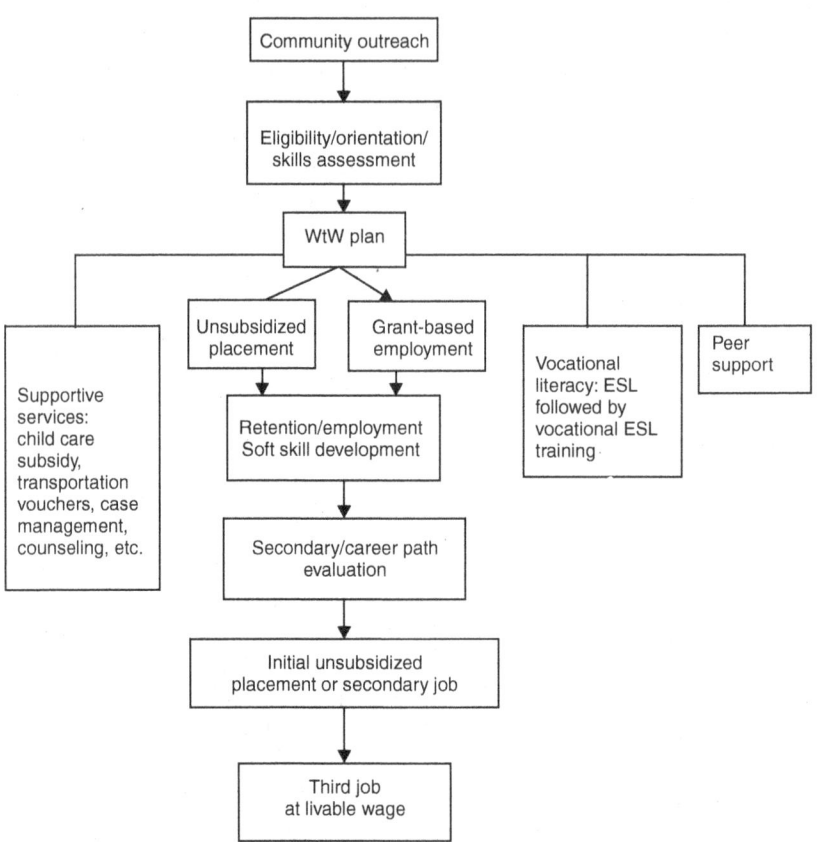

Note: CIRCLES / Lower San Antonio/Fruitvale Comprehensive Integrated Resources for CalWORKs Limited English Speakers (Lower San Antonio and Fruitvale Districts of Oakland, California)

FIGURE 13.2. Oakland Neighborhood CIRCLE Service Flowchart

management, ESL, or VESL classes. A case manager helps to develop a plan, monitors and evaluates progress, and helps reset goals toward self-sufficiency. An employment development plan (EDP) is created for each participant following the initial work-readiness evaluation, which is conducted at intake. In addition to work history, education, abilities, and job preferences, the evaluation includes an assessment of individual need for support services. A plan is created and timetables established based on individual needs. EDPs are reviewed and updated periodically throughout a client's enrollment in the program. Upon placement, clients are involved in a career advancement program for up to two years which helps identify specific skills to be developed.

Participants are scheduled for ESL training at the time of enrollment. The level of training is determined through evaluation of the client's language proficiency. Practice and reinforcement of ESL skills are heavily emphasized in all activities. Case managers incorporate language skill-development activities into the job-readiness courses. For example, the ESL curriculum includes working with job listings and completion of applications. Classes are offered four days per week through partnerships with Oakland Adult Education and the Peralta Community College system. Class times include evening and weekend hours.

Upon enrollment, participants are enrolled in peer support groups with people who share their language. Groups comprise about eight people to ensure participation by all members and are designed to provide a mutually supportive environment that focuses on culturally specific issues related to employment. Participants identify their internal goals and barriers and ways to overcome them as they transition from welfare to work. In addition, the development of support systems allows the clients to deal with the day-to-day difficulties of becoming and remaining employed. Groups remain open to all participants even after they find employment.

Strengths and Challenges

The following strengths were identified by EBALDC and Unity Council staff members:

- The SSA has supported alternative programs targeted at LEP clientele such as the development of a program which circumvents the job club in the standard CalWORKs process and allows LEP clients to access postassessment services.
- Collaborative partnerships were established during the first year of planning which (1) developed commitment to the collaborative, (2) strengthened neighborhood employment efforts, (3) encouraged

sharing of resources, and (4) provided the data and clarity of goals that helped it gain credibility in the eyes of the funders.
- The language capacity of employee support specialists along with the development of assessment tools in relevant languages is essential to the program. The project serves five language groups: Laotian, Mien, Vietnamese, Cambodian, and Spanish, which have organizations in the partnership who share resources and job trainers.
- CIRCLES initiated a staff support group that was initially held weekly, then biweekly, and now is held monthly. This group is effective in facilitating training through the use of modeling as well as providing space for staff to resolve problems and release frustrations through group process.

The following challenges were identified by EBALDC and Unity Council staff members:

- Current funding is based on specific program and service performance measures and does not include support for technical assistance and administration. For example, EBALDC provided technical assistance to increase the capacity of the agencies serving LEP DOL-WtW clients.
- Categorical funding does not facilitate comprehensive, integrated services. Agencies apply for funding under service categories and cannot provide comprehensive services to their clients due to the performance-based nature of the categorical funding. Language and job skills, as well as support services, are necessary for job placement and retention. Moreover, performance-based funding encourages the processing of as many clients as possible under specific categorical services for which the agency is funded. This approach may not be what the client needs or wants and discourages referrals of clients to other needed services.
- The high reliance on coordination between agencies to provide services to clients creates a tension over who has ultimate responsibility. For example, staff may blame another agency for mistakes made or lack of follow-through with clients.
- It is difficult to conduct vocational training with non-English-speaking clients. The clients first must learn English and then they may be trained for employment. Clients are at various levels in their knowledge of English. Some are not literate in their own language and require a comprehensive literacy program to complement the CalWORKs program.
- Access to employment opportunities within the community, but outside the collaborative partnership, is difficult.

- Clients require additional resources to obtain and retain employment such as low-cost housing, parenting skills, and after-school programs for children older than twelve years.

LSAFC has pursued additional resources to help meet some of these challenges. In addition to the Rockefeller Foundation start-up planning grant, CIRCLES has received funding through the SSA and the Hewlett Foundation for postassessment services. The SSA and Federal Transit Administration have provided resources for transportation development and related staff training activities. In addition, the SSA has provided funding for a CalWORKs financial literacy program. Moreover, an electronic infrastructure to enhance network capacity and connection to the Internet is planned. The site is being wired through a demonstration project sponsored by Pacific Bell Telephone. This infrastructure will allow access to the electronic job bank located at East Bay Works (sponsored by the private industry council) and electronic resources such as those provided by the California Employment and Development Department (EDD), as well as facilitate communication as well as documentation, evaluation, and reporting between agencies.

LESSONS LEARNED

Challenges faced by the neighborhoods such as the difficulty in creating and maintaining collaborative partnerships, integrating categorical funding streams to produce more comprehensive services, locating funds for support services, as well as accessing community resources for employment, training, and educational opportunities have produced much learning. Based on their experience with the NJPI, three sets of lessons were identified, categorized under funding, collaboration, and program development.

Funding

1. It is important to locate unrestricted funding to cover capacity building and administrative and start-up costs for pilot projects as well as for services such as outreach, referrals, and follow-up.
2. In the planning process, local needs must be balanced with programs or services that funders will support.

Collaboration

1. High levels of communication and trust are necessary for collaborative partners with different values to pursue common community goals.

2. It is easy to become disheartened with the collaborative vision because program implementation is more difficult than program design.
3. It is important to assess the capacities of potential partners when building a collaborative partnership. There needs to be a balance between providing and receiving technical assistance as well as between demonstrated and potential administrative expertise.

Program Development

1. A comprehensive community needs assessment is essential to effective program design and implementation.
2. Program flexibility is important for integration of clients who have various levels of need, skills, and knowledge.
3. Better coordination and communication need to be fostered among county and community resources to link clients with programs as well as provide opportunities for education, training, and support services.
4. A semiannual, issue-based forum needs to be created for communities to discuss their challenges and to provide technical assistance to one another.

The collaborative partners have maintained high levels of commitment despite their overwhelming challenges. Although they are in different stages of development, all three neighborhoods have leveraged SSA and Rockefeller Foundation support to access additional resources, gain community support, and create new and innovative services for their clientele.

NOTES

1. "The workforce development system generally refers to a broad range of employment and training services whose purpose is to enable job seekers, students, and employers to access a wide range of information about jobs, the labor market, careers, education and training organizations, financing options, skills standards or certification requirements, and needed support services" (Martinson, 1999, p. 2).

2. The Rockefeller Foundation is designing, testing, and evaluating four Jobs Initiatives models to increase employment rates and create "entire communities of work" (The Rockefeller Foundation, 1999, p. 3). The Alameda NJPI is part of the Connections to Work initiative whereby the Rockefeller Foundation is working with public welfare agencies, employment and training providers, and local officials in several cities to establish training and placement services that meet the needs of low-income residents as well as exploring the creation of publicly subsidized community service jobs.

3. ICPC is the county's governing body for the AB1741 Blending Funding Strategies for Youth Project. Membership includes individuals from the county Board of Supervisors, the county Office of Education, health care services, juvenile court, probation, and social services, as well as nongovernmental organizations.

4. The Temporary Assistance for Needy Families (TANF) program was created by the welfare reform law of 1996. TANF became effective July 1, 1997, and replaced what was then commonly known as welfare: Aid to Families with Dependent Children (AFDC) and the Job Opportunities and Basic Skills Training (JOBS) programs. TANF provides assistance and work opportunities to needy families by granting states the federal funds and wide flexibility to develop and implement their own welfare programs.

5. Lead and fiscal agencies are separate entities.

6. The Unity Council was formed in Fruitvale in 1964 as the Spanish Speaking Unity Council. It is a community development organization that aims to attract resources critical to the neighborhood. The Unity Council, through its network of institutions, provides a comprehensive program of physical, economic, and social development aimed at enriching the lives of families in the community. Programs include leadership in community advocacy, social service delivery, housing, and economic development especially for minorities in the community.

7. American Viet League, East Bay Cambodian Council, Former Vietnamese Political Prisoners Mutual Assistance, United Laotian Community Development, Inc., and Unity Council.

BIBLIOGRAPHY

Alameda County Social Services Agency (1997). *Neighborhood jobs program pilot project concept paper.* Oakland, CA: Author.

Alameda County Social Services Agency (1999a). *CalWORKs report: April-September 1999.* Oakland, CA: Author.

Alameda County Social Services Agency (1999b). Dean Curtis. Available at <http://www.co. alameda.ca.us/assistance/calworksI/calwo006.htm >, April 30.

Alameda County Social Services Agency and South Hayward Harder Tennyson Neighborhood Collaborative (1997). *Alameda County Social Services Agency and South Hayward Harder Tennyson Neighborhood Collaborative: Jobs pilot project: The Glad Tidings Community Campus: Four month start up budget.* Hayward, CA: Authors.

Alameda County Social Services Agency and South Hayward Harder Tennyson Neighborhood Collaborative (1999). *Jobs pilot project: The Glad Tidings Community Campus.* Hayward, CA: Authors.

East Bay Asian Local Development Corporation (1999). *Oakland Neighborhood CIRCLES: Comprehensive Integrated Resources for CalWORKs Limited English Speakers.* Oakland, CA: Author.

East Bay Local Development Corporation (1998). *Service plan to the County of Alameda Workforce and Resource Development Department.* Oakland, CA: Author.

Employment Development Department (1997). *California one-stop career center system* (Fact sheet). Sacramento, CA: Author.

Green, R., Zimmermann, W., Douglas, T., Zedlewski, S., and Waters, S. (1998). *Income support and social services for low-income people in California*. Washington, DC: Urban Institute.

Holcomb, P., Seefeldt, K., Trutko, J., Barnow, B., and Nightingale, D. (1993). *One stop shopping service integration: Major dimensions, key characteristics and impediments to implementation*. Washington, DC: The Urban Institute.

Interagency Children's Policy Council of Alameda County (1999). *Rockefeller Foundation report*. San Leandro, CA: Author.

L. L. Brown International Inc. (1997a). *Company brochure*. Renton, WA: Author.

L. L. Brown International Inc. (1997b). *30 days to gainful employment*. Renton, WA: Author.

Martinson, K. (1999). *Literature review on service coordination and integration in the welfare and workforce development systems*. Washington, DC: The Urban Institute.

Nightingale, D., Trutko, J., and Barnow, B. (1999). *The status of the welfare-to-work grants program after one year*. Washington, DC: The Urban Institute.

Northern California Community Development (1999). *Financial plan: Glad Tidings Community Campus*. Hayward, CA: Author.

Northern California Council for the Community (1997). *Alameda County Community Assessment: Executive summary: United Way of Alameda County: Community Assessment 1997*. Oakland, CA: United Way of Alameda County.

Prescott Community Collaborative (1997). *Neighborhood-based family self-sufficiency project: Proposal summary: September, 1997*. Oakland, CA: Author.

The Rockefeller Foundation (1999). *The employment challenge: The Rockefeller Foundation Jobs Initiatives*. New York: Author.

Social Services Agency and Lower San Antonio/Fruitvale Collaborative (1999). *Grant based employment initiative—A demonstration project*. Oakland, CA: Authors.

South Hayward Community Campus (1998). *The South Hayward Community Campus at Glad Tidings: Strategic planning report*. Hayward, CA: Author.

South Hayward Harder Tennyson Neighborhood Collaborative (1997). *South Hayward Harder Tennyson Neighborhood Collaborative: Rockefeller jobs pilot technical assistance budget*. Hayward, CA: Author.

South Hayward Neighborhood Collaborative (1999a). *Assessment center and collaborating agencies utilization plan: June 1999*. Hayward, CA: Author.

South Hayward Neighborhood Collaborative (1999b). *South Hayward Neighborhood Collaborative: Childcare facility plan for Glad Tidings Community Campus: June 1999*. Hayward, CA: Author.

South Hayward Neighborhood Collaborative (1999c). *Welcome to South Hayward: "A living neighborhood of hope, dignity and strength."* Hayward, CA: Author.

Spain, S. (1998). *Lower San Antonio welfare to work partnership: Focus group results*. Oakland, CA: The National Economic Development and Law Center.

Trutko, J., Bailis, L., Barnow, B., and French, S. (1991). *An assessment of the JTPA role in state and local coordination activities.* Washington, DC: U.S. Department of Labor.

Trutko, J., Pindus, N., Barnow, B., and Nightingale, D. (1999). *Early implementation of the welfare-to-work grants program.* Washington, DC: Urban Institute.

Women's Economic Agenda Project (1999a). *Prescott Resource Center local service provider list.* Oakland, CA: Author.

Women's Economic Agenda Project (1999b). *Reuniting and rebuilding the Prescott community: The future of economic development in West Oakland.* Oakland, CA: Author.

Women's Economic Agenda Project (2000). *Quarterly Report for WEAP/Prescott Resource Center: January-March 2000.* Oakland, CA: Author.

Chapter 14

Neighborhood Self-Sufficiency Centers

Christine M. Schmidt
Michael J. Austin

With the signing of President Clinton's 1996 Personal Responsibility and Work Opportunity Reconciliation Act (PRWORA), the goals of the welfare system in the United States changed from job training and economic assistance to a focus on removing barriers to employment and propelling welfare recipients into work. The bill consolidated the Aid to Families with Dependent Children (AFDC), Emergency Assistance, and Job Opportunities and Basic Skills (JOBS) programs into a single block grant for Temporary Assistance to Needy Families (TANF). With the new legislation came time limits on assistance and a demand to the states to develop welfare-to-work programs that could address the needs of those with multiple barriers. In response, California developed its own legislation (CalWORKs) that would both adhere to federal standards and delineate guidelines for county welfare-to-work programs.

In February 1996, Santa Clara County Supervisor James T. Beall Jr. and the Social Service Agency's (SSA) executive team initiated a local planning effort to address the expected welfare reform legislation. Local businesses, community groups, public and private agencies, and public assistance recipients were invited to participate in a collaborative partnership with the SSA to develop a response to the pending changes. The basic vision of this Employment Support Initiative (ESI) was "to strengthen low-income parents' access to the resources they need to care for their children through employment and related services" (Employment Support Initiative, 1996, p. 3). Through this collaboration, SSA hoped to develop a countywide welfare-to-work strategy based on existing funding and resources that could be implemented and operational before any new policy constraints were imposed.

To further this goal, SSA developed a partnership with both NOVA Private Industry Council (NOVA PIC) and Silicon Valley Private Industry Council (SVPIC) and began discussing plans that could both comply with federal guidelines and support the agencies' objectives for community-coordinated service delivery. While the principal tenet of the new welfare-to-work legislation was to move people into employment, the partnership recognized that successful, sustained family self-sufficiency would be obtained only by providing for the needs of the entire family in their own neighborhoods.

Out of this basic idea for addressing family needs came the concept of developing neighborhood centers that would offer family services in areas where CalWORKs participants needed them most. The centers would focus on postemployment support services to CalWORKs participants entering the workforce in an effort to sustain long-term employment and foster advancement. This is a case study of how Santa Clara County SSA, along with both private industry councils, developed and implemented neighborhood self-sufficiency centers to address the multiple barriers to employment and provide neighborhood-based supportive services.

BRIEF LITERATURE REVIEW

Since the 1996 PRWORA was passed, welfare programs in the United States have placed primary emphasis on moving as many welfare recipients as possible into sustainable employment. Helped by the strong economy in most states, many people have left the rolls for work. Nationwide, caseloads have dropped by more than 40 percent, or approximately 2 million families (Tweedie, 1999). This success is due, in large part, to state and county efforts to combine a work-first philosophy with supportive employment and training programs, tailored to the abilities and requirements of clients.

The implementation of the Temporary Assistance to Needy Families program, along with the welfare-to-work (WtW) grant program provided funding to states to be used not only for helping recipients find jobs but also for implementing postemployment services to help them keep those jobs (O'Connor, 1999). Such services help them maintain employment, avoid returning to welfare, and earn higher wages. WtW grants complement TANF in that they are designated specifically for work-related activities and not for cash assistance.

Unlike TANF, which is distributed by the U.S. Department of Health and Human Services (DHHS), the WtW program is administered by the U.S. Department of Labor. WtW funds can be used for training or education once a person has begun work and are targeted toward those who face numerous barriers to employment. Services utilizing WtW funds may also be used to serve noncustodial fathers of children who receive TANF. Some uses of WtW funds include but are not limited to the following (U.S. Department of Labor, 1997):

- Wage subsidies
- On-the-job training
- Job readiness
- Job-placement services
- Postemployment education and services
- Job vouchers for job readiness, placement, or postemployment services, community service, or work experience
- Job-retention services
- Other support services

Seventy-five percent of WtW funds are allocated to states based on a formula that takes into account number of poor individuals and adult recipients of assistance under TANF in each state. States are required to pass along 85 percent of the money to local private industry councils, which oversee and guide job-training programs in specific geographical jurisdictions called service delivery areas.

Changes in the U.S. economy over the past twenty years have led to an increased emphasis on educational achievement and the acquisition of technical skills. Well-paying, low-skill manufacturing jobs have been replaced by low-paying, service-sector jobs (Trutko, Nightingale, and Barnow, 1999). Some researchers estimate that in today's labor market, most welfare recipients will earn between $5.00 and $8.00 an hour (Burtless, 1989). Although these entry-level jobs may provide a starting point for gaining work experience, they are not enough to provide long-term self-sufficiency for the families of low-income workers. Postemployment education and training services can provide the means for low-paid individuals to transition over time into higher-paid career-oriented work (Trutko, Nightingale, and Barnow, 1999).

In response, some welfare agencies are implementing postemployment training and retention services and promoting coordination with WtW programs to provide additional training opportunities and workplace support. This type of service integration features a common intake and a seamless service delivery system that eliminates repeated registration procedures, waiting periods, or other administrative barriers. Advantages to this coordinated system include the following (Pindus et al., 2000):

- *Referrals to more services and to a wider range of services:* Availability of expanded services is often the result of referral agreements or contractual relationships between coordinating agencies.
- *Greater intensity of services to clients:* Linkages with other agencies may reinforce the services that are provided through the welfare agency.

- *Simplified referrals:* A simplified client referral process might mean the client faces fewer obstacles when seeking services from another agency because the agency has already received some basic information about the client.
- *Convenience of having several or all agencies in one location:* In some instances, agencies are colocated in the same building or at a one-stop center.
- *Improved case management:* When staff of coordinated programs share information and communicate regularly, they can better understand and address the client's needs.

Implementation of an integrated system has advantages for those interested in promoting economic development and for the providers of job training and placement who have tended to operate in separate worlds. The efforts to attract industry have rarely been matched with the efforts to appropriately and adequately prepare a workforce.

As a result, it has been rare for either to make use of the tools and experiences of the other, despite the potential benefits (Theodore and Carlson, 1998). However, postemployment education and training are likely to be most effective if developed in conjunction with employers and sensitive to the realities of the workplace. Working closely with employers will not only improve possibilities for enhanced skill development among WtW participants but also help pave the way to identifying an expanded range of job openings, increased chances of job retention, and leveraging of private-sector training dollars (Trutko, Nightingale, and Barnow, 1999).

LAUNCHING THE CENTERS

On October 9, 1998, a request for concept papers (RFCP) was issued and called for agencies to develop plans that would evolve into future neighborhood self-sufficiency centers. These centers would provide employment, reemployment, and skills upgrade services to CalWORKs participants who are able to secure employment. To sustain long-term employment, the centers needed to provide family services to complement employment services. At a minimum, this would require age-appropriate educational and recreational child care activities for the children of CalWORKs participants so that the parents could then use that time for skill-building training or education. In addition, centers would be required to provide additional services such as specialized classes on topics of interest to CalWORKs participants.

In order to receive funding, the applicant providers had to demonstrate a collaborative partnership with a minimum of three providers along with a plan to leverage other revenues or in-kind services. Proposed programs needed to include innovative activities and services that do not duplicate currently available services. Proposals needed to reflect a three-year plan for the use of federal WtW funds based on the contract renewal policy of funding years two and three on the basis of the continued need for services and performance outcomes.

PROPOSAL REQUIREMENTS

Each proposal needed to include a statement of work that reflected the following principles (Silicon Valley Private Industry Council, NOVA Private Industry Council, and Santa Clara County Social Services Agency, 1998):

- *Customer service:* Services that respond to both CalWORKs participants and employers.
- *Family-friendly and family-focused services:* Services that address the needs of the entire family.
- *Leveraging resources:* Services that leverage additional resources to augment the WtW program.
- *Community collaboration coordination:* Services that reflect new and/or expanded community collaboratives that support the WtW program and strengthen the entire community. In addition, services need to be coordinated among the NOVA PIC, SVPIC, and the SSA and the multitude of educational, training, and service agencies that work within the county.
- *The employer is a key customer of the WtW program and a critical partner in its success:* NSSCs need to work with employers to develop on-the-job training and work experience, on-site mentoring, job coaching, and/or skills upgrade training. Service may include assistance in coordinating job listings, improving job matches, and accessing tax credits.
- *Providing services to customers who are currently employed will require new and creative approaches to outreach and recruitment:* Services need to include incentives such as vouchers redeemable with local merchants, free recreational and educational activities for children, or financial incentives for attending educational programs.

In addition to this statement of work, proposals needed a budget and cost analysis outlining financial plans for each partner as well as one for the program as a whole. Funding allocations could not include administrative expenditures, as these costs were to be a matched expense. A bidder identification form would identify each proposed partner, with subcontracts or memorandums of understanding between bidder and partners to be attached. Oversight for the approved programs would be based on the policies and procedures of both PICs in conjunction with all applicable state and federal laws, regulations, and policies, including the application and enrollment policies of the federal WtW program.

Once clients meet eligibility and are enrolled in the federal WtW program, they then meet with a case manager who assists them in completing a family assessment and service strategy form. This form includes personal and family history, assessment of current and needed skills, work history, self-sufficiency/supportive service needs, and a plan for action. Staff members complete monthly activity records, which document the activities and services received by a participant and the dollar value of each service. These records are used for WtW monitoring and reporting to the federal Department of Labor. When clients leave the program or become ineligible under WtW requirements, NSSC staff members file termination of active enrollment forms.

PROGRAM REQUIREMENTS

The four principal partners in the county's welfare-to-work strategy were identified as the CalWORKs participant, the participant's family, the participant's community, and the employer. Service programs need to reflect a plan to provide coordination and services to each of these partners. The following seven basic services were required either directly or through service collaborators (Silicon Valley PIC, NOVA PIC, and Santa Clara County SSA, 1998):

1. Basic skills training
2. Vocational skills and skills-upgrade training
3. Case management
4. Employment and placement services
5. Employment retention and reemployment services
6. Mentoring services
7. Support services

In recognizing the importance of family stabilization in job retention and success, all program components needed to be family focused and community related. Working closely with the employment community was seen as a crucial step in forging better job opportunities and a stable workforce. At the same time, stable family lives and job retention help to strengthen the communities.

While the NSSCs can serve as a complement to and support a one-stop service model, they are themselves a network of services located in the neighborhoods of greatest need. Each center has so many partners that it would be impossible for all services to be colocated, although they are able to provide several of the same benefits of one-stop centers to their participants. For example, multiple collaborative activities simplify referral, and program staff members are able to refer clients to a wider range of services. Case management services are improved through shared information and regular communication among partner agencies.

With the assistance of the local CalWORKs office, NSSCs are responsible for participant outreach and recruitment. The focus is on unemployed and employed persons residing in the NSSCs' surrounding zip codes. All CalWORKs participants who obtain employment and meet eligibility requirements of the federal WtW program are referred to the centers by CalWORKs offices.

Concept papers and work statements were evaluated with the use of the following criteria (Silicon Valley PIC, NOVA PIC, and Santa Clara County SSA, 1998):

1. Innovative retention services
2. Family-centered services
3. Nutrition programs
4. Mentoring
5. Supportive services
6. Work experience and subsidized placement
7. Multilingual employment services targeting high poverty areas
8. Additional services not otherwise provided

After reviewing all submissions, six centers were selected to share in the initial $2 million in WtW funding. In addition, NOVA PIC applied for and was granted an additional amount of $750,000 by the David and Lucile Packard Foundation to be distributed among the centers to provide services to persons not eligible for federal WtW enrollment. Each center ultimately received $100,000 of the foundation grant to supplement their WtW funding, with the remainder of the grant reserved for capacity-building and administrative support services such as in-house evaluation and an independent customer survey.

Based on the incidence of TANF recipients by zip codes as well as community input, three centers were located in San Jose, one in East San Jose, one in South County (Gilroy), and one in North County (Santa Clara). The following sections outline the implementation, operation, and early successes and challenges of three of the NSSCs: (1) North County Consortium, serving Mountain View, Santa Clara, Los Altos, Sunnyvale, Cupertino, and Palo Alto; (2) South County (Adelante Familia), serving Gilroy, Morgan Hill, and San Martin; and (3) Resource Net, serving the entire county.

NORTH COUNTY CONSORTIUM

North County Consortium NSSC provides services to employed CalWORKs participants who are still receiving aid and live in the northern part of Santa Clara County. The consortium is made up of businesses, agencies, and schools that have successfully served CalWORKs participants in the past and offers job-retention services, case management, educational services and skills upgrade, child care and recreation, support services such as substance abuse and domestic violence workshops, and homeless services. The main collaborators in the consortium are the Department of Employment and Development of the City of Sunnyvale, the Housing Authority of Santa Clara County, the Santa Clara City Library, Mountain View/Los Altos Adult Education, Foothill/De Anza Community College, Springboard employment placement agency, YWCA Santa Clara Valley, Scott Lane Elementary School, Kathryn Hughes Elementary School, Santa Clara Unified School District/Educational Options, UC-Berkeley Cooperative Extension, Work Skills Associates, Software Quality Associates, AmeriCorps volunteers, and the City of Santa Clara Adult Education (lead agency). Given the diverse populations of CalWORKs participants in Santa Clara County, each of the NSSCs include a unique mix of service providers, which allows for a wide range of family-oriented services to maximize client support. Multilingual services are available at all centers, and services are accessible beyond business hours, during evenings, and on Saturdays.

The North County NSSC has a total operating budget of $450,000, with WtW funding comprising $350,000, and an additional $100,000 in Packard Foundation money. In program year 1999-2000, the program enrolled a total of seventy customers, thirty-seven into the 70 percent WtW eligibility category and thirty-three into the 30 percent category. Fifty-three of these customers were currently employed (76 percent), with an average wage of $9.08 per hour.

The North County Consortium has four neighborhood outreach centers located in high poverty areas at two elementary schools and two adult education centers. Each center has a site coordinator (SC) who provides case management services by assessing the customer's needs upon enrollment and assisting in developing a plan of action for reaching desired goals. The

SC is responsible for coordinating services and activities of the various agencies and for tracking WtW participants by utilizing the state-mandated reporting system to provide monthly cost and activity reports on each participant.

The adult education teachers in each center provide instruction on basic reading, writing, and math, while volunteers provide individual tutoring. At the elementary school sites, computer-assisted basic skills training is provided, along with an adult education instructor to guide students through the curriculum, monitor progress, and provide assessment and feedback. Families are encouraged to take part in the elementary school program called Even Start that provides child care and instruction for children while parents attend literacy classes. Child care services are provided at all sites during center activities.

SOUTH COUNTY (ADELANTE FAMILIA)

Adelante Familia NSSC is a collaborative serving South Santa Clara County in Gilroy, Morgan Hill, and San Martin. It includes seven primary partners: CET (Center for Employment Training), Community Solutions, ESO (Economic and Social Opportunities), MACSA (Mexican American Community Services Agency), Gavilan Community College, Morgan Hill Community Adult School, and the City of Gilroy Department of Housing and Community Development. The center's budget includes $280,000 in WtW funding and $100,000 in Packard Foundation funding, for services primarily to current CalWORKs participants who are employed but still receiving aid for their families. The program offers family support services, job-retention services, skill upgrades, and job-readiness training, along with classes and workshops available in parenting, making the transition from family to work, anger/stress management, conflict resolution, and assertiveness.

A case manager, working in conjunction with the local CalWORKs office, recruits the participants for the NSSC. As he or she receives the lists of local CalWORKs participants, he or she calls them to describe the NSSC and its services. Although most of the CalWORKs participants called are not yet eligible because they are still unemployed, the case manager describes the services they can receive when they are employed and encourages them to contact him or her as soon as they find employment. The case manager also participates in various welfare-to-work job search presentations and encourages potential participants to call when they become eligible for center-based services. Although the center does not enroll the unemployed, some participants lose their job while receiving services and the center then provides job-search assistance and training.

Since its inception, the Adelante Familia NSSC has had its share of challenges mixed with successes. Start-up of the program was slow due to staff changes and confusion about policies and procedures. In spite of proactive recruiting, the center enrolled a total of forty-seven customers in its first program year, which represented 59 percent of its goal. Stringent WtW eligibility criteria made it difficult to enroll participants, although recent legislation has loosened the criteria for the second year. Only nine of the forty-seven participants (19 percent) were employed at that time, due to an unexpected number of participants losing their jobs while enrolled. Although it was unforeseen that job search and placement would become such an increased need, the center has adjusted accordingly, offering more services to unemployed participants.

Although the center has had many obstacles to face, it has also had some success. One example is an innovative program called Family Fun Night, a weekly program designed to provide a family-oriented educational and recreational activity to promote family unity. At each of the weekly meetings, guest speakers present information on family topics of interest to adults, while separate activities are available for the children and child care is available for the very young. Dinner provided by Adelante Familia and free drawings for prizes for both adults and children follow the short presentation. Participants look forward to these events, as they provide opportunities to develop support groups with other participants. Although customer satisfaction surveying has been sporadic, those interviewed have reported positively about the program, citing Family Fun Night and counseling services from Community Solutions as helpful in meeting their needs.

RESOURCE NET

Resource Net is a collaboration of housing providers, family support agencies, and employers that provides services to CalWORKs and former CalWORKs clients and their families throughout San Jose who are homeless and at risk of becoming homeless. Partners include InnVision (housing), the Emergency Housing Consortium (housing), Second Start (employment services), Santa Clara Adult Education, Head Start, and the county board of education's Homeless Youth Education project. On any given day, Resource Net's two housing partners, InnVision and the Emergency Housing Consortium, provide shelter to eighty TANF families.

Resource Net's primary customer service center, located in downtown San Jose, is inside InnVision's Georgia Travis Center. The center is in an existing multiservice organization that primarily serves homeless single women and homeless mothers with children. It is the only facility in the county specifically designed to meet the needs of homeless women and children seeking respite from the streets during the day. In addition to emergency and respite services, the Georgia Travis Center provides Resource Net participants with:

1. housing search assistance,
2. transportation services,
3. outreach,
4. family recreation,
5. educational enrichment activities for children,
6. school services for homeless children,
7. legal services,
8. tuition assistance,
9. training resources,
10. mental health and substance abuse services, and
11. Internet/voice mail services.

Participants also have access to the training or other employment resources of current Second Start programs. These employment and training services include individualized assessment, customized job matching, on-the-job training, apprenticeship training, employment retention services, and links to the area's private industry councils and community colleges.

One of the successes of the Resource Net NSSC has been its ability to maximize funding for client services. In addition to their $175,000 WtW funding combined with $100,000 in Packard Foundation funds, Resource Net leverages an additional $622,000 in housing, family, and employment resources. These funds help to create a valuable continuum of emergency, transitional, and permanent housing services for its participants. Other signs of success in the first program year are the high number of enrolled persons employed (95 percent) and the average hourly wage of employed customers ($9.89), the highest among the six NSSCs.

Although Resource Net has shown itself to be successful, it also got off to a slow start. Agencies that had never worked together had to quickly familiarize themselves with one another's roles and responsibilities and the goals of the program as a whole. Staff needed to devise a workable system for distributing tasks and paperwork and for making sure they continued to operate under all local, federal, and state guidelines. Although expenditures exceeded the initial budgeted amount, additional leveraged monies and in-kind resources absorbed the overflow.

ADDITIONAL CHALLENGES

Although a number of center-specific challenges have been presented previously, it is important to note several challenges that impact the program as a whole. First, the process of collaboration, a fundamental part of the program model, also provided a major implementation challenge. The partnership at the federal level between the Department of Health and Human Services (DHHS) and the Department of Labor (DOL) was new and difficult to navigate due to very different systems of funding, eligibility, and accountability. In the centers' first year alone, there were three changes in required paperwork, making it hard to keep abreast as well as retrain staff.

Second, during this same time period, a transition from county to city administration caused a considerable staff turnover in terms of county staff assigned to the project. As a result, existing NSSC staff did not receive the level of technical assistance they would have under normal circumstances, making it even more difficult to keep up with complex paperwork. Third, private industry councils are in the process of transitioning to workforce investment boards, in compliance with the Workforce Investment Act (WIA). This further complicates matters in that county staff must familiarize themselves with new or additional WIA guidelines that could negatively affect the three-year project.

FUTURE DIRECTIONS OF NEIGHBORHOOD SELF-SUFFICIENCY CENTERS

Currently all of the NSSCs, in conjunction with the social services agency and county workforce investment boards, are in the process of reviewing the start-up experience and defining future service outcomes. They are looking at ways in which to increase the capacity of service providers to understand the complexities of serving low-income workers and their families. It is anticipated that improved data collection and the use of technology to link the six centers will help to maximize services to all participants. The county is encouraging city administration to follow up on their plan to install a common case-management system for the centers that can be networked with the social services agency and area one-stop centers.

The neighborhood self-sufficiency centers represent a new model of collaboration between provider agencies as well as between cities and the county. Partners are beginning to see the value of working together and sharing successes. The collaborative partnerships are also positively impacting the interagency culture through ongoing dialogue about what works and what does not and how to work together to improve services.

LESSONS LEARNED

The following lessons are derived from the experiences of Santa Clara County and its two private industry councils as they developed and implemented the neighborhood self-sufficiency centers:

1. When working with multiple systems of funding and/or oversight, it may be difficult to keep abreast of changes in eligibility or monitoring requirements. Ongoing training is necessary to ensure compliance with state and federal reporting mandates.
2. It is necessary to identify strong leadership to develop and guide intergency partnerships, especially to help staff understand the purpose and desired outcomes of new service systems. Partnership start-ups that lack central leadership due to staff turnover or other internal issues can often result in role confusion among partners and lack of initial program progress.
3. Whenever possible, it is important to implement centralized information systems for use by program staff. In order to prevent the loss of time and momentum in recruiting participants, technology needs to support the distribution of information to and among centers to aid in identifying potential participants.
4. It is important to blend federal policy and program objectives with local needs and priorities. While the goals of the federal welfare-to-work plan are focused primarily on getting people back to work, priorities of PICs and social service agencies are to help people secure a job with a living wage and services that provide for a stable family life.

The NSSCs build on the success of federal programs in helping people get jobs by providing additional supportive services that can help them keep those jobs. Opportunities for additional skills and education also help participants achieve self-sufficiency by maximizing employability and increasing earning potential.

REFERENCES

Burtless, G. (1989). The Effect of Reform on Employment, Earnings and Income. In Phoebe H. Cottingham and David T. Ellwood, eds., *Welfare Policy for the 1990s* (pp. 103-140). Cambridge, MA: Harvard University Press.

Employment Support Initiative (1996). The Santa Clara Valley Employment Support Initiative: An Agenda for Children and Their Families. Concept Paper. Santa Clara County, CA.

O'Connor, M. (1999). Getting a Job and Keeping It (Window of Opportunity for Welfare Reform). *State Legislatures,* 25:4, 21.
Pindus, N., Koralek, R., Martinson, K., and Trutko, J. (2000). *Coordination and Integration of Welfare and Workforce Development Systems.* Prepared for the U.S. Dept. of Health and Human Services, Assistant Secretary for Planning and Evaluation. Washington, DC: Urban Institute.
Silicon Valley Private Industry Council, NOVA Private Industry Council, and Santa Clara County Social Services Agency (1998). Welfare-to-Work Neighborhood Self Sufficiency Centers (NSSC) Request for Concept Paper (RFCP) Solicitation. Santa Clara County, CA.
Theodore, N. and Carlson, V.L. (1998). Targeting Job Opportunities: Developing Measures of Local Employment. *Economic Development Quarterly,* 12:2, 137-149.
Trutko, J., Nightingale, D.S., and Barnow, B.S. (1999). *Post-Employment Education and Training Models in the Welfare-to-Work Grant Program.* Prepared for the U.S. Department of Labor Employment and Training Administration. Washington, DC: The Urban Institute.
Tweedie, J. (1999). Eight Questions to Ask About Welfare Reforms. *State Legislatures,* 25:1, 33-35.
U.S. Department of Labor (1997). Welfare to Work (WtW) Grants: Rules and Regulations. *Federal Register,* 62(222), 1,6-7.

COMMUNITY-WIDE PARTNERSHIPS

Chapter 15

A Community Partnership Approach to Serving the Homeless

Margaret K. Libby
Michael J. Austin

The Transitional Residential Alliance and Integrated Network (TRAIN) was conceived in June 1996 by a group of community advocates for the homeless. The group included representatives from the Napa Valley County Health and Human Services Agency, the Napa County Housing Alliance, the Napa Valley Shelter Project Advisory Board, and the Nonprofit Coalition of Napa. The program idea was developed out of a community-initiated needs-assessment process. The Napa community participants recognized the increased need for additional transitional housing with case management services specifically designed for individuals with chronic substance abuse problems, survivors of domestic violence, and the street homeless. The county health and human services agency became the lead agency for the TRAIN due to its access to resources, while the community-based nonprofits became the outreach and service providers.

This chapter originally appeared as "Building a Coalition of Non-Profit Agencies to Collaborate with a County Health and Human Services Agency," in *Administration in Social Work*, 26(4): 81-99. Copyright 2002 The Haworth Press, Inc.

This is a case study of the TRAIN program, a successful community-led initiative to provide transitional housing and case-management services to those in great need, and also an example of a successful partnership between the county health and human service agency and community-based nonprofit organizations. This case study highlights the success of this partnership, which is due, in large part, to the TRAIN's ability to effectively capitalize on the strengths of each of its partners. The county provides oversight and resources, and the community-based agencies provide access to and support for the clients. The partnership successes impact directly on those in greatest need of housing and support services.

BRIEF LITERATURE REVIEW

Homelessness is a way of life for growing numbers of Americans, as many as 600,000 on any given night. Factors contributing to the national problem of homelessness have included the closure of state mental hospitals, increase in private development, reduction in the stock of affordable housing, and increases in substance abuse and drug abuse (Schussheim, 1999). In 1998, about 4.9 million units were eligible for HUD subsidies, and 1 million were available through rural housing programs (Schussheim, 1999). Despite the many federal programs designed to address homelessness through the provision of affordable housing, the level of federal housing available has been inadequate to make any real progress in addressing the problem.

Those low-income Americans housed in affordable housing are finding themselves increasingly at risk of becoming homeless. "As of 1995, 5.5 million renter households and 3.8 million owner households are spending more than half of their incomes on housing and/or living in severely inadequate units. Most of these households have extremely low incomes" (Joint Center for Housing Studies, 1998, p. 1). The Joint Center for Housing Studies (1998) also notes that while subsidies are needed to assist low-income households and to build new affordable housing, they are not available at a sufficient level. The demand for affordable housing outweighs the supply. For example, in Alameda County, when the housing assistance waiting list, which had been closed since 1989, was opened for four days, 6,000 families were added (Basgal, 2000).

The Joint Center for Housing Studies (1998) also asserts that for extremely low-income individuals, paying unsubsidized rent remains the most significant housing problem. Approximately 1.5 million low-income recipients of housing assistance also receive income support, two-thirds of which are TANF recipients. This overlap in low-income individuals receiving both income and housing support suggests that these families are at high risk of becoming homeless when their TANF benefits are exhausted. Especially in this welfare reform era, these low-income families are at risk of becoming homeless.

Homeless families, particularly those headed by single mothers, are the fastest-growing population among the homeless (Letique, Anderson, and Koblinsky, 1998). Individual factors such as mental illness and substance abuse increase the likelihood that a family will experience homelessness (Letique, Anderson, and Koblinsky, 1998). Domestic violence is another factor in family homelessness, as mothers fleeing an abusive partner often have no place to go with their children. Research indicates that homeless single mothers often feel isolated, have less contact with friends and relatives, and can rely on fewer people than can housed women. In other words, they have less social support, and they feel less able to trust their social network to provide support in times of need (Letique, Anderson, and Koblinsky, 1996). Due to the lack of social support experienced by homeless single mothers and their children, case management could provide them with referrals that may offer them opportunities to reduce feelings of isolation and build a network of support.

Homelessness also continues to be a problem for the mentally ill. Due to the ongoing process of deinstitutionalization of mental health care service provision, treatment approaches for the severely mentally ill emphasize reduction of long-term hospital care. This is due in part to an increase in availability of community-based services, as well as the belief that these services are beneficial to the clients (McGrew et al., 1999). With increasing numbers of severely mentally ill individuals living in the community, it is essential that appropriate services be available to support these individuals, such as housing and treatment. When beds are lost, community providers must work together to develop treatment options (McGrew et al., 1999).

Case management and transitional housing programs have proven to be an effective way to support severely mentally ill individuals living in the community. Case management can assist the mentally ill in negotiating service systems, which, in most communities, can be described as fragmented and uncoordinated. Case management is ideally driven by the client's goals and not the system's goals, and is necessary regardless of how integrated or coordinated the system (Anthony et al., 2000). Anthony and colleagues (2000) view case management as a process that includes the following four components: (1) connecting with clients, (2) planning for services, (3) linking clients with services, and (4) advocating for service improvements. These steps are beneficial for individuals with a psychiatric disability and are particularly critical when making the transition from the street to transitional housing.

Case management benefits not only the mentally ill but all clients attempting to navigate through a complex and often fragmented service delivery system. This was recognized by the state of New York within the context of housing the homeless. New York State designed a two-pronged approach to homelessness with a program called the Homeless Housing and Assistance Program (HHAP). HHAP meets both the emergency housing needs and the transitional housing needs of homeless people in New York. Established in 1983, it was the first public program to acknowledge the importance of social services in a program that houses homeless people (Travers, 1989). Case management services have been provided and several shelters and transitional housing units have been renovated and/or constructed with these funds.

Although a policy-level approach can be effective, other communities have used a more grassroots approach to homelessness. In DuPage County, Illinois, a church group responded to the growing number of homeless people in their community by raising enough money to cover the housing costs for a single family for one year. A year later the group established Bridge Communities, a nonprofit transitional housing agency, which served a total of eighty-five families in its first ten years, and thirty-five families in 1997 alone (Bendis, 1998). Bridge Communities now owns thirty-five units of transitional housing, for which clients must pay 30 percent of their income after their first sixty days in the unit. The maximum stay for each family is two years, though most secure permanent housing much sooner (Bendis, 1998). Through volunteers and a partnership with the local Catholic Charities, Bridge Communities offers day care, an academic tutoring program for youth, and a mentorship program for the formerly homeless adults. The mentorship program, which is staffed by trained volunteers and supervised by a licensed social worker, includes weekly visits and referrals to community services.

Currently, the typical transitional housing program for homeless families provides housing for up to two years (McChesney, 1990). The programs often provide life skills training, job training, and substance abuse treatment programs. Few studies have examined whether these programs actually help clients secure permanent housing. Still, it is widely accepted that the provision of case-management services within the context of a transitional housing program is critical and can improve outcomes.

Studies have also indicated that it is critical for transitional housing and subsidized housing programs to target specific groups and include services designed to address their particular needs. Early (1998) examined the homeless and housed poor in fifteen U.S. cities and discovered that many programs which offer subsidized transitional housing and services do not actually reach the poorest and most at-risk homeless populations. Early (1998) argues that to effectively address homelessness, such programs must target the most at-risk populations and incorporate strategies to address their individual needs. More specifically, Early (1998) argues that programs should target individuals with substance abuse problems and mental health issues and provide assistance with the task of securing permanent housing and accessing other services, such as training and job placement. Case managers can effectively provide these services to the most at-risk homeless populations.

HISTORY OF TRAIN

There is a long history of support and cooperation from the local community around the problem of homelessness in Napa County. In 1982, a coalition of community agencies which included the Napa County Council for Economic Opportunity (NCCEO), Catholic Social Services, the American Red Cross, the Volunteer Center of Napa, the Napa Emergency Women's Shelter (NEWS), and the Napa County Health and Human Services Agency (HHSA) came together as the Committee on the Homeless. Their purpose was to develop and coordinate a plan to address the increasing needs of Napa's homeless population. Through their advocacy, two emergency shelters were established, the Samaritan Family Center in 1983 and the Sullivan Shelter in 1988 for single adults. These two shelters, which are managed by NCCEO, are referred to as the Napa Valley Shelter Project (NVSP). In 1983, the Committee on the Homeless created an advisory body for the NVSP, the Napa Valley Shelter Project Advisory Board, which has operated successfully since then.

In 1987, the Napa County Board of Supervisors established the Napa County Housing Alliance (NCHA) to develop and coordinate local initiatives around homelessness. The NCHA includes representatives from private and public agencies, churches, and the private sector. They meet monthly and focus on the creation and implementation of policies that will foster the development of affordable housing in Napa. The long-standing presence of these two community-driven bodies in Napa illustrates the community's commitment to addressing homelessness.

CONTINUUM OF CARE FOR HOMELESSNESS

One of the major activities undertaken by the pair of homelessness coalitions was the development of a continuum of care for the homeless population of Napa. In 1994, they conducted a survey of the homeless population to determine their self-identified needs and characteristics. They also involved the community-at-large in the process in order to raise awareness about the homelessness problem and to garner support for their efforts. Homeless and former homeless individuals participated in that planning as well. The results of the survey were as follows:

- The average age for the homeless population is 24.5 years of age. The oldest surveyed was seventy-four and lived along the river, and the youngest was a newborn who lived at Samaritan Family Shelter.
- Twenty-one percent of households in the City of Napa earn between 0 and 50 percent of the median income, and 18 percent earn between 51 and 80 percent. These percentages suggest that many households are at risk of becoming homeless.
- Over 3,500 individuals have used NVSP shelters since 1983 when they were founded.
- Over 500 adults have been housed each year between 1993 and 1996. The average daily census at NVSP is sixty, while the number of homeless families increased between 1993 and 1996. On any given night, there is a waiting list of fifteen to twenty families.
- According to HHSA, at any one time at least twelve homeless mentally disabled individuals are living on the streets who are not served by the shelter or mental health care system.
- As their current source of income, 76 percent at Samaritan Family Shelter listed AFDC, 44 percent at Sullivan Shelter listed "none," and 13 percent listed SSI; at a free lunch table program, 22 percent said "none," 21 percent named SSI, and 12 percent listed social security.

They found the following regarding the needs of the homeless population in Napa County:

- Support services to link them to permanent housing
- Increased level of affordable housing in Napa
- Outreach to the homeless population not living in shelters
- Child care services for homeless families
- Supportive services for homeless individuals living with mental illness

Through these community discussions, the Napa County Continuum of Care was developed in 1995. Beginning in Spring 1996, the members of the NVSPAB and NCHA began meeting as the ad hoc Continuum of Care committee. The primary purpose was to compile the results of the survey, conduct community meetings, and develop a strategic plan for a continuum of care based on prioritizing the identified needs and the need for an action plan. From these discussions, they created the concept of the Transitional Residential Alliance and Integrated Network. Service gaps and funding needs were ranked from high to low by the NCHA committee. The following were the highest-priority items:

1. *Street outreach:* It was estimated that at any one time, between 100 and 250 people are homeless on the street. Outreach was defined as reaching out to these homeless individuals and providing them with case management and referrals to emergency shelters and other relevant services.
2. *Transitional housing for individuals with substance abuse issues and/or dual diagnosis:* Due to HHSA budget cuts in the early 1990s, twelve transitional housing beds for individuals recovering from substance abuse and six residential detox beds were lost. Due to these cutbacks, the need increased for both emergency and transitional housing for individuals with substance abuse issues and/or dual diagnosis. In addition, outreach was needed to refer street homeless individuals with chronic substance abuse problems to existing shelters and transitional housing programs. Transitional housing for substance abusers and individuals with dual diagnosis was defined as the top priority in the continuum of care.
3. *Transitional housing for survivors of domestic violence:* No transitional housing was available for women and children fleeing domestic violence, and there were consistently long waiting lists at family shelters. Transitional housing for survivors of domestic violence was defined as a top priority.

With these identified service gaps and funding needs established as part of the Napa continuum of care, the committee designed the TRAIN to address three populations whose needs were not being met by current transitional housing programs: (1) domestic violence survivors and their children, (2) individuals with chronic substance abuse issues and dual diagnosis, and (3) street homeless. Although other transitional programs and services were available to homeless individuals and families in Napa, none were designed with these populations in mind. The committee designed and drafted the TRAIN program in a matter of days and submitted the HUD grant proposal with the assistance of a professional grant writer in June 1996.

After this quick and intensive program design and proposal-writing process, the group tried to catch their breath while waiting for a response from HUD. In September 1996, HUD approved the initial proposal and requested the technical submissions, which were completed and submitted in December 1996.

TRAIN PROGRAM PROPOSAL APPROVED BY HUD

In May 1997, the TRAIN proposal was approved by HUD, nearly a year after the proposal was first submitted. The county HHSA staff member that had coordinated the proposal submission had left the agency in December 1996 and had been replaced in May 1997. This newly hired county HHSA representative was charged with implementing the TRAIN program without prior involvement in the planning or even a review of the process by the departing county staff member, as their employment did not overlap. He reconvened the group to begin a discussion around implementation of the TRAIN. Because it was nearly one year later and a degree of group memory had been lost, it took four months for the individuals to remember what they had put together and to determine how to move forward. In addition, there was a degree of confusion about the program design, as some significant program elements had changed in the technical submissions phase:

1. Staffing changed from two FTE (full-time equivalents) county and nonprofit staff positions to 2.75 FTE nonprofit staff positions across three agencies.
2. The budget was reduced from $467,000 to $400,000.
3. The program length was reduced from eighteen to twelve months of subsidized housing and services.

These changes presented the group with a significant, but not unusual, challenge: do more for less. Due to the staff change at the county HHSA and the length of time that had passed since the initial planning, it was difficult to determine exactly how these alterations had been made. Assessing the implications of those changes was more important than piecing together an explanation of how these changes occurred.

Although the TRAIN had been conceived as a partnership between HHSA and community-based nonprofits, it had become a county-sponsored program run entirely by community-based nonprofits. This meant that nonprofits would handle the case management, as expected, as well as outreach and referral that had been an HHSA responsibility during the initial planning. The TRAIN had become more of a county-directed, nonprofit-administered program and less of a shared responsibility partnership between nonprofits and the county HHSA. Second, the nonprofits were charged with running a program with more participants than planned for, with fewer funds for staff, no administrative funds, and expectations to achieve the same results regarding transitional housing for all program participants with less money and in less time (twelve months rather than eighteen).

IMPLEMENTING THE TRAIN

Despite the frustration around these changes in the program scope and decreased resources, the group was determined to move forward with the TRAIN program. Due to these challenges, however, it took four months to develop and sign the contracts between the county and the three agencies providing the outreach, referral, and case-management services. Those agencies included the following:

- Napa Emergency Women's Shelter, a shelter for survivors of domestic violence and their children (1.0 FTE case manager to serve its shelter and the Samaritan Family Shelter).
- Napa County Council on Economic Opportunity, which manages two shelters for single individuals (1.0 FTE case manager to serve the Sullivan Shelter for single adults).
- Progress Foundation, a mental health service agency (One .75 FTE case manager to provide street outreach, referrals, and case management).

Although the process of developing contracts and reconvening the group was challenging, another aspect of the TRAIN implementation posed a dilemma for the partnership. The three community-based nonprofit agencies selected to provide case management are very different in terms of their missions, values, and approaches to clients. NCCEO is a large economic and community development agency founded in the 1960s as a social action agency. NEWS is a woman-centered, domestic violence-oriented agency, and the Progress Foundation is a mental health provider. It was a challenge to develop a shared sense of purpose, as the needs of domestic violence survivors differ greatly from those of an individual with a dual diagnosis. In addition, perpetrators of domestic violence could be at other shelters, which could complicate the program. However, the agencies were determined to address these differences as they moved forward with the implementation process.

The TRAIN program was successful in leveraging additional funds to supplement the HUD grant. With the assistance of the director of Napa County HHSA and a local consultant, two organizations (the Health Care for the Poor and the Solano Leadership Council) were encouraged to provide annual matching grants ($100,000 each year for a total of three years). This would bring the total amount to $500,000 per year. This enabled the TRAIN program to (1) raise the rent subsidies budget, (2) increase the outreach position to full time, and (3) add additional services.

In addition to these resources, the local Catholic Charities became involved in providing assistance with housing development, access to a landlord network, and providing a roommate referral service. They had considerable expertise and years of experience in this area. The TRAIN program also brought on board the Napa County Rental Information and Mediation Service to provide tenant education and mediation services to program participants. The Napa Housing Authority also became a TRAIN partner to provide assistance with the recruitment of landlords willing to accept TRAIN clients, inspect housing units identified for the TRAIN, and facilitate the process of securing Section 8 vouchers and/or housing for clients as they exit the TRAIN. The partnerships with these agencies strengthened the TRAIN and ensured that participants would get the range of services necessary to support them as they transitioned into housing and ultimately into permanent housing.

Despite the implementation challenges, the TRAIN partners were committed to working together to address the unmet needs of domestic violence survivors, street homeless, and individuals with chronic substance abuse issues. By October 1997, all three case managers had been hired and the TRAIN officially "left the station."

THE TRAIN PROGRAM

Because the TRAIN is staffed by three case managers who are employees of three different agencies, a biweekly TRAIN staff meeting is attended by the case managers and the representative from the county HHSA. The purpose of these meetings is to provide staff support and solicit feedback from case managers. This feedback mechanism has facilitated the process of identifying and addressing issues around implementation, program design, and general concerns, and has led to improvements and new program activities. For example, based on feedback from a case manager concerning the lack of free meals for the street homeless on Sundays, a new Sunday meals program was created with donations from local restaurants and grocery stores.

The TRAIN is governed in part by a policy committee that includes representatives from both of Napa's homeless advocacy coalitions which created the TRAIN, as well as representatives from the agencies that are part of the TRAIN's integrated network. The policy committee meets quarterly and addresses policy-related issues. For example, the committee makes caseload distribution and program design decisions.

The goals of the TRAIN are the following:

- To assist twenty-four households (seventy-two to ninety individuals) to move from homelessness to permanent housing and self-sufficiency for the three-year grant period (two individuals and six families each year).
- To provide case-management services to the street homeless.
- To be "the only transitional housing program in Napa that targets individuals and families with chronic substance abuse and survivors of domestic violence" (Napa County Health and Human Services Agency, 1996, p. 2).

The TRAIN program is designed to provide the following:

1. *Outreach to the street homeless:* The TRAIN employs one case manager whose sole purpose is to provide outreach and referrals to street homeless. The case manager coordinates programs that assist the street homeless in their efforts to provide for their basic needs and provides case management. The case manager provides referrals to emergency shelters, treatment programs, and the TRAIN program, as well as other community-based services.
2. *Rental subsidies for transitional housing:* NCCEO is the fiscal intermediary for TRAIN subsidies, which follow HUD guidelines. TRAIN clients pay 30 percent of their income for rent and the subsidies cover the rent balance. Because the TRAIN's philosophy is to foster self-sufficiency and reduce dependence, all TRAIN clients make a contribution, however small, to their rent payment. The client's rental expenses are subsidized by the TRAIN program for twelve months. Throughout this period, the client makes an increasingly larger contribution to the rent in order to transition gradually from subsidized to unsubsidized rent.
3. *Case-management services:* TRAIN clients receive intensive case management throughout the first three to four months of the program and gradually receive less case management with the transition "off the TRAIN" in mind. With the assistance of his or her case manager, each client develops a case plan with a series of monthly goals related to building self-sufficiency. Although many of the goals established by the client can be achieved by the client independently with the assistance of the case manager (for example, paying the bills on time,

maintaining a clean apartment), other goals require the assistance of the TRAIN's partner agencies.
4. *Access to a network of other services geared toward building client self-sufficiency:* The TRAIN offers an integrated case-management system that links clients to a range of services to address the multiple needs of homeless families and individuals seeking to become self-sufficient. Those services include mental health treatment, drug and alcohol treatment programs, HIV/AIDS education, life skills training, parenting education, child care, move-in assistance, vocational education, and job-placement services.

The TRAIN program operates in the following way with respect to referrals, intake, locating housing, case planning, rental subsidies, exit transition, and follow-up.

Step One: Referral Process

The referral process happens two ways: street outreach referrals and shelter referrals.

- *Street outreach referrals:* The street outreach worker's referral process has a dual purpose, both referring the street homeless to an appropriate shelter and identifying clients for the TRAIN. She develops relationships with homeless individuals through a long process of building trust, which she calls "the courtship period." During this phase, this case manager attempts to reach out to homeless individuals by providing them with information and basic goods (such as clean socks and food) and care ("respecting them and giving them a reason to believe that I truly care"). She demonstrates her willingness to help and makes her expectations clear. When a homeless individual indicates readiness to "get on the train," she will advocate for the individual and provide the referral.
- *Shelter referrals:* The case managers at the NEWS, Samaritan, and Sullivan shelters receive referrals from shelter staff.

Step Two: Intake Process

- *Street outreach:* During the "courtship period," the case manager has developed a relationship with the client and has made her expectations and the TRAIN guidelines clear. When a client says he or she is ready, the case manager has had the opportunity to assess the client's readiness throughout the courtship. Typically, the first step toward "getting

on the TRAIN" for the street outreach clients and individual shelter clients is completing a substance abuse treatment program. Clients must be clean and sober before they can begin the next step of locating housing. Case managers link the clients to the treatment programs.
- *Shelter intake:* In the shelters, the intake process is more formal. When case managers receive a referral, they set up an intake meeting with the client. The case manager meets with the client to review their expectations and to prepare the client for the next steps. According to clients, "There's lots of work to do when you're on the TRAIN. It's not always easy." The purpose of the intake meeting is for the case manager and the homeless individual to determine whether they are ready to "get on the train." As one case manager put it,

    As a case manager for the TRAIN, you need to be able to do a good screening with respect to their budgeting skills, parenting skills, and most importantly, their readiness for the program. The TRAIN is an intense program; it is not for everyone, especially when it comes to setting goals and being really clear about expectations for each of us.

- *Intake approval:* After identifying a potential client through the intake process, an intake report request is reviewed by the county HHSA representative and the three case managers in the bimonthly staff meeting and then recommended for approval. Upon approval of the subsidy request, the search for housing begins.
- *Orientation:* Upon approval of their subsidy request by the county HHSA representative, the client and case manager attend a tenants' rights orientation provided by Napa County Rental Information and Mediation Service (NCRIMS).

Step Three: Identifying Housing

Once the screening has taken place and a client commits to "getting on the TRAIN," the case manager in both street and shelter programs begins to assist the client in locating appropriate housing. Often the case manager seeks assistance from Catholic Charities. This phase can take a matter of days to a period of six months, depending on the specifications of the housing sought and the shelter case plan goals of the particular client. For example, if a client with a substance abuse problem developed a case plan while in the shelter to stay sober for three months, the TRAIN housing identification process would begin when that goal had been achieved. If a client has a large family and a pet, it may take a longer period of time to secure housing that meets the client's needs. An additional challenge to identifying housing is that the housing market in Napa is very tight; very few quality affordable units are available.

- *Housing inspection and approval:* Once the housing is located, the housing authority will inspect the unit. The TRAIN ensures that no clients are placed in substandard housing, which means that much of the affordable housing stock in Napa is not an option for TRAIN clients. If the housing unit is approved by the housing authority, all documents for subsidies will be completed and NCCEO will be notified, as it is the fiscal intermediary for all subsidies.
- *Landlord outreach:* Case managers have found that the housing situations of TRAIN clients can be improved, or at least better managed, when the case managers establish a relationship with the landlord and make it clear to the landlord that they are available to handle any issues that may arise. For example, if a landlord receives a tenant complaint about the noise level of a TRAIN tenant's apartment, the landlord would contact the case manager so that they could address the complaint together. Otherwise, landlords would usually confront TRAIN clients without the interpersonal or clinical skills to effectively convey the complaint or issue. The relationship-building process should include (1) educating landlords about the clients and their needs as well as the availability of program supports and how to use them if there is a problem, (2) fostering a team approach with landlords by encouraging them to educate clients about their perspective as landlords, and (3) helping to prevent problems between landlords and clients by contacting the case manager, rather than confronting clients in potentially insensitive ways. Attention to the relationship-building process should lead to long-term relationships with landlords willing to provide placements.

Step Four: Case Plan Development

Within one month of securing transitional housing through the TRAIN, the case manager and the client will develop a service case plan for the client. It can include employment training, therapy, and/or parenting classes. The follow-through on this plan is intensive, as case managers and clients meet regularly to track client progress or issues. In the first six months of the program, they meet together weekly, in some cases more regularly, and at six months, the regularity of the meetings is gradually reduced to monthly. Throughout the program a monthly contract for clients helps ensure follow-up on case plan goals and assists clients in managing other aspects of their lives. For example, a monthly goal might be to visit the dentist, pay the bills, or stay within the established budget.

Another aspect of the case plan for individuals with substance abuse problems is family reunification. Many have become estranged from their families but will need the support of their family members to successfully complete their treatment. According to a street outreach staff member,

> many people that I help get on the TRAIN have alienated their family members due to substance abuse histories. One of the first things we do, once they complete their treatment program, is begin the process of reunification with families. I get family input on exactly where they want to see improvement or accountability.

When clients recruited through street outreach return from treatment, they are housed and supported in a variety of ways: (1) placement on the TRAIN, (2) placement with family members, (3) provision of general assistance funding, or (4) placement in halfway houses.

Step Five: Rental Subsidies and Case Management for Twelve Months

The TRAIN transitional housing subsidies last twelve months. Clients pay 30 percent of their income initially and then pay an increasing portion of their rent. This gradual rent increase enables them to transition more easily from subsidized to unsubsidized rent. For example, rather than suddenly jumping from a monthly rental payment of $135 (30 percent of income) to $450 (the total rent cost), the client would be contributing roughly $250 by month six of the TRAIN. In addition, the case manager begins to reduce the number of visits so that by the sixth month the visits will be monthly.

Step Six: Getting off the TRAIN

After twelve months, clients can apply for an extension, but that has rarely happened. The goal is to secure HUD Section 8 vouchers for TRAIN clients through the Napa Housing Authority in order to offer long-term permanent housing. Due to the partnership, many TRAIN clients receive Section 8 vouchers and stay in their current housing, or move into Section 8 designated housing when the twelve months has ended. Some clients have been able to increase their earning power enough to pay market-rate rent when they are moving off the TRAIN.

Step Seven: Follow-Up

As part of the HUD grant requirement, TRAIN staff conduct follow-up with TRAIN program graduates to determine whether they have been able to maintain their permanent housing. At the end of the second year, a follow-up survey indicated that twelve families and/or individuals were still maintaining permanent housing status. Housing status for five families and/or individuals was unknown, as these TRAIN participants could not be located at the time of the survey.

SUCCESSES

- Since its inception in October 1997, the TRAIN program has provided transitional housing and integrated case-management services to twelve individuals and twenty-one families. As mentioned above, nine families (twenty-nine adults and children) and eight individuals have "graduated" from the program and secured permanent housing. The TRAIN has successfully assisted its clients not only with transitional housing, but perhaps more importantly, with permanent housing.
- Because the TRAIN is designed for particular populations, it has been especially successful in meeting their specific needs. For example, one TRAIN client suggested that other programs were not able to provide her with the assistance and support she needed because they did not understand her situation. When she became homeless due to domestic violence, she found herself and her children in an unstable and dangerous situation. She had never worked outside of the home, had focused on raising her children, and had a car that was worth enough to render her ineligible for many services and programs. When she attempted to access other agencies, she received what she called "the runaround" and the feeling that no agency could help her and her children. The TRAIN provided this client with case management and transitional housing subsidies that enabled her and her children to successfully rebuild their lives.
- The TRAIN program is an example of successful county HHSA and nonprofit partnership. The program relies upon the strengths of each: the ability of community-based agencies to reach the homeless and to provide services to them and the county's ability to leverage federal funds. In addition, through the assistance of the NVSPAB and the NCHA, the TRAIN has included more organizations in the partnership.

- The TRAIN has led to systemic changes in the way that landlords approach tenants with dual diagnosis or problems with domestic violence. Due to the efforts of Catholic Charities, the case managers, and the success of the clients themselves, landlords are increasingly willing to rent their apartments to TRAIN clients. One landlord even offered to hire the participating nonprofit agencies to manage a fifteen-unit property in order to make those units available to the TRAIN. This would entail the nonprofit agencies taking responsibility for the management of the building, which would include all of the decision making regarding tenants. The landlord's offer could significantly expand the TRAIN program and is being explored by members of the TRAIN policy committee.
- The TRAIN supervisors have allowed case managers to design innovative programs and activities geared toward their particular target population. For example, the street outreach case manager designed a free Sunday meals program through donations from local restaurants when she learned from street homeless clients that no meals were available to them on Sundays.

CHALLENGES

- How does an organization maintain organizational memory during staff transitions? Had the same staff person handled the TRAIN program from the proposal submission to the implementation, the process would have been, most likely, smoother and shorter. The individual would have been in regular contact with HUD in order to push the process along. The group would have been involved in the alteration process and less time would have elapsed from initial planning to implementation.
- The TRAIN program relies upon three very different agencies to provide case-management services to its clients. Although this is a program strength, it has also proven to be a tremendous challenge. The program seeks to have consistency across the agencies, in terms of the services clients receive and the responsibilities of the three staff members. This presents a continuing challenge given the different missions and values of the three participating agencies.
- Although the TRAIN attempted to develop job descriptions that were consistent, each agency wrote its own and there are differences, despite the equivalent pay. Staff members are bound to have additional tasks and responsibilities assigned that differ from agency to agency.

In addition, there has been some difficulty with staff turnover in the case manager positions.
- Despite efforts to educate Catholic Charities and the landlords about the needs of TRAIN program clients, the landlords do not always respond appropriately. Rather than contact the client's case manager to intervene or provide assistance, landlords have attempted to deal with tenants without the necessary interpersonal and/or clinical skills. It is critical that case managers develop relationships with landlords so that they will feel comfortable contacting them when necessary, instead of confronting tenants themselves.
- The process of client placement has been difficult, as agencies advocate for their own clients to be placed ahead of others. It is important to develop a clear prioritization process, in order to avoid unnecessary tension around who should be placed in the next available apartment.
- The tendency to choose the most desirable clients for apartment placement is another dilemma. It is important that the TRAIN partners assisting with placement understand the purpose of the program and the characteristics of the clients. For example, an agency with long-standing relationships with many landlords has a keen interest in maintaining those relationships. Rather than place a TRAIN client with multiple problems, greater emphasis is sometimes placed on low-income individuals and families without the degree of issues that TRAIN clients face, in order to preserve the landlord relationship. It is critical that landlords and placement partners are informed and educated about the program mission since HUD, as a funding source, requires that all three types of clients be served by the TRAIN (domestic violence survivors, chronic substance abusers, and street homeless). In addition, if placements lag and the whole subsidies portion is not used, future funding of subsidies may be jeopardized.

LESSONS LEARNED

1. It is important to carefully examine and clarify the differences in agency mission, values, and approach within a partnership at the very beginning of a collaborative effort. Glossed-over differences and seemingly small problems can sneak up and derail the project. Therefore, it is critical to uncover differences at the outset in order to prevent larger issues from developing.
2. It is critical to develop relationships with landlords and build a landlord network specifically around the program, rather than relying on one agency's prior relationships developed for different clients. The rela-

tionship-building process should include educating landlords about the clients and their needs, providing program supports and demonstrating how to use them if there is a problem, fostering a team approach with landlords by encouraging them to educate staff about their perspective and responsibilities as landlords, and helping to prevent problems between landlords and clients by contacting the case manager, rather than confronting clients in potentially insensitive ways. Attention to the relationship-building process should lead to long-term relationships with landlords willing to provide placements.

3. An effective intake process is critical to ensuring the success of TRAIN clients. The intake process provides both case managers and potential clients with the opportunity to assess the clients' readiness to "get on the TRAIN" in the form of a serious commitment from clients to work toward self-sufficiency. Case managers must develop an intake process that ensures the sharing of information which will enable staff and clients to determine whether the client is ready.

4. A partnership between the county DHHS and community-based nonprofits needs to build upon the strengths of each partner and needs to recognize that the relationship-building process takes time. It is critical that a collaborative partnership is built upon the strengths of each partner to most effectively deliver the highest-quality services to clients. However, developing a partnership between the county DHHS and community-based nonprofits, especially when the county is providing the funds and assisting with the planning, but not providing services and staff, requires special handling. Given the differences in power and status, it is critical to be aware of the barriers to participating agencies in order to ensure that they engage positively in the partnership with the county.

Building a good partnership takes time and it is an ongoing process that continuously must deal with politics and personalities. For example, when it became clear that the agency providing landlord referrals did not exercise sensitivity when addressing TRAIN clients about problems that arose in their housing situations, other TRAIN agency participants were frustrated and even angry. However, due to the importance of finding landlord referrals, it was essential that the message be communicated in a constructive manner in order to ensure continued collaboration.

5. Efforts to minimize the disruptive aspects of staff turnover are critical. Staff turnover can be disruptive to the development and implementation of a program, regardless of the staff level or the point at which the transitions occur. Whether it is the county staff during the planning stages or the case manager during implementation, staff turnover can

disrupt the process and block progress. Efforts to minimize the disruptive aspects of staff turnover may help to maintain the motivation of the other participants and the success of the program.

REFERENCES

Anthony, W., Cohen, M., Farkas, M., and Cohen, B. (2000). Clinical care update: The chronically mentally ill and case management—more than a response to a dysfunctional system. *Community Mental Health Journal, 36*(1), 97-106.

Basgal, O. (2000). Welfare reform: Should housing have a role? *Journal of Housing and Community Development, 57*(1), 15-24.

Bendis, D. (1998). Bridgework: Work of DuPage County, IL residents to end homelessness. *Christian Century, 115*(18), 598-600.

Early, D. (1998). The role of subsidized housing in reducing homelessness: An empirical investigation using micro-data. *Journal of Policy Analysis and Management, 17*(4), 687-697.

Joint Center for Housing Studies (1998). The state of the nation's low-income housing. *Journal of Housing and Community Development, 55*(6), 19-22.

Letique, B., Anderson, E., and Koblinsky, S. (1996). Social support of homeless and permanently housed low-income mothers with young children. *Family Relations, 45,* 266-272.

Letique, B., Anderson, E., and Koblinsky, S. (1998). Social support of homeless and housed mothers: A comparison of temporary and permanent housing arrangements. *Family Relations, 47*(4), 415-421.

McChesney, K. (1990). Family homelessness: A systemic problem. *Journal of Social Issues, 46*(4), 191-205.

McGrew, J., Wright, E., Pescosolido, B., and McDonel, E. (1999). The closing of central state hospital: Long-term effects for persons with severe mental illness. *Journal of Behavioral Health Services and Research, 26*(3), 246-261.

Napa County Health and Human Services Agency (1996). HUD grant proposal. Napa, CA: Author.

Napa County Health and Human Services Agency (1998). HUD annual progress report. Napa, CA: Author.

Napa County Health and Human Services Agency (1999). HUD annual progress report. Napa, CA: Author.

Schussheim, M. (1999). Housing for low-income families: Problems, programs, prospects. *Journal of Housing and Community Development, 56*(5), 30-37.

Travers, N. (1989). New York launches two-pronged effort: The state meets emergency needs of the homeless while creating transitional housing models. *Public Welfare, 47*(1), 19-22.

Chapter 16

Wraparound Services for Homeless TANF Families Recovering from Substance Abuse

Debbie Downes
Michael J. Austin

Pueblo Del Mar (PDM) is a transitional housing program that offers wraparound services to homeless families recovering from substance abuse. It is located on a former army base near Monterey, California (Fort Ord), and funded, in part, through the U.S. Department of Housing and Urban Development (HUD) Supportive Housing Grant. Sun Street Centers, a community-based organization, operates the program component of Pueblo Del Mar and supervises the programs related to child protection, job training and employment, counseling, substance abuse treatment, child care, recreation, independent living skills, school, retention services, and parent education. The Monterey County Housing Authority is the property manager, property owner, and grant recipient of HUD funding for Pueblo Del Mar.

HISTORY

In 1987, Congress passed the Stewart B. McKinney Homeless Assistance Act. Title V of this act stipulates that the first priority for the use of surplus federal properties should be to serve the homeless. The McKinney Act did not anticipate the large number of military base closures in the 1990s, nor the large number of groups interested in occupying former bases. Therefore, the Department of Defense (DOD), U.S. Departments of Housing and Urban Development, Veteran Affairs (DVA), Health and Human Services (DHHS), General Service Administration (GSA), homeless assistance providers, and other community groups joined to suggest modifications to the McKinney Act. The suggestions led to the Base Closure Community Redevelopment and Homeless Assistance Act of 1994, which regulates the use of surplus federal land, but did not affect Fort Ord which continued to operate under the 1987 McKinney Act.

In 1988, the Monterey County Board of Supervisors formed a task force and launched a study on homelessness, which found that there were over 3,000 homeless in the county. The task force considered the findings of the study and public suggestions in developing the county's first five-year homeless services plan. In 1991, the Coalition of Homeless Services Providers was established to create viable solutions for homelessness. The coalition was made up of representatives from thirteen agencies, including the Monterey County Department of Social Services (DSS), Monterey County Department of Health, Children's Services International (CSI), and the Monterey County Housing Authority. The coalition met every week for two years in order to discuss ideas and develop plans for serving the homeless in Monterey County, and finally they acquired 150 housing units at the former Fort Ord for use by an array of programs.

According to the policies of the McKinney Act, the Monterey County Housing Authority was able to receive the Fort Ord property from health and human services in 1995. The director of the Monterey County Department of Behavioral Health (Robert Agnew) approached the director of the housing authority (Jim Nakashima) with the idea of using some of the land to serve parents in recovery. They contacted the director of the Monterey County Department of Social Services (Marie Glavin) and planned together the development of Pueblo Del Mar. In 1998, the housing authority gave fifty-six housing units to PDM and signed a HUD Supportive Housing Grant to rehabilitate transitional housing units for homeless families. The grant was for $1,185,910 and was signed in January 1998 (22 percent for rehabilitation of the buildings, 18 percent for operating and administration costs, and 60 percent for supportive services). In addition, the housing authority received a State of California HOME Loan for $1,000,000 as a match for the housing rehabilitation funds.

As soon as they had secured the HUD grant and begun thinking about the development of wraparound services for substance-abusing homeless families, the agency directors began to involve other community organizations in the planning process. They included Sun Street Centers and Children's Services International in the development of programs at PDM. Through monthly planning meetings, they formed a team of representatives from social services (child welfare and CalWORKs staff), the housing authority, behavioral health, Sun Street Centers, and Children's Services International. The PDM planning team invited representatives from the Independent Living Program, Salinas Adult School, Golden Gate University (Welfare to Work Retention Program), Office for Employment Training, Monterey Peninsula Unified School District, and the Business and Education Alliance of the Monterey Peninsula (BEAM) to provide services at PDM. Members of the service delivery team made a special effort to acquire teamwork training through the Bay Area Academy.

LITERATURE REVIEW HIGHLIGHTS

Most of the literature regarding families and substance abuse suggests that no one intervention works for everyone because substance abuse is usually precipitated by a number of factors (Azzi-Lessing and Olsen, 1996). The number of low-income, substance-abusing mothers has increased dramatically (Carten, 1996). The increase in maternal substance abuse correlates with an increase in the number of infants born addicted to drugs (Segal, 1991). Parental substance abuse is a potential risk factor in child abuse (Azzi-Lessing and Olsen, 1996), and maternal substance abuse multiplies the possibility that children will be removed from the home (Gustavsson, 1991). Substance-abusing mothers need coordinated treatment that will address all of the factors which led to and support substance abuse in their lives (Gustavsson and Rycraft, 1993).

A few studies on substance abuse focus on the multiple needs of drug-affected families and their treatment. Gustavsson and Rycraft (1993) found that drug-dependent mothers were more likely to experience environmental stress, including domestic violence and inadequate housing. In addition, drug-dependent mothers were more likely to experience financial instability, criminal activity, and health and mental health problems. They concluded that drug-dependent mothers need services which address their varied needs, incorporating drug treatment with financial help, mental health services, domestic violence counseling, housing, and reunification.

Carten (1996) assessed the outcomes of graduates of the Family Rehabilitation Program in New York City, which serves substance-abusing mothers and their families in response to the rising number of drug-related foster care placements. The program offers drug treatment services, counseling, parenting classes, home management skills training, health care, and help in accessing outside services and entitlements. The author found that most of the women were unemployed, despite the fact that the majority had been employed in the past and had received their high school diplomas or an equivalent. Many of the women came from families where domestic violence was prevalent, and 25 percent of the women had been abused. Eighty-five percent of the women had family members who abused drugs or alcohol. The women attributed much of their success in the program to encouraging, nonjudgmental staff, the opportunity to develop their own service contracts with staff members, and the inclusion of family members in the treatment. In addition, the women appreciated the team approach to treatment because they felt comfortable asking any member of the team for help.

The research that has been done on recovery for substance-abusing families supports comprehensive, wraparound services (Borkman et al., 1998; Kaskutas, 1998). Families who are affected by substance abuse have a multitude of needs that must be addressed in order for the recovery process to succeed (Room, 1998; Tracy, 1994). Therefore, a special treatment model is needed. The social model of recovery is based on the idea that when the environment is changed to support a sober lifestyle, the patient is more likely to change as well (Barrows, 1998). It is very different from the medical model which advocates hospital stays and clinical treatment. In the social model, clients take responsibility for their own recovery, while medical-model clients follow a treatment plan laid out by professionals. The social model is the primary focus of PDM, as it seeks to provide a safe and supportive environment for recovery while offering residents a variety of services to meet their diverse needs.

SOCIAL MODEL APPROACH TO SUBSTANCE ABUSE RECOVERY

The main goal of Pueblo Del Mar is to give people who wish to achieve and maintain sobriety the time, security, resources, and support necessary to develop life skills that promote sobriety and self-sufficiency. In order to support people through their own recovery to become self-sufficient in the community, the following supportive housing goals need to be met:

- help participants obtain permanent housing,
- increase their level of income,
- increase living and employment skills,
- promote increased self-determination and empowerment, and
- foster a sober lifestyle and functional family dynamics utilizing effective parenting skills.

As a staff member of the housing authority noted, "Addiction is a family problem. Pueblo Del Mar addresses the family unit in order to deal with the learned behavior of children that may lead to drug abuse."

The programs of Pueblo Del Mar are based on a social model of recovery in which residents are active participants in their own recovery in an environment that is carefully monitored and free of substance abuse. Emphasis is placed on developing an interactive and supportive community environment. PDM is fundamentally a recovery community, and twelve-step meetings and workshops are offered on the property. Many of the principles and teachings of Alcoholics Anonymous are evident at PDM, where all residents have a sponsor and are engaged in a twelve-step program or its equivalent. A staff member of Sun Street Centers noted, "We take people with a desire to recover and place them in an environment where that desire is supported and valued." All staff of the collaborating agencies work with the residents to provide an environment that encourages recovery.

The social model supports experiential learning. Participants are more likely to learn by doing than by just learning something in class. According to one employee, "The only way to learn to live clean and sober is to live clean and sober.... The social model gives people the latitude and opportunity to make mistakes because people learn from their mistakes." Staff members do not tell residents what they must do. The community learns how to keep itself in check as community residents check on one another and offer support and advice. Four housing units make up a "cluster," and the residents in each cluster meet once a week to discuss their progress and improvements.

The residents play a major role in the governance of PDM as required by the HUD Supportive Housing Grant. The PDM program manager provides leadership and support for the resident community council. One member of each cluster is elected to the resident council. The council governs PDM based on a locally created community covenant as noted in the appendix to this chapter. The resident council members meet regularly to discuss issues that arise at PDM, including conflicts and changes needed in the covenant, and develop plans for community events and traditions that support recovery. Bernie, an officer of the resident community council, noted that "Working with others, being involved, being in service to the community—these are some of the things that have helped me the most." The intake review committee, which reviews all applicants, gives the residents a voice by including one representative from the resident community council.

PROGRAM OPERATIONS

Social services and drug and alcohol recovery programs refer families to the intake staff of the behavioral health department, who work with the program manager of Sun Street Centers to assess client eligibility. Eligibility for PDM is based on giving priority to families who are homeless and living on the street or in places not meant for human habitation as noted in the appendix to this chapter. While a family must include a child, children, or a pregnant mother, couples and single fathers are eligible. Residents must meet the following eligibility criteria:

- Currently receive CalWORKs and Medi-Cal, based on a welfare-to-work plan or work full time.
- Must be legal U.S. residents.
- Show proof of graduation from a certified Monterey County drug and alcohol program (parents only).
- Show proof of ninety days abstinence from alcohol and drugs and regular attendance at a recovery group.
- Written verification from a counselor or sponsor that the parent is involved in a rehabilitation plan, including the elements of the twelve steps of Alcoholics Anonymous/Narcotics Anonymous.
- Agree to a background check related to past violent crimes or sexual offenses.
- Meet income eligibility requirements.

If a family meets all of the eligibility criteria, they must appear before the review committee to explore the appropriateness of the program and demonstrate a commitment to sobriety. If the family seems to be appropriate for the program, a review committee member explains the community covenant as well as the community expectations and house rules. The rules of PDM include the prohibition of alcohol and illegal drugs on the premises and limited guest visiting hours with no overnight guests. If the family agrees with the goals and rules of PDM, they sign all of the forms and schedule one final meeting with the housing authority to sign the lease and inspect their new home. Residents pay 30 percent of their adjusted gross income to PDM as rent. In commenting on all the rules, Kim, a PDM resident, noted that "Anything that they ask you to do in order to stay here in the program is minimal. You have to do it all to stay sober anyway."

Pueblo Del Mar is a truly collaborative service program. Sun Street Centers operate PDM, under contract from the Department of Behavioral Health, who in turn is in a contract relationship with the housing authority. Sun Street Centers employ three full-time staff at PDM. The resident program manager oversees the case management program, the resident council, the monthly program coordinating committee meetings, and the monitoring of PDM goals and outcomes. Two case managers organize and train residents for peer outreach to local agencies, assist residents in creating and maintaining family recovery plans, and provide documentation in resident case files regarding activities. In addition to the full-time staff, two half-time PDM residents train as clerks and assist the program manager and case managers with tasks related to the resident council, classes, groups, workshops, day care, and recreation. An on-site police officer receives a housing unit rent-free in exchange for living on the premises to discourage any illegal activities. The following list describes the full array of PDM support services:

- *Case management* provided by the Monterey County Department of Social Services
- *Family recovery plan* developed by the resident and the program manager; outlines the resident's goals, objectives, and tasks for achieving sobriety and self-sufficiency in three educational phases
- *Educational curriculum* corresponds with the educational phases outlined in the family recovery plan
- *Resident community council* governs PDM
- *Independent living program* prepares PDM teens for future self-sufficiency
- *Parenting classes* provided by the Monterey Peninsula Unified School District
- *Child care* provided by Children's Services International
- *Job training and education* prepares parents to enter the workforce
- *Support groups* based on the social model of recovery help maintain sobriety
- *Counseling* provided for residents as needed

Each adult PDM resident develops a family recovery plan with the help of the resident program manager. The plan describes goals, objectives, and tasks for improving the legal, familial, vocational, social, and recreational areas of each family member's life as well as maintaining sobriety. The tasks and objectives match the state and federal timelines for achieving self-sufficiency. The family recovery plan also outlines all of the classes and groups that require resident participation. Residents and PDM case managers review and update the family recovery plan monthly. Residents pass through three phases of the plan by attending all of the classes and groups on the following topics:

1. *Early sobriety and stabilization:* Residents must attend classes and demonstrate an understanding of topics, including the etiology of addiction, relapse prevention, withdrawal, sober coping skills, attachments to unhealthy interpersonal relationships, communication skills, conflict resolution, anger management, grief processes, and sober parenting.
2. *Middle recovery and achieving lifestyle in balance:* Residents study health in recovery, relapse prevention, family systems, relationships

and codependency, human sexuality, communication, conflict resolution, anger management, time management, goal setting, budgeting, building social support networks, gender discrimination, and sexual harassment.
3. *Late recovery and maintenance:* Residents learn to maintain a recovery program, cope with stuck points in recovery, expand their social networks, continue growth and development, develop a life plan, cope with life transitions, find and maintain housing, and find closure to their time at PDM.

Sun Street Centers and the collaborating agencies work with many other organizations to ensure that PDM residents receive all of the services they need to maintain sobriety and regain control of their lives. At the beginning of the planning process, representatives from Children's Services International were invited to planning meetings for PDM in order to evaluate and accommodate the need for child care. CSI is a private, nonprofit organization that provides child care to 1,500 children daily through eight CSI centers and 600 licensed child care providers in Monterey County. An on-site nurse works at each CSI center to refer families to care, immunize children, and respond to the immediate needs of the children. CSI centers offer day care from birth through elementary school, preschool education, transportation for each child to and from the center, a nutrition program including three meals a day for each child, and monthly parent meetings that cover topics suggested by the parents. In addition, CSI will pay for licensed family child care providers, if the parents prefer, through the state alternative payment plan. Currently, CSI is serving all children of appropriate ages from PDM (fifty-three) at a CSI center.

The Independent Living Program (ILP) offers PDM teens, ages thirteen and over, life skills training through games that explore incomes, housing, rent, cars, bank accounts, and credit. In addition, ILP helps teens identify their school and career goals through an educational and career assessment process. BEAM also helps teens, ages fifteen and over, to identify their career goals through job-shadowing activities. While ILP and BEAM both prepare teens for the future, BEAM also trains teens for job interviews related to finding after-school jobs.

The Monterey Peninsula Unified School District conducts parenting classes at PDM. The classes focus on discipline, communication, and limit setting. The school district would like to offer PDM children Healthy Start services, but a three-year minimum commitment is required for a child to be included in the Healthy Start caseload, so most PDM children do not qualify. However, the school district offers counseling, parent activities, and teacher home visits to young PDM students.

The Department of Social Services provides PDM residents with case-management services. The behavioral health department refers clients to PDM and works with them through the Employment Assistance Program. Children's Services International offers child care. The Office for Employment Training, Golden Gate University (Welfare to Work Retention Program), and Salinas Adult School ensure that PDM residents receive the education and training necessary to enter the workforce.

PDM tracks residents who transition out of the program. They offer referrals when necessary and monitor the progress of families. Residents who become self-sufficient and leave Pueblo Del Mar are still encouraged to participate in PDM support group meetings. As Bernie, a PDM resident, noted, "The groups helped me a lot in my recovery." To assist with transitions to self-sufficiency, the housing authority is seeking more housing units at Fort Ord for low-income housing, whereby PDM residents could move to another house in the vicinity and keep their connections in the PDM community.

SUCCESSES IN PROGRAM IMPLEMENTATION

In 1999, Pueblo Del Mar served forty-nine families, comprised of fifty-five adults and ninety-five children. In total, eleven families were discharged from the program, including twelve adults and sixteen children. There were six relapses (12 percent) among the forty-nine families. "That is an incredibly small number of relapses, given the population," noted a staff member at Sun Street Centers. "Most of our residents have been through multiple drug treatment programs." In addition, two families have graduated from the program and are living successfully on their own. Based on their PDM work experience, two women are in school to become drug and alcohol counselors. The remaining residents are working hard to maintain sobriety and remain active in the PDM community during their eighteen-month stay at PDM. The first families arrived at PDM in the fall of 1998, and most residents completed the eighteen months required to graduate from the program.

Staff members of the housing authority have seen positive changes in family cohesiveness and self-esteem as a result of PDM. For example, Kim, a resident, was able to reunify with her children and improve her relationship with her sister. Kim noted that

> This is exactly what a mother in recovery needs. Pueblo Del Mar offers me a place to stay and the freedom to be responsible for the choices I make. There is always someone to talk to here, a neighbor. And I always have the support of the staff and my sponsor. You have to

open your mind to live in a community like this, change the way you think. I've become friends with a lot of women who are very different from me. I recommend Pueblo Del Mar for anyone who wants their family and their life back.

PDM residents take many small steps forward each day. Many of them are living in a safe environment for the first time, and they are taking time to make the right choices for their families. As one of the counselors of Sun Street Centers noted, "We have people at Pueblo Del Mar who are clean and sober every day and that is a major success." As Bernie, a PDM resident, states, "This place is a miracle. It has helped me be a stronger person in recovery. It really does work, but you have to make a commitment."

CHALLENGES IN PROGRAM IMPLEMENTATION

Some of the challenges and difficulties that the Pueblo Del Mar staff face are watching residents decide to leave prematurely or relapse. One resident, who had recently received custody of her child, left PDM in the middle of the night with no explanation. She never returned and the Department of Social Services has been unable to locate her. PDM staff does not feel that she was ready for self-sufficiency, so they are concerned about her welfare. Another difficulty for PDM staff is trying to help residents make their own plans for progress. Parent-child reunification is one of the primary goals for each resident, so as soon as it occurs the entire family recovery plan changes. PDM staff must be flexible as they help each family make the necessary adjustments to their plan.

Another major challenge for PDM staff is helping residents follow the rule that forbids overnight guests. Women have a difficult time obeying this rule because their boyfriends frequently do not have a safe place to stay, so the women want to invite them to PDM. The rule is designed to protect the other PDM residents. The first overnight guest who was caught was a known sex offender. PDM staff and residents feel strongly that the rule is necessary, yet it is the primary reason that residents are asked to leave PDM. In 1999, four families were asked to leave after hosting guests overnight.

The planning team for PDM encountered some logistical difficulties, including working with the outside community to establish PDM as a respectable community project. Some Monterey residents, who had relied on Fort Ord for their livelihood, feared that low-income residents would spend less money in town than had military personnel. In addition, some town residents associated low-income housing with contributing to unsafe neighborhoods which would be close to their homes. The housing authority convinced the city council and staff that PDM would make extra efforts to integrate its residents into the community. The housing authority also spent considerable funding to assure members of the community that the houses at PDM were aesthetically pleasing and were not simply warehouses for homeless people. The community slowly began to accept the idea. The timeline for completing the physical rehabilitation of the houses presented another logistical challenge, as the opening date was delayed over a year due to construction delays and the need for extensive housing rehabilitation.

LESSONS LEARNED

1. It was critical to invite all relevant participants to the planning meetings from the beginning. Ensuring that representatives from all of the involved organizations participate in the meetings, especially local government officials who need to support such a new idea, decreases opposition and increases support. The PDM planning team said that communication was an integral part of its success, especially attending the teamwork training sponsored by the Bay Area Academy. As one of the supervisors of reunification at Monterey County Family and Children's Services noted, "Teamwork, communication and consistent training are essential for success in a collaborative effort like this. There are lots of bureaucratic service issues which can be simplified by working together."
2. Representatives from different public and private agencies need opportunities to build teamwork. Attending teamwork training together provided the key element in the successful start-up of PDM.
3. It is important to have a comprehensive knowledge of the population to be served, especially their needs and the different ways to address them. In working with families, it is important to take into account the needs of each member of the family because they are all affected by the substance abuse.
4. It is important to give clients choices related to program entry, participation, and exit. PDM needs to be seen as one option that leads to family reunification, not the only option.
5. Successful programming requires a wide array of supportive services including coordinated intake, a clearly defined service model, family recovery plan, educational curriculum, resident council, independent living program, parenting classes, job training, case management, and support groups.

APPENDIX: PROGRAM PARTICIPATION FORMS

Residency Covenant—Pueblo Del Mar

I, _____, am committed to maintaining my recovery. To do this, I desire to live in an alcohol- and drug-free environment with others who are willing to share experiences, strengths, and hopes with one another to overcome our addictions. Therefore, I make this covenant with the members of the Pueblo Del Mar community.

I understand that this covenant is for the duration of my stay at Pueblo Del Mar.

1. I commit to comply with all terms of my Housing Authority Lease Agreement, Pueblo Del Mar Transitional Housing Program Rules as determined by the Community Council, and the Pueblo Del Mar Residency Covenant.
2. I commit to abstaining, at all times, from alcohol and/or illegal drug use and/or any misuse of any prescribed or over-the-counter medicine. I will voluntarily submit to a drug test if there is any question concerning my sobriety. I understand that if I, my children, or my visitors bring alcohol and/or illegal drugs onto the premises, I will be immediately discharged from the program.
3. I commit to strengthening my sobriety through participation in a twelve-step recovery program, regular twelve-step meeting attendance, and working the steps with my sponsor.
4. I commit to actively pursue the goals of my Family Recovery Plan that includes my Welfare to Work Plan.
5. I commit to regularly participate in all scheduled Pueblo Del Mar community events.
6. I commit to abide by decisions made by the majority of my cluster and/or the Community Council.
7. I commit to encourage and support the recovery efforts of all community members.
8. I commit to respect the rights of all Pueblo Del Mar residents, including the children.
9. I commit to provide a safe and living environment for my children by instructing them on program rules and accepting responsibility for their compliance.
10. I will refrain from any type of physical, emotional, verbal, or sexual abuse of any Pueblo Del Mar child, including my own.

11. I commit to refrain from use of threatening language, violent behavior, gang-related behavior; use of racial, sexual, or ethnic slurs and/or other verbal abuse; and participating in or contributing to gossip and rumors.
12. I commit to inform the Resident Program Manager and the Behavioral Health EAP of any relapse and to abide by the means that they determine appropriate to help me address my relapse issues. I understand that failure to disclose a relapse will result in my immediate discharge from the program.

By signing this Covenant, I understand that I am entering into a community and lifestyle based on the twelve-step concepts of recovery, unity, and service. Should I fail to abide by the terms of this Covenant as determined by the Community Council, I commit to voluntarily leaving the Pueblo Del Mar program and terminating my lease.

_____   _____
Resident   Date

_____   _____
Pueblo Del Mar Staff   Date

_____   _____
Community Council Representative Date

We, the Pueblo Del Mar Community Council, respect your commitment to sobriety. In order to help you attain your goals, we commit to the following:

1. We will provide an alcohol- and drug-free environment for you and your children.
2. We will provide orientation to and understanding of Community Council procedures.
3. We will govern in a fair and just manner that fosters equality and betterment of the community and all of its members.
4. We will respect the rights of you and your children at all times.
5. Along with you, we will continually pursue our recovery efforts in order to share experiences, strengths, and hopes with each other.
6. We will provide a safe, welcoming, and nonabusive environment at all times.

Homeless Status Preferences

The Supporting Housing Grant regulations give first priority to those living on the streets, in their cars, parks, sidewalks, or other places not meant for human habitation (HUD excludes as homeless those heads of households existing in jails or prisons). Therefore, the following preferences, in addition to the eligibility criteria established for the program, are applicable to Pueblo Del Mar.

The highest preference is giving to applicants with the most rating points, and the applicant family is evaluated along with the date and time stamped on the housing application. The earliest date of an eligible family is considered along with the priority for homeless status.

Categories of Homeless	Priority	Rating Points
1. Staying in a public or private place not designed for or ordinarily used as a regular sleeping accommodation for human beings.		
2. Family or head of household is within one week from release of a hospital or other institution for drug/alcohol recovery and lacks resources and support networks needed to obtain access to housing.		
3. Family is living with someone in an overcrowded situation or unsafe situation (e.g., domestic violence or child abuse) and must move for the safety of the children, has no housing identified, lacks the resources and support networks to obtain access to housing, and is being forced out of the dwelling unit by circumstances beyond their control.		
4. Family is referred by an emergency shelter or referral agency.		
5. Family is living in substandard housing that has been condemned as unfit for human habitation.		
6. Family is exiting a transitional housing program, has no housing identified, and lacks the support networks needed to obtain access to housing.		
7. Family is within one week of being evicted from their dwelling unit and lack the resources and support networks needed to obtain access to housing.		

REFERENCES

Azzi-Lessing, L. and Olsen, L. (1996). Substance-abuse affected families in the child welfare system: New challenges, new alliances. *Journal of Social Work,* 41, 15-23.
Barrows, D.C. (1998). The community orientation of social model and medical model recovery programs. *Journal of Substance Abuse Treatment,* 15(1), 55-64.
Borkman, T.J., Kaskutas, L.A., Room, J., Bryan, K., and Barrows, D.C. (1998). Resident self-governance in social model recovery programs. *Journal of Substance Abuse Treatment,* 15(1), 7-17.
Carten, A. (1996). Mothers in recovery: Rebuilding families in the aftermath of addiction. *Journal of Social Work,* 41, 214-223.
Gustavsson, N. (1991). Chemically-exposed children: The child welfare response. *Child and Adolescent Social Work Journal,* 8, 297-307.
Gustavsson, N. and Rycraft, J. (1993). The multiple service needs of drug-dependent mothers. *Child and Adolescent Social Work Journal,* 10, 141-151.
Kaskutas, L.A. (1998). Methodology and characteristics of programs and clients in the social model process evaluation. *Journal of Substance Abuse Treatment,* 15(1), 19-25.
Room, J.A. (1998). Work and identity in substance abuse recovery. *Journal of Substance Abuse Treatment,* 15(1), 65-74.
Segal, E. (1991). Social policy and intervention with chemically dependent women and their children. *Child and Adolescent Social Work Journal,* 8, 285-295.
Tracy, E. (1994). Maternal substance abuse: Protecting the child, preserving the family. *Journal of Social Work,* 39, 534-540.

Chapter 17

Building a Coalition of Nonprofit Agencies to Collaborate with a County Health and Human Services Agency

Margaret K. Libby
Michael J. Austin

It is rare that a group of community-based nonprofit social service providers can successfully develop a coalition that includes not only a range of providers but the county health and human service agency as well. It is more common for nonprofit service providers to compete with one another for clients, status, and reputation within the community and for scarce resources. In addition, their relationships with the county agency are typically characterized by tension and even mistrust, and often resemble a grant-maker-recipient relationship, rather than a partnership. This is a case study of a coalition of nonprofit agencies in Napa County that has come together in an attempt to plan and implement a comprehensive service delivery system to address the needs of Napa residents. The case study is based on the coalition's first five years, and the first three years of its behavioral health committee.

The Napa nonprofit coalition came together to address a multitude of issues that presented barriers to the delivery of high-quality and effective services to residents. These barriers included the following:

1. fragmentation of services in nonprofits,
2. competitive relationships between nonprofits,
3. dependence upon the county health and human service agency for funds,
4. lack of collaboration among nonprofits and between nonprofits and the county,
5. no sense of shared destiny, and
6. little understanding about shared client populations.

267

A BRIEF HISTORY

In 1980, the first incarnation of the nonprofit coalition of Napa was formed by a small group of agency directors interested in forming a coalition in order to increase their potential for sharing resources and skills and for leveraging funds. The directors asked the county to support them in a revenue-sharing program. The county health and human services director encouraged the directors to organize themselves and to be as inclusive of other agencies as possible. With this support from the county, the directors expanded the group of nonprofit agency directors from three to six and began to discuss the benefits of working together. Once organized, the county asked the six members to assist with the county decision-making process as advisors in ranking the importance of a group of capital expenditure projects totaling $500,000. These projects related to funding nonprofits through revenue sharing. This experiment in shared decision making was deemed a political failure by some and was short-lived. The group folded after a year and a half.

In 1995, another group of agency directors began to discuss the need to work more cooperatively and to nurture younger directors, as many of the current directors were nearing retirement. The group included the executive director of Napa County Council for Economic Opportunity, the director of Napa County Health and Human Services, and the executive director of the Napa Volunteer Center. It met monthly for several months to determine how best to address the following goals: (1) find ways to empower agencies and clients, (2) explore ways to share resources among agencies, (3) identify ways to consolidate efforts to serve the needs of Napa clients, and (4) search for joint grant-writing opportunities. Despite the past failures, they decided to try to build a coalition. As one director put it,

> It was clear that the world was changing at this time. We could see welfare reform, health care reform, managed care, realignment, and capitated costs coming. The trend was moving toward block granting, consolidating, and local control. We were looking to empower the community agencies as a political, economic, and social force for change.

Their vision was to develop a seamless system of health and human services in Napa County managed and delivered collaboratively by community-based nonprofit agencies and the county health and human service agency. This rebalancing of responsibility for health and human services between the county agency and the nonprofit sector is the central theme of this case study. With the behind the scenes support of the county health and human services director, these nonprofit agency directors began to actively discuss and plan for the future direction, scope, and design of the county service delivery system.

It is important to note that, in addition to the vision of the agency directors and the coalition leader, another factor contributed to the development of a coalition of nonprofits focused on systematically changing service delivery. It was the decision by Napa County Health and Human Services to shut down two critical programs due to changes in state funding: the twenty-four-hour walk-in crisis clinic in 1992 and the residential detoxification program for alcohol and drugs in 1995. Those changes caused concern about whether the county health and human services agency was equipped to fulfill its obligation to provide these services. Both losses had a major impact on the landscape of health and human services in Napa County and increased the burden on Napa's nonprofits without any increase in funds or resources. The loss of these programs motivated the behavioral health committee of the fledgling nonprofit coalition to develop a plan for a twenty-four-hour system of care that ranged from education and prevention to outpatient services to crisis hotlines to residential care.

The group of agency directors felt that a coalition of nonprofits was necessary to shift from a reactive to a proactive posture in order to bring about changes in the local service delivery system. In 1995, they invited other nonprofit health and human service agency directors to participate, and fifteen directors showed up for the meeting. Many were meeting one another for the first time, despite their long-term involvement in their particular agencies and in the community. Clearly, establishing trust and moving beyond turf issues would be a challenge for this new coalition, as it began its ambitious attempt to radically transform the way that services are designed and delivered in Napa County. After competing with one another in the community for funds and for status, these agency directors found themselves struggling to move beyond the business as usual approach in order to construct together a whole new way of doing business in the form of a seamless service delivery system. However, it is important to place the developments within a larger context and the experiences of others around the country.

BRIEF LITERATURE REVIEW

Although much of the recent literature about behavioral health services integration and agency collaboration focuses on examples of managed care organizations, this brief literature review highlights the challenges and benefits of service integration and coalition building in the nonprofit context. This review focuses on the benefits of service integration and collaboration to clients, related to service accessibility, early intervention, and increased resource allocation.

The behavioral health care delivery system tends to be fragmented and difficult to navigate (Jensen, Hoagwood, and Petti, 1996). Negotiating the various types of providers and their specialized services and eligibility not only challenges but also discourages some clients from pursuing the services they or their family members truly need. Awareness of this problem has caused a shift in resource allocation in recent years from funding public mental health providers to funding community-based services. The rationale behind this shift in values is the belief that community-based care is best for delivering services to those populations which face barriers to accessing services, for example, low-income clients, homeless clients, etc. (McGrew et al., 1999).

Despite the support for community-based approaches, the effectiveness of community-based services has been called into question. Research suggests that community-based delivery systems can be hampered by the ideological differences of diverse community-based agencies, and that these differences have created a splintered and decentralized system at the grassroots level with range of client and treatment philosophies (Rosenheck, 2000).

Research indicates that not only community-based but also integrated service delivery systems are more effective for children and families than fragmented service delivery systems. For example, the most successful mental health interventions for youth appear to involve not only youth but their parents, as well. These integrated systems and interventions that treat the whole family not only reduce negative behaviors and improve school outcomes for youth but also can improve the functioning of the whole family. In addition, integrated services are preventative in nature. For example, integrated youth interventions have been shown to reduce the likelihood of out-of-home placements in families at risk for involvement with the child welfare system (Jensen, Hoagwood, and Petti, 1996).

Although a community-based integrated system of care provides an alternative, it also presents challenges. Developing a coalition comprised of agencies that have traditionally competed for funds with staff members distrustful of interagency collaboration is a tremendous challenge for any community leader (Schmieg and Climko, 1998).

Interest is growing in integrated community-based mental health service delivery models that rely on community coalitions or advocacy groups, but little research documents those few attempts that have been made; even fewer have systematically collected data or followed theoretical models (Nelson, 1994). Although models are available for communities to follow, it may prove difficult to apply a single coalition-building framework to a range of communities with diverse stakeholders and community contexts. The challenge of developing coalitions may overwhelm leaders, causing them to experiment with what might appease members rather than emulating other successful models (Nelson, 1994).

Jenkins (1983) found that the success of a coalition is related to two key factors: organizational bases of support (resource allocation and policy developments) and the political climate (the politics of decision making and who is involved). To relate this framework to community mental health coalitions, success could be defined as client and community-based provider participation in shared decision making linked to securing adequate resources and relevant policies to support community-based mental health efforts.

For example, Nelson (1994) described a coalition of mental health reformers in Vermont that was successful, in part, due to Vermont's progressive government, a well-developed community support system, relative consensus among stakeholders regarding their values and philosophy, and the access to resources needed to shift them to community-based programs. In Maryland, major stakeholders were recruited toward the goal of shifting resources into community mental health. A diverse group of agencies came together to form a statewide coalition. The prior informal relationships of these key players was instrumental to the development of the coalition and its success in obtaining increased resources for community mental health services and other policies (Nelson, 1994).

Timing and personalities can be critical, as well. A group of community-based care advocates in Connecticut were not as successful in their fight for a regionalized community mental health system. Although some progress was made, the implementation of the plan was blocked by the state mental health commissioner. When this commissioner retired, he was replaced by an individual that supported the group; soon after they were able to redirect funds to community care (Nelson, 1994).

Based on these case examples, it is clear that the support of local officials is critical to the success of community coalition building. Success is also related to a favorable political climate, as well as the importance of public awareness and familiarity with the issues. Finally, these cases demonstrate the importance of relationship building in coalitions, both within the coalition and outside. It is clear that a coalition can achieve its goals and change the service delivery landscape of mental health services if it is able to build relationships and public awareness of the issues.

COALITION LEADERSHIP AND GROWTH

A recently retired health care professional (the retired county health and human services director) was recruited by some agency directors to provide the leadership and the facilitation necessary to begin the process of coalition building. In 1995, the group of fifteen adopted the name Napa Coalition of Nonprofit Agencies. It opted not to formally incorporate, in order to allow the collaboration to evolve and not constrain it with formal policies and procedures. Their monthly meetings soon became the "meeting not to miss" in the nonprofit community. As the size of the group grew from fifteen to thirty by 1996, it became clear that some formalized policies and procedures needed to be in place, especially to share responsibilities for agenda development and policy formation.

The membership of the coalition grew quickly, and by November 1996 they decided to reevaluate their purpose in order to formalize their group process. One of the newest members was the newly appointed director of Napa County Health and Human Services. The coalition had invited her to be an associate member of the coalition, which meant she could attend meetings but not vote; only directors of nonprofit organizations could vote as members of the coalition. The coalition sought to extend this welcome to the health and human service director to keep her informed of their plans, include her in the process, gain access to county resources, and develop and maintain a relationship with the county.

In February 1997, the coalition appointed a committee to clarify the coalition governance, mission, goals, and objectives. Out of that effort came a new name, Napa Valley Coalition of Nonprofit Agencies, and a mission statement: "working together to strengthen and support nonprofit service providers and their health and human service mission in the Napa Valley." At a planning retreat in early 1997, the coalition refined its purpose, which was "to develop a partnership between the public and private nonprofit sectors that would lead toward the development of a single system of health and human service in the Napa community." By 1998, the coalition was operating with a formal process and had policies and an evaluation process in place.

THE COALITION'S MENTAL HEALTH COMMITTEE

During the first few years of the nonprofit coalition (1995-1997), most meetings were characterized by a degree of informal group process, which included discussion and debate among the agency directors about the types of services and delivery system that would work best. The dialogue featured discussions about the effectiveness and relevance of current services, which were deserving of increased funding, or whether consolidation was an option to be explored. The coalition leader and facilitator was critical in keeping the coalition members involved and focused on the mission of strengthening and supporting nonprofit service providers.

While these discussions were taking place, two members of the coalition, the executive director of the Volunteer Center of Napa and the executive director of Lutheran Services, volunteered to submit a proposal for a three-year service planning grant from the Blue Cross Foundation. The grant proposal addressed the gaps in mental health services created by the closure of the county's twenty-four-hour crisis center and the long-term vision of a seamless system of mental health services available to all Napa residents, regardless of ability to pay (Napa Nonprofit Coalition Behavioral Health Committee, 1995).

In 1996, when a $400,000 three-year grant was awarded, the coalition members, as well as other nonprofits in the community, took notice. This successful fund-development effort proved to the coalition members that their vision of a single system of care might actually have a chance of being implemented.

The two directors that wrote the grant sought to bring together a group of mental health care providers to participate in the grant-funded planning process. The agencies selected were primary mental health service providers. It was difficult to select this group of agencies, as many agencies that provided mental health services, in addition to other services, were interested in participating. Many agencies wanted to become committee members, those that had been involved with the coalition but not the mental health committee, as well as agencies that had not been involved with the coalition. Whether they were attracted by the grant funds, by the opportunity to be involved in an important project, or by the fear of being left behind, more agency directors became interested in joining the committee. It had become clear that if a social service agency sought to stay relevant in Napa, it needed to become part of a coalition that was leveraging new funding and building a single system of care.

Although there was a degree of political fallout in terms of how the agencies were selected and which agencies were left out, the process of pulling together a group of agencies to begin to fill service gaps marked a significant turning point in the long process of developing a seamless system of care that included primary outpatient and crisis agencies (Aldea, Family Service of the North Bay, Community Counseling, the Napa Walk-in Center, Child or Parent Emergency [COPE], and the Volunteer Center). The planning process began in early 1996 and became known as the mental health committee of the nonprofit coalition. The mental health committee coalesced around the process of implementing the first year of service planning which was part of the three-year planning grant from the Blue Cross Foundation.

Overall, the purpose of the planning grant was to begin the process of building the capacity of each agency member to contribute to a full continuum of care to meet the mental health needs of Napa County residents, with an emphasis on outpatient care. The group of primary mental health care providers comprising the mental health committee identified the array of existing mental health services provided by each participant in the community, the level of client demand, and the steps needed to begin the process of redesigning the system. Several gaps in services were identified (including the underserved populations of low-income families, children, and the Latino population) along with increased capacity needed to fill those gaps.

These conversations were not always easy, as committee members had difficulty moving beyond turf issues to address the needs of clients for comprehensive and integrated services. The diverse group of mental health agencies reflected an array of values and services, each with deeply held beliefs about the effectiveness of their services. Another factor which complicated the discussions was the fear that service integration might lead to the consolidation of existing programs and/or agencies. Throughout these discussions, committee members attempted to stay focused on a client-centered and services system-centered vision. Ultimately, the focus on the mental health needs of Napa County residents helped committee members to move beyond their own agency's funding needs or their personal investment in a particular program.

Although the planning grant signaled the official inauguration of the coalition, members had serious concerns about the ambitious plan to integrate nonprofit community services. For example, some agencies might receive reduced reimbursements for their services or none at all; others feared that delayed reimbursement could jeopardize their limited cash flow, resulting in the need for different levels of staffing (more low-cost staff). However, the group was determined to weather the challenging process for the benefit of the clients who deserved and needed integrated services.

Although the grant term was three years, the Blue Cross Foundation that awarded the grant stopped its grant-making activities after fulfilling one year of the grant term, leaving the mental health committee without the prospect of funds to assist with streamlining mental health services. Due to their success in their first year of planning, the committee was able to secure additional resources through the efforts of coalition members, the coalition leader, and the county health and human service agency director. The Queen of the Valley Hospital's Health Care for the Poor Fund awarded the committee a $200,000 grant in 1997 for the continuation of planning and implementation and encouraged them to incorporate behavioral health service agencies into the process by requiring their participation as a condition of the grant funds (Napa Nonprofit Coalition Behavioral Health Committee, 1997). This presented a challenge to the committee, as they had undergone an assessment of existing services and had identified gaps, had built trust, and developed relationships between six agency directors. Including a new group of agencies meant they had to begin building once again. The mental health committee became the behavioral health committee and brought in behavioral health and substance abuse providers to round out the array of services for the new grant. In addition to the original six, the additional group of five included the following organizations:

- Our Family (outpatient services)
- Head Start (early childhood services)
- Jammin Company (youth job readiness)
- Los Ninos (early childhood services)
- Nuestra Esperanza (outpatient services)

The purpose of this local grant was to continue the process begun by the Blue Cross Foundation grant. While the committee faced the challenge of rebuilding trust and reframing its purpose, it simultaneously attempted to continue working toward the establishment of the following goals: (1) service protocols, (2) a referral system, (3) a quality-assurance system, (4) a utilization review process, and (5) an evaluation of the planning and implementation. In addition, the purpose of the new grant was to provide subsidies for the provision of professional mental health services for poor and uninsured individuals. In addition to the funded agencies, many directors of agencies not receiving funds were invited to participate in the planning and design of the system of care. They understood that the vision of the committee was based on addressing the service needs of clients, not the funding needs of agencies and programs. A director who worked closely with the committee and never received any funds at all explained it this way: "The clients they serve are also my clients. Whatever we can do to improve those services helps my client and makes my job easier. It's really not about the funds. This is a client-centered vision." Although this perception was shared by others, all members agreed that it took time to get there.

COMPONENTS OF THE NEW SYSTEM OF CARE

The purpose of the planning has always been to provide a continuum of care that is accessible to the poor and uninsured residents of Napa. All services are designed to be available at no or low cost to residents. The committee also sought to emphasize services for children, as they viewed this as a way to intervene early in an individual's life, in order to prevent more serious problems later. The committee also emphasized the need for supportive crisis services, due to the absence of adequate crisis services in the community. Interventions including crisis hotlines and weekend and evening access were viewed as ways to address problems early and prevent escalation of issues. Not only would this provide residents with needed services and assist them in avoiding major family or individual crisis, but it could also reduce the number of hospitalizations and law enforcement emergency calls. By 1997, the behavioral health committee had coordinated the provision of the following services:

- Subsidized outpatient psychotherapy (limited to fifteen sessions, with possibility of extension)
- Paraprofessional lay counseling and crisis counseling
- Suicide prevention crisis line
- In-home support services
- Group counseling

Building capacity was another priority. In the initial planning process, the committee found that not enough services existed to meet the needs of seniors, children, and bilingual and bicultural populations. Agencies used their own funds to fill some of these gaps by hiring counselors that specialized in senior services as well as bilingual/bicultural counselors. By the end of 1997, due to the committee's focus on capacity building and support from local funders, the system of care grew to include the following:

- Psychological assessments and evaluations
- Core training program for volunteers and nonprofit staff
- Increased availability of subsidized outpatient psychotherapy sessions
- Internship committee and subsidy for stipends and supervision
- Increased services to Latino community, including colocating therapists at Nuestra Esperanza facility
- Implementation contract with Napa County Health and Human Services Agency for EPSTD (Early and Periodic Screening, Diagnosis, and Treatment Program) billing of Medi-Cal clients
- Potential colocation of two mental health service provider agencies
- Contracted counseling and consulting services to other nonprofit agencies
- Plans to consolidate crisis hotlines

HOW THE NEW SYSTEM OF CARE WORKS

The Volunteer Center is the fiscal agent for the new service system. As fiscal agent, the center reviews all requests from participating agencies for reimbursement for services provided. Agencies are reimbursed by the Volunteer Center with grant funds on a monthly basis. In order to ensure that the reimbursement claim will be approved by the fiscal agent, all agencies thoroughly reviewed client eligibility to ensure no other avenues for reimbursement or service provision were available, such as Medi-Cal or school-based services. In other words, the participating agencies screen carefully and request approval to utilize grant subsidies only as a last resort.

Napa's new system of care operates in the following way with respect to assessment, referrals, treatment, and utilization review:

1. *Assessment:* When a client contacts one of the agencies, a therapist does an assessment of the client's needs. After assessing the client, the therapist fills out an intake form, which includes basic client information and a *Diagnostic and Statistical Manual of Mental Disorders* (DSM) code. Therapists first review all other avenues of payment before and requesting authorization for subsidies from the Volunteer Center as a last resort.
2. *Referral, if necessary:* If the therapist recognizes that another agency could better serve the client's needs, a referral is made. If the client could benefit from family or children services, the therapist would inform the client about those options and make the appropriate referrals. For example, a low-income, recently divorced mother with two children can get counseling for her own depression, a children-of-divorce group for her children, and referrals for school-based support or tutoring for her children.
3. *Treatment:* When the approval is received from the Volunteer Center (that same day), the authorization for service from the appropriate agency is made. Each client receives fifteen sessions of free therapy through the new service delivery system without any delays or waiting lists. Clients copay from two dollars to five dollars per visit or pay nothing if they cannot afford to pay. The types of treatment include the following:

   - Subsidized outpatient psychotherapy (limited to fifteen sessions, with possibility of extension)
   - Paraprofessional lay counseling and crisis counseling
   - Suicide prevention crisis line
   - In-home support services
   - Group counseling
   - Family and play therapy
   - Youth development services
   - School-based supportive services
4. *Utilization review:* After twelve sessions of therapy, a therapist can request an extension for the client. The utilization review committee reviews requests for extensions and can grant another fifteen sessions of

therapy. This system is remarkable for two reasons: (1) the convenience for the client of not waiting after the assessment and referrals for high-quality services to treat the whole family in one place, and (2) services provided at no cost or low cost depending on the client's ability to pay. This means that services are accessible and available to all residents and that no one is left to fall between the cracks. Prior to this program, many of these clients were not served, due to service barriers such as language, financial difficulties, and waiting lines. In addition, barriers around scheduling existed, as appointments were not available after regular business hours for working parents. To date, participating agencies have been so conscientious about their assessments and funding considerations that the lead fiscal agency has never turned down a request for services.

THE "FRONT PORCH" PROGRAM

In December 1999, the behavioral health committee, in partnership with the county health and human service agency, was awarded a $2 million planning and implementation grant from the California Endowment for its "Front Porch" program, which will reestablish Napa's twenty-four-hour walk-in crisis center. The Front Porch will be a "twenty-four-hour integrated system of care and a full continuum of client-centered services promoting the mental health and behavioral well-being of the people of Napa County through public and private interagency collaboration" (Napa Nonprofit Coalition Behavioral Health Committee, 1999, p. 1). The Front Porch will accomplish this in the following four ways:

1. Napa's crisis hotlines, which include the suicide prevention, stress, and phone-friend support lines, are consolidated and housed at the Front Porch. The lines are staffed by student interns and trained volunteers from the participating nonprofit agencies. Licensed supervisory staff members are provided by a nonprofit agency and the county health and human service agency. This consolidation helps to improve the quality and coordination of crisis support services.
2. The Front Porch offers a range of behavioral health, mental health, prevention, and substance abuse services that include the following:
   - Information
   - Drop-in services
   - Peer counseling
   - Brief mental health counseling
   - Drug and alcohol intervention

- Groups (self-help, support, and therapy)
- Walk-in crisis response
- Psychiatric evaluations
- Emergency psychiatric services

In addition to these services delivered on site, there is outreach to people in crisis, and eventually crisis prevention and response services will be delivered to hard-to-reach communities.
3. Respite care is provided to prevent escalation and reduce the need for crisis intervention.
4. The Front Porch also provides a range of other critical services, including adult protective services, child protective services, sexual assault response, and emergency aid, such as food vouchers, baby formula, and other essential items.

In addition to offering clients an integrated truly one-stop mental health, social, and substance abuse service delivery system, the Front Porch program expands the after-hours access for Napa residents. Its services are available after regular business hours five days a week in order to address the needs of residents who would not otherwise be able to access services. The goal is to eventually expand the hours further in order to become a twenty-four-hour integrated system of care. The implementation of the Front Porch program brings Napa closer to achieving its ultimate goal: a sustainable twenty-four-hour integrated human service delivery system for Napa residents.

SUCCESSFUL COMPONENTS

System of Care

- The committee has successfully implemented a system of care that includes high-quality outpatient services ranging from information to group therapy to psychiatric assessment for all residents of Napa regardless of ability to pay.
- The system of care has treated an average of 300 clients per month through the subsidies—individuals and families who otherwise would not have access to counseling services.
- The behavioral health committee's ultimate goal of developing a twenty-four-hour system of care has become a reality with a $2 million California Endowment grant to plan and implement, in partnership with the county health and human service agency, the Front Porch program.

- The committee, in partnership with the county, has been able to leverage increased resources for other important projects related to behavioral health, such as a large-scale family home-visiting program and a program for school-based counseling in partnership with the state Medi-Cal program.

Coalition-Building Process

- Agencies have put funds back on the table for other agencies to use; this level of sharing and trust between participants and commitment to the project reflect a willingness to first consider client service needs and coalition support, rather than agency turf and ego.
- The leadership of agency directors proved to be a critical part of the committee's work. Many on the committee have worked in Napa for years and know their organizations' strengths and histories well enough to understand how they could link with other agencies. Each one had also been around to witness the failure of the prior attempt to develop a coalition. They were determined to make this attempt successful. Agency directors demonstrated a high level of commitment to staying at the table through extremely difficult discussions and debates.
- The insistence that directors are able to make decisions at the table without conferring with their boards of directors has been another key to success. The boards placed final authority over decision making related to the single system of care in the hands of the directors so that decisions could be made quickly. This also demonstrates the level of board commitment to the new service system.
- Leadership of the committee facilitator was also essential when it came to procuring resources, bringing in new participants, and keeping everyone focused on the goal/vision. Some participants felt that the role of the outside facilitator, someone who was not an agency director, was helpful, while others perceived his connections to his former employer (the county health and human service agency) as a sign that he was not a totally independent facilitator.
- The coalition has been able to influence long-term and systemic changes in Napa through its involvement in local decision making; for example:
  —The county director asked the coalition for input for Napa's welfare reform plan submitted to the state of California.
  —The coalition was asked to recommend one of its members to sit on the advisory board of the Partnership HealthPlan of California.

—The coalition radically transformed the City of Napa's Community Development Block Grant (CDBG) decision-making process to include nonprofit agencies as recipients of funds, resulting in $700,000 for Napa nonprofits.
—The coalition provided leadership in successful community establishment and adoption of an inclusionary zoning ordinance for the City of Napa.
—The coalition provided direction in the distribution of county trust monies for the development of low-income and special-needs housing for the city and county of Napa.
—The coalition has been asked to designate a representative to fill several permanent coalition seats created by local task forces, boards, and commissions, including the Health Care Task Force, Proposition 10 Commission, and City of Napa Affordable Housing Task Force.
—Several foundations, including California Endowment, Marin Family Trust, United Way, Headlands Foundation, and Gasser Foundation have requested the coalition's assistance and input in the decision making about the distribution of their funds in Napa.

DEALING WITH THE CHALLENGES

The most significant challenge faced by the committee was linking the collective vision to a shared sense of responsibility for services that address client needs. The committee's relationship with the county has also become a challenge, especially when communication breaks down or disagreements do not get addressed. As the committee grows and succeeds, the role of the county becomes less clear. When is the county a funder, partner, advisor, or nonparticipant?

Although some committee members felt that the coalition facilitator's ability to generate interest, resources, and publicity for the committee was a strength, some also felt it slowed the committee's progress, especially when unannounced guests arrived or extra agenda items were added at the last minute. On many occasions, sensitive/confidential agenda items had to be postponed, due to the presence of an unexpected visitor. While new agency directors were regularly invited to expand the partnerships and scope of services, committee meetings had to devote more time to review the past in order to bring new members up to date and include their services/programs into the continuum.

The committee has struggled with its identity. It shifted from mental health to behavioral health and, with the Front Porch program, may shift back to mental health. In addition, although its focus is on nonprofit agencies, the county health and human service agency has become increasingly involved as a partner in recent projects. How can the committee and the coalition as a whole maintain an identity that is separate from the county, while acknowledging its role as a partner?

Maintaining licensed staff members has posed a challenge for most participating agencies. Although the system relies upon its well-trained community volunteers, student interns, and paraprofessionals, licensed professional staff are essential.

LESSONS LEARNED

1. *Coalition building takes time* and will most likely be difficult. It helps to have a respected leader and facilitator with a clear vision, the ability to remind members of that vision as regularly as is necessary, and the capacity to help group members build trust and relationships. When resources and funds are involved, interest follows.
2. *It is critical to establish, as early as possible, policies and procedures for managing meetings,* so that all coalition members understand and work within those policies. A key policy is to ensure that minutes are thorough and complete so that information can be shared.
3. *It is critical to involve as many community agencies in the process as possible.* Increased membership and agency buy in strengthens the system of care. It is essential that new members understand and support the vision and not just search for more funding to support their own agencies.
4. *County health and human services agency support is essential,* not only for financial resources but also for the encouragement and partnership development. It is possible for nonprofits, local funders, and a county agency to develop a sustainable partnership based on addressing the needs of the community.
5. *A coalition of nonprofits can wield much economic, social, and political power in a community.* In terms of numbers alone, its current membership is fifty agencies; with their boards of directors, staff, and clients, it is clear that the coalition impacts thousands in Napa. As a result of its visibility and growing degree of influence, the coalition has continued to grow in membership and is increasingly called upon to provide input on a range of city and county issues. Coalition members have written letters, attended city council meetings as a group to demonstrate support and advocate for issues that interest them, influenced funding decisions at the county level, developed alliances with other

coalitions, and raised funds through local foundations. Coalition participation in local decision making has led to systemic and long-term changes in Napa County.

BIBLIOGRAPHY

Jenkins, J. C. (1983). Resource mobilization theory and the study of social movements. *Annual Review of Sociology, 9,* 527-553.
Jensen, P., Hoagwood, K., and Petti, T. (1996). Literature review and application of a comprehensive model: Outcomes of mental health care for children and adolescents, part 2. *Journal of the American Academy of Child and Adolescent Psychiatry, 35*(8), 1064-1078.
McGrew, J., Wright, E., Pescosolido, B., and McDonel, E. (1999). The closing of central state hospital: Long-term effects for persons with severe mental illness. *Journal of Behavioral Services and Research, 26*(3), 246-261.
Minutes from the Napa Nonprofit Coalition. (2/18/97, 11/19/97, and 11/20/96).
Napa Nonprofit Coalition Behavioral Health Committee (1995). Blue Cross Grant Proposal.
Napa Nonprofit Coalition Behavioral Health Committee (1997). Queen of the Valley Health Care for the Poor Grant Proposal.
Napa Nonprofit Coalition Behavioral Health Committee (1999). California Endowment Grant Proposal.
Nelson, G. (1994). The development of a mental health coalition: A case study. *American Journal of Community Psychology, 22*(2), 229-256.
Rosenheck, R. (2000). The delivery of mental health services in the 21st century: Bringing the community back in. *Community Mental Health Journal, 36*(1), 107-125.
Schmieg, G. and Climko, B. (1998). Strategies to preserve public-private partnership practices. *Behavioral Health Management, 18*(3), 32.

Chapter 18
Collaborative Partnerships Between a Human Services Agency and Local Community Colleges

Kirsten A. Deichert
Michael J. Austin

The events that led to the collaboration between the human services agency and the community colleges in San Mateo County are a mixture of legislative and agency-based circumstances. In the 1980s, the initiation of community-based care led the California State Department of Mental Health (DMH) and Department of Rehabilitation (DR) to develop partnerships to ensure that individuals with psychiatric illnesses were given appropriate supports to gain employment and rehabilitation. However, a study conducted by the DMH/DR's Cooperative Programs and BEST (Building Employment Service Team) networks revealed a lack of trained staff to aid in such job placement and retention efforts.

Around the same time, Tim Stringari, at the College of San Mateo Psychological Services, developed a "supported education program" designed to increase the retention of and services for college students with psychiatric illnesses by providing them extra support and guidance. Mental health managers and consumer groups in San Mateo County began collaborating with Stringari, hoping they could convince local community colleges to develop a vocational program that would give mental health providers the training they needed in rehabilitation and employment support strategies. Unfortunately, the projected number of student enrollments was insufficient to convince the colleges of the merits of developing such a program.

By the mid-1990s, the passage of welfare reform legislation and the Workforce Investment Act made job development and employment outcomes the common objective of all human services providers. The Workforce Investment Act reformed the nation's job training system and established local one-stop centers to provide job seekers with convenient access

285

to employment services and direct referrals to job training and education. In addition, the one-stop centers established partnerships with programs authorized under welfare-to-work and vocational rehabilitation. One-stop centers mandated that diverse human service providers begin working together in one location to help clients attain the common goal of employment success.

At this time, Edie Covent (employment systems specialist with the state Department of Mental Health) and Tim Stringari concluded that a community college curriculum which responded to the system changes and training needs of mental health services, in addition to the needs of all human service providers, might gain sufficient support of community college faculty and administration. Not only would mental health and vocational rehabilitation providers have a community college training program to prepare them for providing rehabilitation and employment support, but any human services provider could use the program to train staff in developing the employment and self-sufficiency of clients. In addition, human service clients and others interested in a career in human services would have an inexpensive, accessible program in which to participate.

With these new prospects, Edie Covent formed the Human Services Educational Collaboration (HSEC) and invited the participation of major stakeholders. They included the state Department of Mental Health, county Department of Rehabilitation, Poplar ReCare, and local community colleges (College of San Mateo, Cañada College, Skyline College, Solano Community College, and Riverside Community College). In the spring of 1997, Madelyn Martin, director of planning and development of the San Mateo County Human Services Agency, met with the Human Services Educational Collaboration to discuss the possibility of including her agency in the collaboration. At this point, the human services agency had just begun implementing a new model of service delivery (i.e., SUCCESS) that created new staff roles and responsibilities and necessitated the training of almost 200 staff members in case management and employment outcomes. The agency immediately recognized the potential benefits of participating in the collaboration and helping design a human service curriculum that would meet their training needs. All stakeholders in the collaboration were able to recognize the limitations of their own agencies and that partnering would help each of them serve clients more effectively.

DEVELOPMENT OF THE HUMAN SERVICES CERTIFICATE CURRICULUM

Utilizing the human services agency's training funds and responding to its immediate training needs, the Human Services Education Collaboration began developing the vocational curriculum at once. Through an evolving partnership between the human services agency of San Mateo County and the College of San Mateo, a survey was administered, a community forum with human services providers was held, and interviews with employers were completed. Essentially, employers wanted a curriculum that was very practical and differed from other programs which had been previously tried in the community. The programs at the College of San Mateo and Cañada College were also reviewed to be sure that a new program would not duplicate curricula already offered. Other counties in California were also consulted to learn about similar certificate programs. The final steps in establishing the certificate's curriculum at the College of San Mateo and Cañada College included approval by the college's chancellors, the Bay Area deans of community colleges, and the state of California.

By spending a great deal of time collecting information, the planners were able to translate the training needs of the agency into practical and realistic courses. The goal of the curriculum development process was to design learning opportunities that could be translated immediately into new approaches to delivering services and improving on-the-job work performance. One student reported that the content learned in the classes "goes hand in hand" with the work she performs at the human services agency. She reports that the classroom learning has "sharpened the tools" she has gained through work experience. It was agreed early on to closely monitor the classes so that the curriculum would always stay current and relevant to employers.

This process was facilitated by the establishment of a human services curriculum advisory board comprised of representatives of local human services providers who meet quarterly with program directors and curricula coordinators of the colleges to provide suggestions for improving the program and reviewing student performance. The advisory board oversees the human services certificate program curricula for both the College of San Mateo and Cañada College.

In addition to the input from local providers, the program also benefited from the Human Services Educational Collaboration work group that included administrators from the human services certificate programs in San Mateo, Solano, and Riverside counties, and its facilitator, Edie Covent of the state Department of Mental Health. In addition to assisting with the development of the certificate programs, its functions include monitoring, refining, and disseminating program innovations through bimonthly meetings.

The successful launching of the human services certificate program can be attributed to the shared benefits of increased community college enrollment and increased low-cost and convenient staff training for agency personnel. Community colleges can provide more cost-effective training than many other institutions or agencies based on their experience in providing technical training related to employee needs (Hirshberg, 1995).

Holub (1996) notes that successful community college programs use community-based programming to become familiar with and respond to the needs and problems of their constituents, including community leaders and community-based organizations. Community-based programming includes "environmental scanning," which involves identifying the training needs of local businesses (Morrison and Held, 1988).

An example of business-community college collaboration can be seen in the partnership between Hyundai, the automotive corporation, and Los Angeles Harbor College (Evaluation and Training Institute, 1993). Interested in developing a training program for technicians, Hyundai saw Los Angeles Harbor College as a resource for the training. Together, the business and the college developed the training materials and modules. Hyundai performed the training and certification of the Los Angeles Harbor College instructors and supplied the equipment, while the college sought additional grant funding. Similar to the Hyundai example, the human services certificate program was very much employer initiated and supported.

DESCRIPTION OF THE HUMAN SERVICES CERTIFICATE PROGRAM

The Curriculum

The human services certificate program is designed to train human services personnel to provide services for individuals and families in need of temporary social, health, and economic assistance. It prepares students for various occupations, such as mental health case manager, job coach/employment specialist, social service intake specialist, community health worker, and other entry-level human services agency positions. The target populations for the certificate program include potential human services employees, the employees of mental health and human services agencies, and human services customers who are interested in entering human services occupations.

In addition, the program is customer friendly because it not only responds to customers' needs, but also makes itself accessible to customers who want to pursue human service careers. Persons with disabilities, as well as former welfare recipients, are encouraged to participate, and, wherever possible, the program is linked to existing supported education programs at the colleges.

The four primary goals of the curriculum are as follows:

1. To respond to the training and staffing needs of the Bay area health and human services community by developing a community-sponsored, value-based human services certificate and degree program with specialties in mental health case management, job coaching, job development, and other areas.
2. To provide human services career opportunities for citizens leaving the welfare rolls and for persons with disabilities seeking self-sufficiency.
3. To further develop the community referral base and partnerships with state and local community agencies that will enhance the ability to serve and support at-risk and special populations by creating a coordinated system of supports with those agencies.
4. To develop a human services curriculum model that includes a community needs assessment and implementation plan that can be disseminated statewide and will respond to system changes in health and human services which result from welfare reform, managed care, and one-stop models.

In addition, all courses included in the curriculum are based upon the following six fundamental values of human service delivery:

1. Belief in the employment and educational potential of all persons, when provided the appropriate supports, accommodations, and skills.
2. Commitment to a client-directed approach to service, partnering with customers to attain their chosen goals.
3. Focus on the strengths of clients as opposed to deficits and functional limitations.
4. Coordinated services that smooth and accelerate client success.
5. Appreciation of ethnic and cultural diversity in identity, customs, and worldviews.
6. Assisting individuals and families to achieve self-sufficiency, requiring community-wide support and commitment.

As noted in Table 18.1, the curriculum is comprised of five core courses, an internship, and four electives, with the issues of case management and employment assistance reflected in all the courses. At the colleges, each course includes forty-eight to fifty-four hours of instruction completed in sixteen to eighteen weeks, meeting once a week for three hours. Specially developed agency-based training sessions for approximately 150 staff were used in August 1997 to pilot the first two courses of the certificate program, "counseling and interviewing" and "employment support strategies."

TABLE 18.1. Program Curriculum for Human Services Certificate

Core Requirements Course Title	Units	Electives (4) Course Title	Units
Introduction to human services	3	Employment support strategies*	3
Introduction to counseling and interviewing	3	Job development*	3
		Business writing and presentation methods	3
Introduction to case management	3	Rehabilitation and recovery**	1
Public assistance and benefits programs	1	Child development	3
Computer applications	1.5	Child, family and community	3
Human services internship	3	Psychosocial rehabilitation**	3
Total units	14.5	Infant development	3
		Psychology of ethnic minorities	3
		Mexican-American culture	3
		Social problems	3
		Diverse racial/ethnic cultures	3
		Interpersonal communication	3
		Total units	12

* Required for employment specialization
** Required for mental health specialization

The Instruction

A distinguishing feature of the human services certificate program is the use of instructors who are practicing professionals in the human service field. This increases the credibility of the program not only in the eyes of employee participants, but also from the perspective of employers who want to ensure that employees participating in the courses are learning pragmatic skills. In addition, staff trainers from the human services agency have been given the opportunity not only to teach the agency's on-site classes, but also to instruct the certificate courses held at the community colleges.

The Students

A majority of students attending the courses are employed full- or part-time in the human service field. Only a few students in each class are not employed or are employed in other fields. The following classifications of San Mateo County Human Service Agency staff have attended classes as part of their job training: (1) screening and assessment, (2) income employment service specialist, (3) employment service specialist, and (4) eligibility technicians/benefits analyst. Approximately 150 employees of the San Mateo County Human Services Agency and about 200 other adults have attended courses in the human services certificate program, demonstrating an eagerness to learn new skills related to their new work roles.

Students come from a wide range of backgrounds, work experience in the human services field, and preparedness for college course work. Some students have not been in a classroom for over twenty years. The diversity in skill level and occupational background is both valuable and challenging for meeting everyone's training needs.

The Community Colleges

All three community colleges in the San Mateo County district (College of San Mateo, Cañada College, and Skyline College) were invited to develop the human services program. Initially, Skyline College decided not to actively participate in the collaboration. During its first year, the certificate program was launched at the College of San Mateo and Cañada College. Today, most of the courses are administered at Cañada College. To better serve the needs of the community, courses will eventually be located at all three community colleges in San Mateo County as well as other community and agency sites in the county.

THE VALUE OF THE COLLABORATION

The human services certificate gives human services employers in the county the opportunity to train their employees inexpensively and conveniently. As long as employment and case-management skills are needed, the current curriculum will provide San Mateo County human services providers with an effective way to learn them. Because the curriculum is dedicated to responding to the needs of the community and its employers, any shifts in the service delivery of human services will be reflected in the certificate's curriculum. Because the human services certificate program is now a part of permanent curricula, the community college can also offer any resident of San Mateo County an accessible, low-cost opportunity for career advancement in human services occupations.

Although the courses taught in the human services certificate program are designed to be as relevant and practical as possible, a trainer for the human services agency reports that its employee training events have also become more purpose directed and relevant to the work performed at the agency than earlier training. For example, staff members are invited to bring real case examples to class for instruction purposes. Assisting in the development of the human services curriculum also gave the agency a chance to further articulate the competencies they require from staff.

The development of a human services certificate program emerged at a time when providers of human services needed to be more skilled than ever before. With lifetime restrictions on the receipt of welfare benefits and the need to assist the hardest to serve, providing skillful employment assistance and case-management services related to client self-sufficiency requires the acquisition of increasingly complex intervention methods. For example, making thorough assessments of each client's employability, job readiness, and planning for long-term self-sufficiency requires case managers to demonstrate considerable interpersonal skills to assist clients facing multiple biological, psychological, or social obstacles. One student in the program reported that the skills she has learned in the courses would easily transfer to any human services agency since, "you need to do case management and know how to interact with others anywhere."

Challenges

As noted, instructors are challenged by the diversity of students' abilities. Students generally attend the program for one or more of the following reasons: (1) it is a mandated part of their employment, (2) desire to advance their service delivery skills, and/or (3) to pursue specialization with a particular client population (e.g., mental health, substance abuse). Although instructors frequently remind students that the course is based on general models of service delivery, students sometimes challenge the instructors by stating that the course content does not reflect "what happens in my agency" or "what we do in my unit."

Another area of diversity is the students' readiness for community college course work. Many students in the program have not been in a classroom for as many as fifteen or twenty years. Simply dealing with the basic skills required to successfully complete a college course can consume a great deal of classroom time. Study habits, note taking, organizing materials, coping with stress, and test taking are all areas with which many students need assistance. As a result, instructors make an effort to include these basic skills throughout course materials. In addition, some students must deal with their own mental illness or learning disabilities.

Because many students are also employed full-time, they often feel overwhelmed by completing course requirements in addition to their work responsibilities. For example, employees of the human services agency were learning a completely new computer system at work, while also expected to learn new intervention strategies in the courses. One student also reported that in the intensive six-week courses such as "case management," it is difficult to learn so much material in a short period of time. Therefore, instructors often play a supportive and motivational role, reassuring the overwhelmed students and reminding them about how they are growing professionally.

Finally, instructors are challenged by the contradictions that sometimes emerge while teaching students about current service delivery methods. For instance, one instructor reported that, although his students from the San Mateo County Human Services Agency believed that the concepts being taught (e.g., extensive assessment of client needs) were valuable and important, their high caseload would prevent them from really practicing the concepts. Fortunately, the agency was very responsive to this feedback and actually decreased the caseloads of workers to make the service delivery goals more attainable and the new learning more achievable.

In the fall of 1999, courses from the curriculum were offered for the first time on-site at the San Mateo County Human Services Agency. Obviously, this contributed to the program's convenience and its responsiveness to both employees and clients. The human services agency is also offering employees a 50 percent compensation for attending the courses, whereby half of the time in class is considered on the agency's time and the other half on the individual's own time. Employees report that this convenience would increase their likelihood of enrolling in the courses. The human services agency also offers tuition reimbursements to employees who enroll in the certificate courses. The goal is to encourage more employers to offer courses on their own premises.

Similarly, current and former welfare clients are encouraged to supplement their work-first experiences with these learning opportunities as a way to advance their careers. In addition, course credits earned in the program may soon become transferable to other colleges in the state, thereby promoting the importance of educational advancement. In addition, interest is growing in developing a practice-based internship to augment the human services certificate program.

The curriculum advisory board has been expanded to involve a larger number of community members and human services employers. This will not only contribute to the responsiveness of the curriculum to employers' needs, but also encourage other employees in the community to participate in human services certificate courses. The additional members may also serve as guest lecturers and provide future internship or apprenticeship sites. Finally, grants are being actively pursued to further develop and disseminate both the curriculum and a manual of best practices that promote quality and consistency in human services instruction.

LESSONS LEARNED

1. The extensive investment in curriculum development by the community colleges, the county human services agency, and a wide variety of human services agencies throughout the community helps to make the curriculum relevant and timely. Curriculum developers need to invest substantial time to design a program that truly meets the training needs of employers throughout the community and does not replicate training opportunities already offered.
2. The involvement of agency-based professionals as instructors in a human service certificate program contributes to its credibility in the eyes of the students, the agencies, and the community. Staff members of human services agencies, particularly familiar with the work-based situations confronted by students, are instructors who help to ensure that course content is reality based and pragmatic.
3. Fostering collaborations and community involvement contributed greatly to establishing a successful human services certificate program as a permanent part of the local community colleges' curricula. The individuals and agencies involved in the development of this program were willing to recognize the limitations of their own services and the value of partnering with others to meet the training needs of staff and better serve human services clients in the county.
4. Human services staff need an increasing level of training and professionalism to effectively meet the changing and complex needs of clients. The curriculum will need to reflect these changing needs if the human services certificate program is going to survive and thrive.

REFERENCES

Evaluation and Training Institute (1993). Industry-education partnerships: Vocational education resource package. ERIC Digest No. 357796. Eugene, OR: Educational Resources Information Center.

Hirshberg, D. (1995). The role of the community college in economic and workforce development. ERIC Digest No. 339443. Eugene, OR: Educational Resources Information Center.

Holub, J. (1996). The role of the rural community college in rural community development. ERIC Digest No. 391558. Eugene, OR: Educational Resources Information Center.

Morrison, J. and Held, W. (1988). Developing environmental scanning/forecasting systems to augment community college planning. Paper summarizing a session from the Annual Meeting of Virginia Community Colleges Association, Williamsburg, Virginia, November 18.

*SECTION IV:
PROMOTING AGENCY
RESTRUCTURING*

Chapter 19

Introducing Organizational Development (OD) Practices into a County Human Service Agency

Andrea DuBrow
Donna Wocher
Michael J. Austin

It is rare that a county human service agency has the opportunity to incorporate an internal organizational development (OD) function to assist with managing organizational change. This is a case study of one such agency that hired an internal OD specialist to facilitate organizational restructuring related to the implementation of welfare reform. The case study is based on the first three years of implementation (1996-1999). It is organized into the following sections: highlights from the literature, the assessment-center approach to hiring an OD specialist, an array of agency-based OD start-up initiatives, and a concluding section on some of the lessons learned from this work in progress.

Organization development is one approach to managing organizational change. Although many definitions of OD have been put forth, the following definitions are most relevant to this case study:

> Organization development is a top-management-supported, long-range effort to improve an organization's problem-solving and renewal processes, particularly through a more effective and collaborative diagnosis and management of organization culture—with special emphasis on formal work team, temporary team, and intergroup culture—with the assistance of a consultant-facilitator. (French and Bell, 1990, p. 17)

This chapter originally appeared in *Administration in Social Work* 25(4): 63-83. Copyright 2001 The Haworth Press, Inc.

> Organization development focuses on assuring healthy inter- and intra-unit relationships and helping groups initiate and manage change through primary emphasis on relationships and processes between and among individuals and groups to effect an impact on the organization as a system. (McLagan, 1989, p. 7)

Rothwell, Sullivan, and McLean (1995) provide a brief description of the following key steps in an OD intervention:

1. *Entry*—A problem is discovered and the need for change becomes apparent in the organization. Someone in the agency looks for an individual who is capable of examining the problem and facilitating change.
2. *Start-up*—The change agent begins to work with agency staff to identify issues surrounding the problem and to gain commitment from staff for participating in the change effort.
3. *Assessment and feedback*—The change agent gathers information about the problem and provides feedback about the information to those with a stake in the change process.
4. *Action planning*—The change agent works with decision makers and stakeholders to develop an action plan to correct the problem.
5. *Intervention*—The action plan is implemented and the change process is carried out.
6. *Evaluation*—With the change agent, decision makers and stakeholders assess the progress of the change effort.
7. *Adoption*—Members of the agency accept ownership of the change, which is then implemented throughout the agency or work unit.
8. *Separation*—The change agent is no longer needed for the change project because the result has been incorporated into the agency. Staff will assume responsibility for ensuring that improvements continue.

These steps are then carried out using a variety of OD interventions, or activities, such as those identified by Stacey (1992): diagnostic data collection, team building, intergroup communications, survey feedback, training and education, restructuring, process consultation, coaching and counseling, and strategic management and planning.

Given the definitions of OD, the major steps in an OD process, and the array of OD techniques, it is important to note the following observations of Rothwell, Sullivan, and McLean (1995) when it comes to developing realistic expectations for what OD can and cannot accomplish:

- OD is long range in perspective and not a quick-fix strategy for solving short-term performance problems.
- Although OD efforts can be undertaken at any level within the agency, successful OD interventions need to be supported by top managers.
- OD expands workers' perspectives so that they can apply new approaches to old problems, concentrating on the work group or organization in which these new approaches will be applied.
- OD emphasizes employee participation in the entire process from diagnosing problems to selecting a solution to planning for change and evaluating results.
- The process of organization development is most effective when facilitated by a consultant who is either external or internal to the agency.

With these caveats and guidelines in mind, the human services agency of San Mateo County, California, began the process of envisioning the involvement of an internal OD consultant. Before describing the process, it is important to note the highlights from the limited literature on OD in the human services.

LITERATURE REVIEW HIGHLIGHTS

Although the OD literature reflects many more examples of applications from the private sector than from public human services, this brief review highlights some of the challenges of using OD practices in a human service agency. The bureaucratic nature of public social service agencies and the general absence of leadership familiar with innovative processes for accomplishing change have created closed systems that are often inflexible and resistant to change. OD requires an open system in order to succeed (Norman and Keys, 1992). The organizational culture of maintenance and survival, along with the unique constraints imposed on public social service agencies, creates unique challenges for OD interventions (Resnick and Menefee, 1993; Golembiewski, Proehl, and Sink, 1982). Successful change processes in human service organizations require mechanisms and models that can deal with the organizational complexity as well as guide diagnosis, action planning, and implementation (Martinko and Tolchinsky, 1982).

Burke (1980) noted that "most OD consultants find working with bureaucracies, especially public ones, to be difficult at best" (p. 429). Documented applications of OD in the public sector tend to focus on resolving racial tension; conflict between individuals, specialties, and organizational units; community conflict; and tensions emanating from reorganization (Golembiewski, Proehl, and Sink, 1982). Research indicates that OD in public organizations can work particularly well with modest goals, acceptance of unexpected setbacks, and willingness to tackle manageable issues as opposed to attempting to change an entire system at one time. OD may be more useful for fine-tuning and improving operations rather than bringing about massive change (Stupak and Moore, 1987).

While OD may confront unique challenges in the public sector, it is important to identify some of the reasons for these challenges before exploring specific OD applications in the human services. French, Bell, and Zawacki (1989) and Golembiewski (1989) pointed out the following major factors that impact the application of OD to the public and service sectors:

- Public and private organizations have different measures of organizational effectiveness than the for-profit sector, especially the lack of clear-cut, verifiable outputs that lend themselves to objective measurement (in contrast to the financial bottom line in the for-profit sector).
- The public sector places greater emphasis on regulatory constraints and a diffusion of power (legislative directives, civil-service rules, confidentiality requirements) due to the complex system of checks and balances which make it difficult for top management to make long-term commitments (as is the case in the private sector).
- The conditioning of executives in the public sector favors management styles that maximize sources of control and minimize the discretion of subordinates. As Golembiewski (1989) noted, the chain of command characterized by competing identifications and affiliations, often producing a fragmented management hierarchy and old public sector management habits, favor patterns of delegation that maximize the sources of information (as seen in the term "direct reports") and minimize the control exercised by subordinates.
- There is far more public scrutiny of the decision-making process in the public sector related to open meeting laws and the role of the media. As Golembiewski (1989) noted, there is multiple access to an array of decision makers (political and managerial) which seeks to assure that the public's business gets looked at from a variety of perspectives. He also observed that a greater variety of individuals and groups are involved in decision making, each with its own set of interests, values, and reward structures, than in the for-profit sector.
- There are outdated views of professionalism and change (e.g., taking the position that staff training is unnecessary if employees are hired who have the abilities to do the job or using old fiscal procedures that include practices which no longer made sense) (Golembiewski, 1989).

These constraints clearly document the challenges facing the introduction of OD strategies into public-sector organizations. Although it is important to keep these constraints in mind, it is also useful to look more closely at a few case studies of the use of OD in public social service agencies to provide some specific examples of OD applications. Norman and Keys (1992) describe their external OD work in the Department of Public Social Services in Riverside, California, where they used process consultation and team building to address the lack of teamwork and peer consultation, and to change management capacities. It concluded with OD training for supervisors.

A second case, described by Martinko and Tolchinsky (1982), takes place in a state department of social services where a training needs assessment led to the planning and implementation of the following activities: (1) a role-clarification process for all levels of management; (2) training activities designed to foster greater integration of service delivery in a matrix organization; (3) performance review training; and (4) first-line supervisory training. During the intervention process, the consultants found that legislative action at the state and federal levels often superceded program and managerial decisions (e.g., legislative mandates requiring uniform salary increases and mandated program reporting procedures). Considerable sensitivity and flexibility is needed from the OD practitioner to successfully conduct meaningful interventions in a highly politicized, bureaucratic system.

A third case, described by Glassman and McCoy (1981), features the Los Angeles County Bureau of Social Services (BSS) and its efforts to deal with budget cutbacks, increasing caseloads, and a loss of a sense of control among workers and administrators. In an effort to shift the culture of an organization from a crisis-oriented perspective to one that is forward looking and proactive, the external OD consultant teamed up with an internal change agent. Together they assessed organizational goals and programs, agency resources, existing managerial systems, staff training needs, staff commitment to the profession and the department, staff participation in decision making, and job satisfaction. With this information, the change agents observed and facilitated staff meetings by assisting with defining goals and objectives, improving communication processes, and assessing group behaviors and identifying areas of influence. This work culminated in an OD plan developed in consultation with the bureau's executive committee to work extensively with line supervisors as well as foster improved relationships between all managerial personnel and line workers.

The common themes emerging from these case examples relate to the need for an external OD consultant to provide technical assistance with goal setting, shared decision making, conflict resolution, work group cooperation, and staff training on OD techniques (Norman and Keys, 1992). Similar themes are illustrated in the following case study of the San Mateo County Human Services Agency.

DEFINING ORGANIZATIONAL DEVELOPMENT AND THE NEED FOR A SPECIALIST

Numerous factors contributed to the creation of a permanent, full-time organization development staff position within the San Mateo County Human Services Agency. In 1992, a newly reorganized agency and a new director, followed by a new strategic plan completed in 1993, marked the beginning of a comprehensive organizational change process. All aspects of the agency were impacted, including service delivery, increased use of teams, organizational structures, and community relationships. In 1995, following the implementation of many changes, the agency conducted a self-assessment involving all levels of staff in order to take the pulse of the agency and identify staff needs and perceptions. The self-study indicated that agency staff were struggling to keep up with the myriad of changes and needed more (1) understanding of the strategic plan; (2) feedback on how staff were doing in implementing the plan; (3) honest and open communications from bottom up and top down; (4) attention to concerns about customer service and productivity; and (5) attention to job performance and workplace stress (Borland and Kelley, 2001).

Throughout this change process, an external OD consultant had been working with the agency to involve external community groups and internal agency stakeholders in the agency's strategic plan. This consultant worked with a group of staff who were to become internal change agents skilled in strategic planning, facilitation skills, and change methodology. In addition, the external consultant worked with the executive staff to expand their views beyond managing their particular job functions to assume new roles as agency-wide leaders. Because the strategic plan called for agency-wide change, the external OD consultant recommended the hiring of a full-time internal OD specialist who the agency director saw as a more cost-effective strategy for the agency. Such an individual would be available to work with staff on a regular basis, engage in hands-on problem solving, acquire and use an insider's view of the agency's future directions, and contribute to the skill base of staff at all levels with respect to learning and applying OD techniques.

The idea for creating an internal OD specialist was further helped by increased attention throughout the county in 1996 to the field of organization development. For the first time, the county sponsored an eighteen-month OD course for representatives from each county department to prepare them to work periodically as OD consultants throughout county departments. This development helped the director of human services present a convincing case to the county manager for the creation of an internal OD position. The director documented the need for internal OD services to help implement a new model of service delivery (the SUCCESS program and school-linked service teams). The director also assured the county manager that creating this staff position would complement the county system by involving the OD specialist in teaching county OD courses and consulting with other county departments.

HIRING PROCESS

Because of the high stakes associated with bringing a change agent into the agency through the creation of this new position, the executive team devoted considerable efforts to developing a job description, recruiting, and using an assessment-center strategy to pick the best candidate. The position called for designing and facilitating processes to help the agency deal with significant change and required experience in process design, workflow analysis and reengineering, along with knowledge of OD theory and practice and public-sector management systems. The major skill sets included the ability to establish collaborative relationships, build consensus, and foster effective intra- and intergroup communication, as well as demonstrated ability in effectively utilizing an array of OD interventions. After an unsuccessful effort to recruit through local newspapers and informal human resource networks, it became clear that a national search was needed. By accessing the Organization Development Network and university OD programs, a pool of qualified applicants was developed by identifying persons with OD training and experience.

The assessment-center strategy included the process of presenting to top candidates an array of agency problems and role-plays in order to observe the candidates in a simulated OD consultant role. Table 19.1 reflects a matrix of the assessment criteria and activities. Candidates also engaged in private consultations with the agency director and were asked to develop and present a plan to senior staff that addressed specific agency problems. The assessment-center approach included an opportunity to observe candidates in a leaderless group where they worked together to solve a problem, while being observed and evaluated by the executive staff and consultants. Another activity required applicants to facilitate a meeting of staff members who were intentionally resistant to having a successful meeting, based on prescribed roles. Third, each candidate met with various senior managers to review different presenting problems and, based on limited data, provide

TABLE 19.1. Human Services Agency Senior Organizational Development Consultant Assessment Center Exam Matrix

Dimensions	Application screening	Panel interview	Facilitation exercise	Leaderless group experience
Adaptability	X	X	X	
Analytical	X	X	X	X
Awareness of political ramifications		X		
Career orientation	X			
Decision making	X		X	
Interpersonal relations		X	X	X
Leadership				X
Oral communication		X	X	X
Teamwork		X		X
Technical experience	X	X	X	X
Written communication	X			X

a response by framing the issues. Finally, the candidates were required to make a presentation to the executive staff about a previous client, reviewing his or her process of start-up, data collection, feedback, intervention, and evaluation in working with this client.

The OD specialist who was selected came to her position with two master's degrees, one in counseling and the other in organizational development. Her primary OD experience was in a large state university and included (1) organizational assessment (using focus groups, needs assessment surveys, team effectiveness surveys, action research related to sources of conflict and service inefficiency, and executive assessment and feedback); (2) inter- and intradepartmental team building and small group facilitation related to fostering collaboration, facilitating strategic planning, team start-up, and program design; (3) organizational training related to management development, diversity training, organizational change management, and quality management, and (4) individual coaching and consulting. Since her move to San Mateo, she is concurrently pursuing a doctorate in OD and is interested in developing a research focus in organization development in order to complement her work as an OD practitioner.

OD ENTRY

The entry phase for new managers is complex under the best of circumstances (Austin, 1989). Learning about a new organizational culture, clarifying one's job description, and assessing realistic start-up activities can be totally consuming. This process becomes even more complex when the senior management role is new and not well understood by other senior managers, let alone staff at other levels of the organization. This was the case for the first OD specialist hired by the agency. It took some time to fully develop a comprehensive OD job description and then find ways to communicate the OD function to the rest of the staff. Box 19.1 includes the updated job description as of 1999.

In the midst of this entry phase, the organization was going through a culture change of its own, in which the vestiges of centralized autocratic management processes and scapegoating among staff were being replaced with a strong decentralized community focus based on teamwork and collaboration. It became apparent to the OD specialist that the organizational culture reflected significant capacities to identify problems but fewer skills in problem solving. It was not easy for senior managers to incorporate OD approaches into their domains because OD symbolized the potential for redistributing power within a unit or division, whereby staff could be empowered to voice their concerns without fear of retribution.

As a result of concerns about the loss or gain of power, early OD efforts were primarily framed as projects that would impact more than one unit or department in the agency. Line supervisors were most responsive to this approach. Out of projects grew opportunities for individual coaching and consulting as staff at all levels became more comfortable with the role of an OD specialist.

The OD specialist was gradually introduced throughout the agency, in order to minimize staff resistance to her position. In recalling this period of her work, the OD specialist said that staff often did not welcome her because they saw her as "a spy for the management team." Yet she viewed her main objective as helping the "client," which she defined as the entire agency, rather than serving an individual supervisor or worker. Her primary responsibility was to assist the client (agency) in accomplishing changes that were identified as desirable. Specifically, her first goal was to help staff change the service delivery system into a seamless, one-stop model, which required

BOX 19.1. Program Service Manager Positions— Organization Development

Current Classification: Organization Development Manager

Current Position Title: Organization Development Manager

Report to: Agency Director

Primary Functions

Supervision

Supervise organization development work of internal and external consultants.

Consultation Services—Organizational and Group Levels

- Consult to the agency directors, managers, and supervisors on organizational structure, system and policies (reward, performance, and career systems), organizational procedures (decision making, communications), job design, practices, and procedures that impede efficient functioning, leadership behaviors, and group processes.
- Provide action research services to the agency directors, managers, and supervisors about structure, technology, culture, performance management, and organizational feedback systems.
- Provide consultation, training, and education on process improvement to process improvement teams and self-directed work teams where applicable.
- Design organizational and group-level questionnaires and focus group interview schedules.
- Conduct organizational and group-level diagnosis using questionnaires and focus groups.
- Summarize and analyze data for agency directors, managers, supervisors, teams, and community partners.
- Prepare and present status reports for purposes of action planning by the agency directors, managers, supervisors, staff, and community partners.
- Design, develop, implement, and evaluate interventions to address agency needs as identified through organizational and group-level diagnosis, i.e., role negotiation intervention for agency directors, program and support managers, and supervisors.
- Design, develop, implement, and evaluate team start-up, team development, and team maintenance retreats with agency directors, managers, supervisors, staff, and community partners to decrease intergroup competition and enhance collaborative work efforts.
- Educate the Success Advisory Strategic Planning Committee regarding the elements of strategic planning and implementation.

(continued)

(continued)

- Conduct an environmental analysis for the welfare reform industry and the agency's environment, as well as external and internal stakeholders through research, focus groups, and surveys in conjunction with the Success Advisory Strategic Planning Committee.
- Research and educate the agency directors, managers, supervisors, staff, and community partners about new methods of change management, planning, and organization development processes.
- Design, develop, instruct, and evaluate curriculums to support ongoing interventions, i.e., coaching, change management, etc.
- Deliver process consultation to intact teams and work groups including the executive team, regional implementation teams, etc.
- Develop and implement evaluation tools and instruments to measure the effectiveness of organization development and interventions.

Consultation Services—Individual Level

- Mentor and instruct directors, managers, and supervisors through on-the-job training how to do short- and long-term planning, strategic planning, process improvement, succession planning, and performance analysis.
- Provide performance coaching to agency directors, managers, supervisors, and staff.
- Assess performance of agency directors, managers, supervisors, and staff through the use of psychological tests, questionnaires, and checklists.
- Administer instruments (see above item for complete listing), score, interpret, and feedback data to client for performance-related action planning.

Consultation Services—Countywide

- Design, develop, instruct, and evaluate San Mateo County's organization development curriculum for directors and managers in San Mateo County departments and other county agencies.
- Design, develop, instruct, and evaluate course components, related to interdisciplinary practice for the Bay Area Social Services Consortium.
- Design and develop a case study, related to changing management for the Bay Area Social Services Consortium.
- Consult to other agency directors, managers, and supervisors on organizational structure, system and policies, organizational procedures, job design, and practices and procedures that impede efficient functioning, leadership behaviors, and group processes in conjunction with the San Mateo County organizational development consultants. This work is to be performed quid pro quo.
- Present at local, regional, and national meetings and conferences on the organization development work performed for the agency.

(continued)

> (continued)
>
> **Other Areas of Responsibility**
>
> - Coordinate and write quarterly implementation report.
> - Write articles for the newsletter.
> - Attend implementation team meetings.
> - Attend executive and management team meetings and provide process consultation.
> - Special projects and assignments.
>
> Source: San Mateo County Human Services Agency Personnel Manual, 1999.

substantial change in the agency's culture. She viewed her responsibility as helping the agency identify "points of leverage for the changes" and developing resources to sustain organizational changes, rather than as advocating for specific changes. As she was gradually introduced throughout the agency, she used many of the classic OD skills related to gaining acceptance, gathering and analyzing data, framing complex issues, developing options, and educating staff about OD principles and practices (Blake and Mouton, 1970).

The OD specialist applied these skills throughout the agency as illustrated in the following examples:

- *Fostering acceptance:* While some staff resisted efforts to address feelings about the workplace and difficulties in dealing with changes, other staff welcomed the opportunity to discuss their feelings with her. The OD specialist worked first with the executive team so that staff and top management could see how she operated to help improve staff meeting processes and priority setting by gathering the perceptions of individuals, aggregating the findings, and collectively developing guidelines to deal with shared needs. The outcome was a new structure for presenting new ideas at meetings, a sponsor system to assist outsiders make presentations, and increasingly productive meetings based on sharply focused agendas and reduced interpersonal friction. Other outcomes included the annual review of performance objectives (key results areas linked to the agency's strategic plan) and the establishment of a new policy group related to human resources focusing on issues related to succession planning (powerful demographics related to a wave of future retirement), leadership development, career development, and mentoring.

- *Collecting data and information:* Valuable data were available when the OD specialist assisted staff in their preparation to work in multifunctional teams through the use of team start-up activities. Staff concerns simply bubbled up to the surface. For example, she sought to create a shared understanding between management staff and line workers about implementation of new job functions (e.g., assisting income/employment services specialists identify the new case-management responsibilities). In performing this type of assistance, the OD specialist was able to gather data and information based on what management staff wanted to know and what line staff needed in order to function effectively, thereby helping identify gaps in understanding between the groups.

  Other OD-led data-collection activities included the use of internal process evaluation to identify implementation issues. These efforts complemented the external program evaluation of service outcomes. The major benefit of these two approaches to evaluation was to demonstrate to staff that the evaluation of what is to be accomplished needed to be balanced with an ongoing evaluation of how objectives are being implemented. These are two key elements of continuous process improvement. These efforts have led to the development of a comprehensive guidebook to facilitate the linkage between contract agencies providing client services and the agency's automated case-management information system.

- *Framing difficult issues:* Through the process of data collection and information gathering, the OD specialist determined that staff was not responsive to the term "strength-based services" (e.g., building on client strengths) which had been promoted by senior management. This was an area of disconnect between the expectations of management and the understanding of line staff. Management staff assumed that the staff had understood and adopted the concept of strength-based services, while staff members were generally not familiar with the skills sets needed to implement this service delivery approach. By pointing out the tension between the various conceptual frameworks for the provision of services held by management and line staff, the OD specialist helped to create a readiness to engage collaboratively in effective issue identification and problem solving.

- *Developing options for group decision making:* Although OD specialists are positioned to identify many areas for improvement, the goal of an internal OD specialist is to provide senior management with a range of options for the effective implementation of change. The framing of options, and the shared thinking about additional options, maximizes flexibility and creativity. Being overly prescriptive can deprive staff of the ultimate ownership of their problem-solving process. In essence, the OD specialist developed recommendations in partnership with management staff. For example, creating the new matrix management structure (see Figure 19.1) required senior managers to shift from managing one service (e.g., child welfare) to an array of services in a region of the county linked to implementing the new geographically based service delivery system. The OD specialist assisted the group of managers to identify potential challenges, established new accountability processes, facilitated the work of new cross-staff policy teams, and created communication systems related to improving information systems and meeting management through electronic calendaring.

- *Demonstrating OD principles and practices:* Before presenting data collected from staff focus groups regarding their responses to agency changes, the OD specialist prepared staff by focusing on how individuals commonly react when they receive survey results about themselves. The goal was to minimize defensiveness. Then, if they did respond defensively, the OD specialist worked with the staff to explore their reactions by demonstrating OD principles and practices.

The OD specialist also engaged in a great deal of process consultation to help staff members improve their capacities to function as team members. In particular, she helped staff deal with significant organizational change by validating their understandable resistance and framing problems as systems issues related to organizational change instead of personal issues related to job performance. It was striking to find so much internalization of change directives where the need for change was seen as related to poor worker performance. Facilitating open exchange between management and staff in meetings for all staff to attend began to model OD approaches for fostering open communications. One of the significant outcomes of these efforts was the staff realization that they had more operational control of their areas of activity than they had realized and that they could take responsibility for initiating change.

ONGOING OD CONSULTATION

Beyond these major activities, the OD specialist is also available as a consultant to respond to requests for assistance in dealing with team functioning or individual staff issues. These requests included the following:

- *Periodic strengthening of team building:* assist team members in examining methods and procedures for working more effectively on problems and issues (offered to teams that have worked together for four to six months).
- *Expanding meeting management skills:* work with committee chairpersons to design effective meeting processes and procedures that accomplish the charge of the committee and motivate committee members to continue working together.
- *Developing an OD training course:* foster OD skills and techniques among key staff throughout the agency.
- *Coaching:* support staff in learning how to acquire the skills to get the desired results from others.

Given the successful completion of the first three years of introducing OD into the agency, the agency director decided it was time to fully integrate organization development into all aspects of human resource development by promoting the OD specialist to manager of human resource and development (all staff development and personnel functions). The primary purpose of this change was to train and coach current trainers into new roles as internal consultants engaged in assessing organizational issues and providing coaching and training on workplace issues. This transition was completed with the assistance of an external OD consultant. A second purpose was to create a human resource policy team that would oversee the implementation of a leadership and management development structure consisting of orientation, succession planning, multisource feedback, career development, and recruitment and retention strategies. All these elements are part of a new human resource strategy to be implemented by the new OD/HRD division and manager.

LESSONS LEARNED FROM A WORK IN PROGRESS

The executive staff considered numerous issues before hiring an OD specialist, given the high stakes associated with creating a staff position for someone whose primary job was to facilitate organizational changes. Although many of the executive team members were interested in filling the position, they were also aware of the potential for negative staff reactions to an internal OD specialist. One common concern among staff was that the OD specialist was hired by top administration to enforce change, especially related to implementing the SUCCESS model. Anticipating this reaction, the executive team gave careful consideration to selecting a supervisor for the OD specialist and selected the agency director so that every area of the

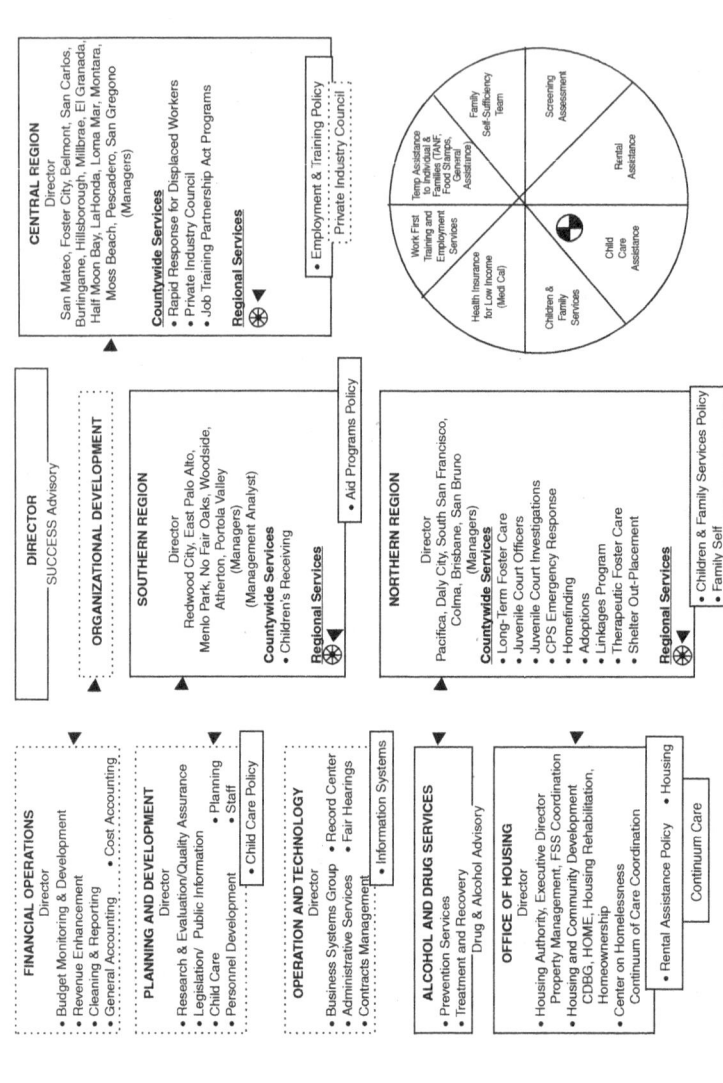

FIGURE 19.1. Management Structure of the Human Services Agency

agency could be open to OD consultation. In an effort to anticipate the feeling of being spied on, staff were told that although the agency director would have a general knowledge of the projects and units utilizing the services of the OD specialist, the details of these projects would remain confidential. For example, if a supervisor requested the OD specialist's services, the director could be informed of the length of time required to complete the task and the geographic location where the OD specialist would be working. However, the details surrounding a particular problem or conflict would not be shared with the director.

In retrospect, few occasions have required completely confidential services. Although the executive staff may make referrals to the OD specialist, asking her to evaluate functioning of teams when there is rumored to be a problem, they do not ask for the details of the intervention. This highly professional and confidential process was necessary to minimize staff resistance to the OD specialist within the agency.

After three years of operation, several preliminary lessons can be gleaned from the experiences of the San Mateo County Human Services Agency. It is important to be cautious about applying them to other agencies, since each agency responds to organization development in a unique way.

1. *It is important for the internal OD specialist to invest the necessary time and energy in developing a close working relationship between staff and management.* The OD specialist described this relationship as "co-partnering," explaining that there must be constant efforts to continue to build trust and communication and to share information between the two groups.
2. *The internal OD specialist does not develop change recommendations for the agency.* Although it is appropriate for external OD consultants to be prescriptive, by recommending specific changes that should be made, the internal OD specialist needs to help staff sort out their options by documenting feelings and needs, collectively developing action plans, and demonstrating how to confront and deal with problems.
3. *Provide information to all levels of staff, preferably at the same time.* Guaranteeing staff input and feedback on data collected from staff, prior to sharing the data with the executive team, has given staff members a sense of assurance that they can share their experiences more openly with the OD specialist. It also allows them to make any changes in how their feedback is portrayed, helping them control its presentation to management.
4. *Organization development is not a solution to all of the agency's problems.* There are limits to changing individual behaviors, and the orga-

nization development process cannot address every problem within the agency. Some staff feel threatened by OD practices and are not interested in using them as tools for changing organizational processes.
5. *Relationship building and sustaining has several levels: (1) creating and nurturing; (2) trusting and supporting; and (3) risk taking and new learning.* Early on in establishing the OD function, it became apparent to the OD specialist that relationship building and sustaining (worker-client, worker-worker, and worker-manager) were essential ingredients in successful agency service delivery (as well as in successful OD). Acquiring new risk-taking behaviors may require new learning experiences in order to transform bureaucratic organizations into learning organizations.
6. *While OD specialists are in a unique agency position to see both sides of an issue since they are not in the chain of command to manage or deliver agency services, they need to help others expand their capacities to see and sense.* OD specialists are in a position to use their antennae or radar to sense the level of interest or disinterest in promoting change. Based on these capacities, they continuously focus on readiness and thereby circle and come back to issues where there is disinterest or resistance. The capacities to see and sense need to be introduced and cultivated among all levels of staff. OD specialists can demonstrate seeing and sensing through their role-modeling in nearly all OD interventions. Another approach is to develop an informal OD network inside the agency based on staff completing in-service training on OD procedures and processes.
7. *It is crucial to monitor the changing and multiple staff perceptions of the OD function.* OD specialists need to continuously monitor their work in order to identify the different ways in which staff perceive their interventions, both the formal and informal as well as the planned and unplanned. Positive and negative staff feedback is an extremely important ingredient for improving the agency's OD operations. Because staff feedback may not be plentiful or continuous, the OD specialist also needs to find outside sources of support and learning related to ethical issues, confronting one's own biases, and avoiding the blame game often rampant in organizations undergoing massive change. OD colleagues (OD Network) and OD educators (graduate programs) are two of the most frequently used sources of outside support.
8. *Moving from project learning to individualized learning requires time and patience.* Most of the OD activity in the first three years of operation involved projects that addressed issues in more than one area of the agency. As the trust level rises, it should be possible to increase the

amount of individualized coaching and consulting to foster more staff learning and expand the ability to change old behaviors.
9. *Communication and collaboration with staff development is essential for the future viability of OD.* Because many of the organizational issues identified indicate needs for additional training, ongoing communication and collaboration between OD and staff development personnel are crucial.

REFERENCES

Austin, M.J. (1989). Executive entry: Multiple perspectives on the process of muddling through. *Administration in Social Work, 13*(4), 55-71.
Blake, R. and Mouton, J. (1970). *Consultation.* Reading, MA: Addison-Wesley Publishers.
Borland, M. and Kelley, J. (2001). How are we doing? San Mateo County's organizational assessment and service survey. In Austin, M. J. (Ed.), *Guiding organizational change: A casebook for executive development in the human services,* Eighth edition (pp. 97-105). Berkeley, CA: Bay Area Social Services Consortium.
Burke, W. (1980). Organization development and bureaucracies in the 1980s. *Journal of Applied Behavioral Science, 16,* 429.
French, W. and Bell, C. Jr. (1990). *Organization development: Behavioral science interventions for organization improvement,* Third edition. Englewood Cliffs, NJ: Prentice-Hall.
French, W.L., Bell, C.H., and Zawacki, R.A. (1989). *Organizational development: Theory, practice, and research,* Third edition. Homewood, IL: BPI Irwin.
Glassman, A. and McCoy, S. (1981). Organizational development in a social service agency: Preparing for the future. *Public Personnel Management, 10*(3), 324-332.
Golembiewski, R.T. (1989). Organizational development in public agencies: Perspectives on theory and practice. In French, W.L., Bell, C.H., and Zawacki, R.A. (Eds.), *Organizational development: Theory, practice, and research,* Third edition. Homewood, IL: BPI Irwin.
Golembiewski, R., Proehl, C. Jr., and Sink, D. (1982). Estimating the success of OD applications. *Training and Development Journal, 36*(4), 86-95.
Martinko, M. and Tolchinsky, P. (1982). Critical issues for planned change in human service organizations: A case study and analysis. *Group and Organization Studies, 7*(2), 179-192.
McLagan, P. (1989). *Models for HRD practice.* Alexandria, VA: American Society for Training and Development.
Norman, A. and Keys, P. (1992). Organization development in public social services—The irresistible force meets the immovable object. *Administration in Social Work, 16*(3), 147-165.

Resnick, H. and Menefee, D. (1993). A comparative analysis of organization development and social work, with suggestions for what organization development can do for social work. *Journal of Applied Behavioral Science, 29*(4), 432-445.

Rothwell, W., Sullivan, R., and McLean, G. (Eds.) (1995). *Practicing organization development.* San Diego, CA: Pfeiffer and Company.

Stacey, R. (1992). *Managing the unknowable: Strategic boundaries between order and chaos in organization.* San Francisco: Jossey-Bass Publishers.

Stupak, R. and Moore, J. (1987). The practice of managing organization development in public sector organizations: Reassessments, realities, and rewards. *International Journal of Public Administration, 10*(2), 131-153.

Chapter 20

Preparing Human Service Workers to Implement Welfare Reform: Establishing the Family Development Credential in a Human Services Agency

Judie Svihula
Michael J. Austin

The need to empower families in their quest toward self-reliance has become critical in the wake of welfare reform. In 1996, the president signed the Personal Responsibility and Work Opportunity Reconciliation Act (PRWORA) into law and fundamentally restructured the nation's safety net for low-income families with children. PRWORA gave states broad authority to restructure welfare programs within the confines of strict time limits and work participation requirements. The employment philosophy of WorkFirst has encouraged those with job skills to find work but has left behind individuals with multiple barriers to self-sufficiency. In an attempt to assist hard-to-place individuals, many states have sought to link agencies and programs to expand the range and availability of support services such as transportation, child care, housing, substance abuse services, and domestic violence services (Trutko, Pindus, and Barnow, 1999). Other states have integrated their programs into one-stop career centers which might include employment services, education, and other services (Martinson, 1999). The new strategies have created a need for strength-based, interdisciplinary service delivery approaches to replace the traditional entitlement/problem-based system.

This case study describes an approach taken by a county human service agency to train human service workers in collaborative case management to deliver strength-based services within a new interdisciplinary system. It begins with a brief literature review of strength-based, interdisciplinary service delivery and the history of the training model developed by Cornell Uni-

317

versity for New York State. It then focuses on the start-up and implementation of the family development credential (FDC) in San Mateo County, California. The final sections identify the strengths and challenges that emerged as well as the lessons learned from the process.

STRENGTH-BASED INTERDISCIPLINARY SERVICES

Strength-based case management practice has been developed for many populations, including those with mental illnesses, older people, troubled youths, addictions, as well as communities and schools (Chamberlain and Rapp, 1991). Rather than focusing on client dependency as a result of pathology and deficits, the strength-based social service delivery approach seeks to foster client self-sufficiency. Through listening to the clients' stories, workers enable clients to identify personal strengths and resources such as families, friends, neighborhoods, and subcultures that empower them to change their environments and foster personal growth (Simon, 1994; Parsons and Cox, 1994; Sullivan and Rapp, 1994; Weick et al., 1989).

Most welfare recipients do not perceive themselves in terms of strengths, but instead identify themselves as deficient and needy (de Shazer, 1991; Holmes and Saleebey, 1993; Lee, 1994). To shift from a deficits to a strengths perspective, human service workers need to learn how to help clients capitalize on their resources, talents, knowledge, and motivation, as well as a supportive environment (Saleebey, 1996). This requires the formation of mutually respectful and collaborative relationships. Empowering clients involves (1) accepting the client's definition of the problem, (2) actively involving the client in the change process, (3) teaching specific skills, and (4) mobilizing resources and advocating for clients (Gutierrez, GlenMaye, and DeLois, 1995). The core concepts include (1) the reduction of self-blame, (2) the assumption of personal responsibility for change, (3) the development of a group consciousness (not alone), and (4) enhancement of self-efficacy. Gutierrez, GlenMaye, and DeLois (1995) found the following four barriers and three supports for agency-based empowerment practice:

Barriers

- *Funding:* the empowerment method is more time consuming than traditional methods, resulting in reductions in clients able to be seen. In addition, it is difficult to measure empowerment as an outcome for funding.
- *Social environment:* differing agency philosophies and competition impede interagency cooperation and client access to resources.

- *Interpersonal:* clients with mental and physical challenges progress incrementally, which is potentially frustrating to the worker.
- *Intrapersonal:* encouraging choice may require a worker to let go of outcomes or responsibility when the well-being of the client is at stake.

Supports

- *Staff development:* four aspects of staff development were important in maintaining an empowerment approach: (1) provision of advanced training and in-service training, (2) entrepreneurial support (e.g., encouragement and opportunities to develop programs and professional skills), (3) being rewarded through promotions and salary increases for pursuing self-learning, and (4) provision of flexible hours and encouragement toward self-care.
- *Enhanced collaboration:* an atmosphere of empowerment in an agency or organization is needed that includes (1) sharing of power and information among all levels of staff, (2) peer supervision and review which serve to build relationships and support systems among staff, (3) a sense of safety to take risks (e.g., confronting one another, developing new ideas), and (4) a shared empowerment philosophy.
- *Administrative leadership and support:* the advocacy and encouragement of the empowerment orientation by the leadership of the agency or organization is fundamental (Gutierrez, GlenMaye, and DeLois, 1995).

These findings emphasize the importance of a supportive organizational culture to help staff engage in strength-based practice. The practice principles and concepts, as well as the research findings, provide the foundation for a training program on family development that helps to strengthen communities (Kretzmann and McKnight, 1993).

HISTORY OF THE FAMILY DEVELOPMENT CREDENTIAL IN NEW YORK

The family development credential is a training program that enables paraprofessionals from a wide range of human service agencies (HSA) to help families solve problems and achieve enduring self-sufficiency. The approach utilizes a common language, skills set, and competencies that emphasize prevention, interagency collaboration, and a greater role for families in determining services. The FDC program was developed as part of a major New York State multiagency initiative to redirect the way its health, education, and human services are delivered to families. Developed and implemented by Cornell University, the FDC program begins with a one-week training institute for future FDC program facilitators from county human service agencies. The goal of the institute is to prepare participants to return to their agencies to teach line staff the twelve-month, 110-hour FDC "Empowerment Skills for Family Workers" curriculum, through which workers can earn college credit. Figure 20.1 describes the FDC training sequence and intended worker outcomes. The FDC is currently offered in every New York county and at least nine states (Dean, 2000; Lang, 1999).

The expected staff outcomes of the FDC curriculum are to enable families to

- regain their sense of responsibility and hope;
- become more self-reliant in caring for their own needs and less dependent on government programs;
- develop healthier interdependence with their communities;
- learn how to assess their own strengths and needs;
- learn how to set and reach their own goals for self-reliance;
- learn skills to reach these goals;
- learn how to get access to services they need to reach these goals;
- learn to serve as their own "case managers"; and
- develop stronger informal support networks, in combination with enabling communities to develop such support networks (Crane and Dean, 1999, p. 3).

START-UP OF THE FAMILY DEVELOPMENT CREDENTIAL IN SAN MATEO COUNTY

The idea for implementing the FDC in San Mateo emerged from changes in services fostered by welfare reform and the interest of the HSA to redesign its service delivery and training approach. This section outlines these major forces.

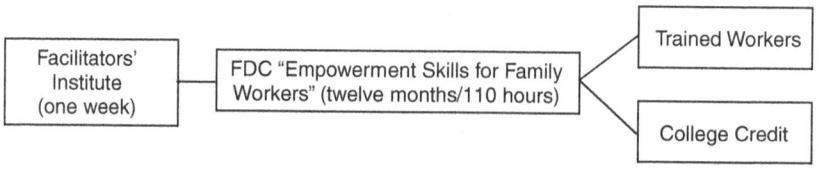

FIGURE 20.1. FDC Training Sequence and Intended Outcomes

Welfare Reform and Organizational Change

A state waiver granted to San Mateo in 1997 gave the county special permission to operate the Shared Undertaking to Change the Community to Enable Self-Sufficiency (SUCCESS) program (San Mateo County Human Services Agency, 2000). The SUCCESS model was developed by the county as a demonstration project under the Aid to Families with Dependent Children (AFDC) program. The model required considerable staff training in order to create a comprehensive, interdisciplinary service delivery system (DuBrow, Wocher, and Austin, 1999). As a result of the new model, job functions changed. For example, SUCCESS divided the eligibility staff into four service categories: (1) eligibility technicians (ET) who work in Temporary Assistance to Needy Families (TANF) children services, Food Stamps, and Medi-Cal, (2) income and employment services specialists (IESS) who work with families and participate in the SUCCESS interdisciplinary team meetings (the Family Self-Sufficiency Team), (3) employment services specialists (ESS) who focus only on preparation for employment, and (4) screening and assessment (SAS) specialists who provided initial assessments and developed preliminary case plans and made referrals. An interdisciplinary team, the Family Self-Sufficiency Team (FSST) was established in every region of the county to review and formulate comprehensive service plans for the increasingly complex and multidisciplinary cases. Human service workers began an in-service training program in multidisciplinary case management to address the complex and multiple barriers of individuals and families.

Education and Retraining

When the SUCCESS service system was implemented, many front-line staff members were not trained in case management. For these staff members, in-service training began with the implementation of SUCCESS. HSA designed and developed in-service training programs in cooperation with a new community college human services certificate (HSC) program on multidisciplinary case management methods.

The Human Services Credential

Soon after the implementation of SUCCESS, HSA developed a partnership with the College of San Mateo to create a two-year human services certificate program (Deichert and Austin, 1999). Because of the new family assessment responsibilities required of line staff in the SUCCESS service delivery model, the first course developed for HSA was "Interviewing and Counseling." Other core courses include introduction to human services, introduction to case management, public assistance and benefits programs, and an internship in human services work experience. Courses are offered on-site at HSA as well as at the community colleges. Staff members receive college credit for all training attended and satisfactorily completed. With permission from their immediate supervisor, staff may attend courses on HSA time (College of San Mateo, 2000; San Mateo County Human Services Agency, 1998).

FDC

It soon became clear that more training was needed because many staff who were trained in case management lacked the collaborative skills necessary for the interdisciplinary SUCCESS model. To build skills in collaborative case management, HSA implemented the FDC to complement its in-service training program and the community college certificate program. Units earned in the FDC and the human services certificate may be applied toward an accelerated associate of arts degree in human services as well as a four-year college degree. Figure 20.2 describes the array of HSA case-management training venues.

The start-up of the FDC in San Mateo was a collaborative effort. The HSA training specialist was searching for a strength-based case-management model that could supplement and/or replace many of the agency's in-service components. Concurrently, the Community College Foundation (CCF) was seeking to develop a human service credential program that would meet the needs of untrained community workers (with or without a high school diploma), who desired further education. The Community College Foundation and HSA had learned of the successful FDC program that New York State had developed in conjunction with Cornell University in 1996.

By August 2000, with the support of the Community College Foundation, HSA decided to begin FDC training for all its front-line human service workers, as well as interagency collaborative partners. Inserted into the staff development program as a link between case management training and the community college human services certificate, the FDC will increasingly incorporate the case-management content into the credential program. As a result, the FDC curriculum is becoming the core of case-management train-

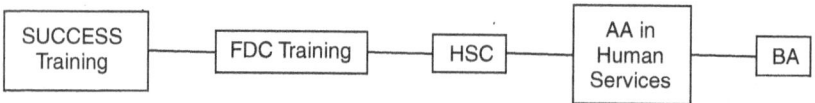

FIGURE 20.2. Case Management Programs Eligible for Community College Credits

ing. The following list outlines the content of the case-management training programs that are eligible for credits and certificates.

1. SUCCESS multidisciplinary case-management training
   - Interdisciplinary case management
   - Mental health overview
   - Alcohol and drug services
   - Employment support strategies
   - Advanced case management
   - Domestic violence
   - Culturally sensitive assessment of risks and strengths
   - Home visitation
2. Family development credential collaborative interdisciplinary case management training
   - Family development
   - Worker self-empowerment
   - Building mutually respectful relationships with families
   - Communicating with skill and heart
   - Cultural competence
   - Ongoing assessment
   - Home visiting
   - Helping families access specialized services
   - Facilitating family conferences, support groups, and community meetings
   - Collaboration
3. Human services certificate
   - Introduction to human services
   - Introduction to counseling and interviewing
   - Introduction to case management
   - Public assistance and benefits programs
   - Human services work experience

FDC PROGRAM IMPLEMENTATION

The Community College Foundation collaborated with Cornell University to bring the FDC program to California. In March 2000, Christiann Dean from Cornell trained thirty lead facilitators from across California at Cabrillo College in Aptos, California. Three facilitators from HSA were trained at the Aptos institute. Community College Foundation members as well as HSA staff attended the facilitators' institute in August 2000. In September 2000 and again in May 2001, the Community College Foundation trained and the HSA sponsored additional facilitators from various HSA disciplines as well as agency partners. The Community College Foundation oversees all aspects of the facilitators' institute.

The primary goal of the FDC training is to empower human service workers to provide services in ways that are family focused and strength based and which help families develop their own capacity to solve problems and achieve self-reliance. The following three FDC components were designed to meet this goal: a facilitators' institute, field instruction, and the training program.

The Facilitators' Institute

The institute is a highly interactive learning experience. The process begins by helping the facilitators establish their own set of ground rules, and then enables them to teach new ideas and principles through group discussion and role-plays, as well as shared experiences, ideas, and feelings. The institute leaders model the role of the facilitator for the facilitators-to-be. Participants gain facilitation experience with helpful guidance and group feedback. The week-long institute builds on the FDC training curriculum and its commitment to two related concepts: empowerment and family support. The role of the institute leaders is to enable participants to demonstrate the empowerment approach in their teaching and class exercises. For example, one exercise included an analysis of the costs and benefits of mutually respectful behavior between worker and client. The exercise demonstrated that the extra time and effort workers spend building respectful relationships could produce better outcomes for both clients and workers.

The institute focuses on empowerment as a developmental process that begins at the personal level. It concentrates on fostering an awareness of the knowledge and skills the participant already possesses and then helps each one acquire new knowledge and skills. The FDC facilitators learn how to guide group processes so that the FDC participants can view themselves as competent and effective. In addition, the facilitators learn to create an engaging learning environment utilizing room arrangements and the use of refreshments.

Field Instruction

Field advisors with master's degrees in social work were selected from HSA staff to provide support and guidance for workers who are working toward the FDC credential. They help workers create portfolios that demonstrate the workers' knowledge and application of their family development skills. Field advisors are expected to understand the curriculum and help workers gain skills and understanding in how it is applied through course exercises. Their responsibilities include the following:

- reviewing the workers' application of the curriculum as demonstrated by their responses to "activities to extend your learning";
- providing assistance for planning, reflecting on, and giving feedback for "skills practice";
- reviewing the three "family development plans" that complete the portfolio;
- providing feedback on what the worker has learned and how it applies to the family development approach; and
- being a resource and mentor for the worker in developing solutions to problems.

The field advisors typically consult with the participants before or after class, by special appointment, or by phone.

The FDC Program

In October 2000, HSA began with two groups of FDC program participants, with twenty-five participants meeting in the morning and twenty-five in the afternoon, twice a week. The first participants were volunteers, but the program will be mandatory in the future for all front-line staff. This section describes the FDC program, participation characteristics, and transformation outcomes.

Program

The FDC program is built on eleven core principles:

1. All people, and all families, have strengths.
2. All families need and deserve support. The type and degree of support each family needs varies throughout the life span.
3. Most successful families are not dependent on long-term public support. Neither are they isolated. They maintain a healthy interdependence with extended family, friends, other people, spiritual organizations, cultural and community groups, schools and agencies, and the natural environment.
4. Diversity (race, ethnicity, gender, class, family form, religion, physical and mental ability, age, sexual orientation) is an important reality in our society and is valuable. Family workers need to develop competence in working effectively with people who may be different

from them or come from groups that are often not respected in our society.
5. The deficit model of family assistance, in which families must show inadequacy in order to receive services (and professionals decide what is best for families), is counterproductive to helping families move toward self-sufficiency.
6. Changing from a deficit model to the family development approach requires a whole new way of thinking about social services, not simply more new programs. Individual workers cannot make this shift without corresponding policy changes at agency, state, and federal levels.
7. Families need coordinated services in which all the agencies they work with use a similar approach. Collaboration at the local, state, and federal levels is crucial to effective family development.
8. Families and family development workers are equally important partners in the empowerment process, with each contributing important knowledge. Workers learn as much as the families from the process.
9. Families must choose their own goals and methods of achieving them. Family development workers' roles include assisting families in setting reachable goals for their own self-reliance, providing access to services needed to reach these goals, and offering encouragement.
10. Services are provided in order for families to reach their goals, and are not themselves a measure of success. New methods of evaluating effectiveness are needed to measure family and community outcomes, not just the number of services provided.
11. In order for families to move out of dependency, helping systems must shift from a "power over" to a "power with" paradigm. Human service workers have power (which they may not recognize) because they participate in the distribution of valued resources. Workers can use that power to work with families rather than use power over them. (Dean, 2000, p. 29)

The FDC differs from other training programs for human service workers in the following ways:

- It calls for a new kind of relationship between families and workers.
- It builds on the strengths of families and communities.
- It recognizes that important changes are needed in human service delivery systems.

- It is based on an understanding of how power is used by agencies either to help families out of dependency or keep them dependent on programs.
- It values diversity.
- It prepares and supports front-line workers through a combination of classroom study and support from a field advisor to help workers apply what they learn to their work with families.

Through HSA's partnership with the College of San Mateo, the FDC participants are enrolled for two semesters at the college. Upon completion of each semester, the participants receive seven semester credits: three for the FDC course work and four for the FDC fieldwork (a total of fourteen units). All units completed by FDC participants enrolled at College of San Mateo can be applied toward the twenty-five-unit human services certificate and are transferrable to the California State University system.

HSA began with two sections of the FDC program held twice a week on Tuesdays and Thursdays. One section was held in the morning and the other in the afternoon. Two primary facilitators from HSA worked with each section throughout the program duration. In addition, adjunct facilitators from community partner agencies taught sections in their areas of expertise.

Participation

The Cornell model encourages interagency participation in the FDC on the premise that agencies frequently work with the same families or similar challenges. It is anticipated that when staff from different agencies attend the FDC program together, they are able to work together to promote family development in their agencies so that families hear a similar empowerment message from all agencies. They learn much more about other services available to families and build networking relationships that will strengthen interagency understanding and referrals to develop a community support system for family development workers.

The first thirty-four FDC graduating participants to receive both the credential and certificate were a diverse group of interdisciplinary human service workers from HSA (thirty-one) and community partners (three). In addition, all facilitators (nine) and one field supervisor received the College of San Mateo certificate. The classes contain group exercises to enhance group relations and develop interpersonal and networking skills. Participants are taught facilitation and family case-management tasks through example as well as group feedback. Feedback is framed in positive, nonjudgmental language. Problems are solved through group interaction and exploration. Box 20.1 provides an outline of the ten FDC modules.

BOX 20.1. Ten FDC Modules

1. *Family development: A sustainable route to healthy self-reliance*
   - Restoring a sense of self-reliance
   - Beyond provision of services
   - Core principles underlying an empowerment and family support approach to family development
   - Understanding family development
   - Empowerment: The opposite of the deficit model
   - Family support
   - Family forms and family systems
   - Families in communities
   - Putting it all together as a family development worker
2. *Worker self-empowerment*
   - "How do I work in empowering ways with families when I don't feel empowered myself?"
   - Developing a personal vision for your work
   - How to spend your time doing what is important (not just what is urgent)
   - Creating a support system for yourself
   - Balancing work and family life
   - Creating your own stress-management and wellness program
   - Staying sane on "soft money"
3. *Building mutually respectful relationships with families*
   - Effective outreach strategies
   - Establishing mutually respectful, trusting relationships with families
   - Helping families build on their own strengths
   - Confidentiality
   - How to avoid families becoming dependent on you
   - When and how to end the relationship
4. *Communicating with skill and heart*
   - Empathy: Putting yourself in their shoes
   - Finding a good balance between listening and expressing yourself
   - Listening well
   - Saying what you mean clearly and respectfully
   - Handling blame and criticism constructively
   - Promoting cooperative solutions to conflicts
   - Confronting people constructively when needed
   - Communicating about "hot topics"
   - Understanding nonverbal communication
   - Working with families with language barriers or low literacy
5. *Cultural competency*
   - What is culture?
   - What is cultural competence?
   - Why is cultural competence important for family development workers?

(continued)

(continued)
- Language and cross-cultural communication
- Displacement and immigration
- Barriers to a culturally competent society
- Exploring your own culture
- Expanding your understanding of and ability to work respectfully with other cultures
- Helping your agency to develop multicultural competence
- Family development and cultural competence

6. *Ongoing assessment*
    - What is assessment?
    - Basic principles of empowerment-based assessment
    - The family development plan
    - The family circles assessment
    - Helping your agency choose empowerment-based assessment tools

7. *Home visiting*
    - Home visiting: A unique relationship
    - A family development approach to home visiting
    - How to enter a family's home respectfully: The first time and on future visits
    - How to establish the purpose of the home visit
    - Safety issues
    - TV, dogs, and another cup of coffee: Handling the practical matters of home visiting
    - Home visits in child protection or other domestic violence situations
    - Ongoing visits

8. *Helping families access specialized services*
    - Helping families use specialized services in order to become self-reliant
    - Identifying specialized services and helping families gain access to them
    - Recognizing the need for specialized services
    - Making and following through on referrals
    - Supporting family members in specialized programs
    - Recognizing, referring, and supporting families needing specialized services
    - Recognizing the need for, referring, and supporting families in other specialized services commonly needed by the families your agency works with

9. *Facilitating family conferences, support groups, and community meetings*
    - The importance of community
    - Helping families identify and strengthen their informal helping networks

(continued)

> *(continued)*
> - Family conferences
> - Support and advocacy groups
> - Facilitation skills
> - Teaching leadership skills to family members
> 10. *Collaboration*
>   - What is collaboration?
>   - Why collaboration?
>   - Coordination and cooperation: Individuals, front-line workers, and systems
>   - Keys to successful collaboration
>   - Practical pitfalls of collaboration (and how to turn them into advantage)
>   - Does case management empower families?
>   - Major functions of a family development worker
>   - The bigger picture: How agency, state, and national policies affect your work
>   - Interagency training: A key to interagency collaboration

HSA developed many incentives for attendance: college credits and a college certificate, a university credential, full salary for classes taken on agency time, tuition reimbursement, and overall agency support. Through partnership with the College of San Mateo, all participants in the program receive a FDC certificate and semester units that may be applied toward a human service certificate, an associate of arts degree, or a four-year college degree. In addition, recent graduates received a family development credential through the Community College Foundation. The credential is accreditation for graduates that is separate from the community college certificate and may be useful for individuals with college degrees or those without a high school diploma. Discussions are in progress for University of California Extension to issue the credential in the future.

The half-day classes are held twice a week for two semesters on agency time at full salary with tuition reimbursement. Moreover, HSA supervisors are requested to provide support to the participants so that their workloads will not accumulate during their time in training. Most participants agreed that the incentives played a large part in their decision to volunteer for the program. Participants gave three main reasons for attending the program: (1) to participate in a formal human service education program, (2) to improve their skills in helping clients, and (3) to advance their careers. It is unclear how these incentives will be perceived when participation in FDC becomes mandatory.

Transformation

The FDC is an empowerment-oriented case-management model and is relevant at many levels. Personal transformation was evident throughout the FDC course as well as at the institute for facilitators. Participants, their families, and colleagues told numerous stories of improvements in their personal attitudes and values, and consequently in their family and professional lives. For example, one participant noted that one of her biggest successes has been the way in which she interacts with her teenage son. One time he left the house without telling her where he was going. When he returned, she treated him like an adult and with respect. She spoke calmly, letting him know that she was concerned about him. She told him that adults communicate this information as a common courtesy. In the past she would have spoken angrily at him, but the program has changed her perspective.

Many participants spoke of how they are spending more time listening to their clients, enhancing their self-awareness, and encouraging them to participate actively in pursuing their goals. Some workers mentioned they are more capable of responding to irate clients. Moreover, workers are more willing to go out of their way to help clients. One participant told an especially poignant story. She enabled a woman who had a severe anxiety disorder and was unable to leave her home to obtain a part-time job, simply because she initiated a home visit by placing a call to the client when she did not show up for two appointments.

All of the participants, from HSA as well as community-based organizations and at various professional levels, noted the value of building a network of trusted, qualified service providers. One community participant indicated the program has been beneficial in helping HSA staff understand his program as well as building collaborative relationships. He noted that more people are aware of his program, make more referrals, and have a better working relationship needed to help clients. In addition, his program is accepting a greater diversity of clients than before.

HSA has sought to create a transformative environment. Although some participants felt they knew much of the course material and that classes were mostly a means toward earning college credits and a certificate, they had ample opportunity to express their ideas for improvement. HSA adjusted modules along the way in response to the needs of the participants. For example, the cultural competency module was extended because of its popularity and perceived importance. In addition, participants have experienced enhanced communications with their clients and supervisors and are eager to provide face-to-face feedback to the agency director. Facilitators encourage participants who demonstrate leadership potential in the FDC classes to become facilitators themselves.

SUCCESS AND CHALLENGES

The successes of the FDC program far outweigh its challenges. Responses from staff, facilitators, and participants are summarized in three categories: program, work, and relationships.

Successes

Program

- The quick six-month program start-up and implementation was a tremendous accomplishment which is a tribute to the successful collaborative partnership among HSA, the Community College Foundation, and the College of San Mateo. It immediately addressed the training needs of line staff.
- HSA is committed to the program and has developed agency support and incentives for participation by (1) conducting the training on county time; (2) reimbursing participants for tuition and mileage; (3) collaborating to provide credentials and college credits; and (4) requesting that supervisors support their participants.
- Facilitators have built a nurturing, spirited, and interactive environment. Facilitators and participants learn from one another and build on one another's knowledge and experience. One participant stated, "I feel as if I'm in a room full of wisdom."
- Learning the strength-based approach and the network of services enhances the ability of workers to provide family support. One participant said, "It opens the mind to a holistic view of family needs and the exploration of different options."
- Active listening skills have increased workers' understanding of clients which enables them to develop positive relationships and build a better perspective of the agency.
- The empowerment model has contributed to positive transformations in the personal as well as professional lives of participants.

Work

- Participants' enthusiastic application of the FDC principles to their work has increased their productivity. Participants shared many stories of how changes in their approach have led to successful client outcomes. Moreover, as case managers, workers are able to provide a higher level of service to families.
- Increases in education and skills have enabled workers to attain their career goals (e.g., one participant applied for and attained an advanced social work position). The county has indicated that, based on their

training, FDC participants will have top priority with regard to promotions.
- Feelings of personal empowerment and positive relationships built with family, clients, supervisors, and co-workers have reduced feelings of worker burn-out and have reinvigorated their work. Participants have stated that although implementing the new concepts is time consuming, happier clients and positive outcomes have improved their work attitudes.

Relationships

- Overall, supervisors have been supportive and accommodating while the participants attended the program. Most participants reported that their supervisor encouraged them to participate and reinforced the importance of attending the classes.
- Facilitators have monitored the reactions of participants to the pace and content of the course work and have adjusted it as needed. They have created a supportive environment for learning and a safe environment for open communication.
- The first FDC cohort has built professional relationships that have resulted in greater networking, greater awareness of services and programs, and more client referrals.
- In general, field advisors have been accessible, supportive, and understanding of the difficulties that participants face in working and going to school. They have been helpful when participants needed to talk about such sensitive topics as cultural competency.
- Greater contact and respectful relationships built with families are resulting in positive outcomes (e.g., successful transitioning to work, greater utilization of supportive services, better oversight of and provision for children's needs, greater client responsibility for their actions, and increased client satisfaction based on the perception that the agency is helpful).
- Participants are spreading the successes of the FDC to their co-workers and peers in other counties. Several of their peers are now attending FDC program and others are advocating for the program in their counties.

Challenges

Program

- The quick program start-up precluded preparatory time for facilitators and field advisors, and it was difficult to ensure that HSA promises

were kept (e.g., tuition reimbursement, college credits). For example, there was confusion initially about when portfolios were due and when field advisors were to meet with participants, as well as whether HSA was going to pay the tuition or reimburse the participant after course completion.
- Participants need assistance in resolving time-management issues and possible lack of support in their job environment. Facilitators have been attempting to help participants negotiate these difficulties during class time. One participant stated she has difficulty giving up her clients to other workers and that she works overtime to keep from being overwhelmed.
- It has been difficult for the three field advisors to assist an average of thirteen participants.
- The homework (e.g., portfolios and reading) required by the program can be overwhelming for participants, as it takes additional time outside class and work.
- Outcome evaluation is needed to assess the impact of FDC on CalWORKs families.

Work

- Because they require additional time, it is difficult to implement the new FDC concepts on the job under current caseload demands and time mandates. Participants need time to become familiar with the new concepts as well as allow the time needed to learn empowerment methods such as active listening. The reductions in the number of clients that are seen may impact departmental staffing and funding. Moreover, applications must be approved or denied within a set period of time. One participant indicated that she used a new approach with every other client until she became comfortable with it.
- It is difficult for supervisors to ensure client coverage and maintain staff morale while their workers attend the FDC classes. It can be difficult to find temporary staff coverage within HSA. For example, because screening assessment specialists are union members, they cannot be temporarily replaced with nonunion workers. As a result, co-workers become burdened with extra work and client service may be delayed.
- The strength-based approach does not always match intake and assessment forms or the work environment. For example, the approach is not as effective when workers have only one or two meetings with the client, or for workers performing risk assessments (e.g., child protective services). In addition, community-based agencies function

very differently than HSA. Community workers may provide greater hands-on client assistance from contact through termination, such as performing counseling, working with clients as they go through court, and guiding them toward their goals.

Relationships

- Although HSA's commitment to the program is apparent to workers and their supervisors, it has not always been communicated to middle and top managers. Moreover, although the supervisors received a letter of support from the HSA director, at times there has not always been a connection between the supervisors' verbal support and their behavior toward the participant.
- Some participants had difficulty arranging meetings with their field advisors, especially those who did not work at the location where the courses were held. Conversely, sometimes field advisors have difficulty collecting homework from participants.
- Co-workers have become upset when they were required to carry an extra workload while participants were away attending the course.

LESSONS LEARNED

The following lessons were derived from the start-up and implementation process:

1. Commitment is essential at all levels of the agency. It is critical to communicate the agency's commitment to all levels of management and to educate them on the program content. It would be beneficial for supervisors to receive education on the program content and perspective; provide strong written support of the FDC to the participants and their co-workers; and inform co-workers that they will be attending FDC classes in the future and will need the assistance of others to handle the workload.
2. Time management emerged as a critical work and program issue for facilitators, field advisors, and participants. In addition, facilitators and field workers needed to problem solve with their participants. Training on time management and problem solving could be added as a half-day component to the facilitators' institute. Moreover, it would be helpful to begin the FDC program with information on time management, how participants may obtain support from supervisors and co-workers, and what coverage is available when they are absent. Furthermore, ongoing semiannual meetings would facilitate peer support.

3. Agency supports (time, tuition, field supervision, etc.) clearly enhance program participation and can reduce resistance to mandatory training. Educational and monetary incentives have been successful in encouraging volunteer participation. However, it is important to ensure supervisor support and staff coverage while participants are attending FDC classes. Additional support might be provided to field advisors in the form of reductions in their caseloads to improve the amount of contact between them and the participants. Moreover, maintenance of a safe environment for learning and program feedback is vital.
4. It is necessary to address the potential disconnect between the strength-based concepts of the FDC and HSA forms as well as barriers in the workplace. Changes need to be made to intake and case-management assessment forms so that they match the interdisciplinary, strength-based FDC content. Program modules might be adjusted to address the difference between the strength-based empowerment approach and risk assessment.
5. It is important to allow adequate time to apply concepts learned in the facilitation and training sessions. Facilitators require preparation time between the institute and leading the FDC classes. Moreover, participants need time to practice their newly learned skills.
6. Diversity of participants and facilitators from different service units and community agencies is essential to learning and future collaboration. The diversity in participants (e.g., from different HSA departments, divisions, job classifications, as well as community partners) and adjunct facilitators enhances the collaborative process. In addition, selecting participants from diverse areas helps decrease coverage issues within HSA (e.g., fewer workers are missing at one time from the same area). More participants from community agencies should be included.
7. High levels of satisfaction among FDC graduates may help with future staff recruitment and retention as well as increased productivity with HSA. The FDC participants reported they are more satisfied with their work. Moreover, some reported job advancement and improvements in productivity and client outcomes as a direct result of the FDC program.

CONCLUSION

On May 2, 2001, San Mateo County HSA sponsored their first FDC graduation, which was also the first FDC graduation on the West Coast (a barbecue-style lunch in a local park for participants, friends, and families).

Many personal stories of transformation were shared by the participants, as well as by those who knew them. A new FDC participant from another county was so moved by the enthusiasm and poignancy of the moment that she stood up and sang the song "You Are My Hero."

The FDC program has been an overwhelming success from inception to implementation. Moreover, the transformations have included personal renewal, work satisfaction, and increased productivity, as well as an improved agency environment. HSA plans to enroll fifty human service workers in the FDC program every sixteen weeks. When 500 workers have been trained, the FDC program will be offered on the College of San Mateo campus and possibly on-site at other agencies. HSA plans to coordinate with community colleges and agencies statewide to achieve core training standardization, career pathways, and transferable job certification.

REFERENCES

Chamberlain, R. and Rapp, C. (1991). A decade of case management: A methodological review of outcome research. *Community Mental Health, 27,* 171-188.
College of San Mateo (2000). *College of San Mateo Human Services program brochure.* San Mateo, CA: Author.
Crane, B. and Dean, C. (1999). *Empowerment skills for family workers: Trainers manual.* New York: New York State Department of State, Division of Community Services.
de Shazer, S. (1991). *Putting difference to work.* New York: W. W. Norton.
Dean, C. (2000). *Empowerment skills for family workers: The comprehensive curriculum of the New York State Family Development Credential.* New York: New York State Department of State, Division of Community Services.
Deichert, K. and Austin, M. (1999). *Collaborative partnerships between the San Mateo Human Services Agency and local community colleges.* Berkeley: University of California at Berkeley School of Social Welfare, Bay Area Social Services Consortium.
DuBrow, A., Wocher, D., and Austin, M. (1999). *Introducing organizational development (OD) practices into a county human service agency.* Berkeley: University of California at Berkeley School of Social Welfare, Bay Area Social Services Consortium.
Gutierrez, L., GlenMaye, L., and DeLois, K. (1995). The organizational context of empowerment practice: Implications for social work administration. *Social Work, 40*(2), 249-258.
Holmes, G. and Saleebey, D. (1993). Empowerment and the politics of clienthood. *Journal of Progressive Human Services, 4,* 61-78.
Kretzmann, J. and McKnight, J. (1993). *Building communities from the inside out.* Evanston, IL: Northwestern University, Center for Urban Affairs and Policy Research.

Lang, S. (1999). First recipients of Family Development Credential to help families achieve self-sufficiency. *Human Ecology Forum, 27*(1), 24.

Lee, J. (1994). *The empowerment approach to social work practice.* New York: Columbia University Press.

Martinson, K. (1999). *Literature review on service coordination and integration in the welfare and workforce development systems.* Washington, DC: The Urban Institute.

Parsons, R. and Cox, E. (1994). *Empowerment-oriented social work practice with the elderly.* Pacific Grove, CA: Brooks/Cole.

Saleebey, D. (1992). *The strengths perspective in social work practice.* White Plains, NY: Longman.

Saleebey, D. (1996). The strengths perspective in social work practice: Extensions and cautions. *Social Work, 41*(3), 296-305.

San Mateo County Human Services Agency (1998). *Human services certificate program.* San Mateo, CA: Author.

San Mateo County Human Services Agency (2000). *Revised CalWORKs plan for SUCCESS in San Mateo County.* San Mateo, CA: Author.

Simon, B. (1994). *The empowerment tradition in American social work: A history.* New York: Columbia University Press.

Sullivan, W. and Rapp, C. (1994). Breaking away: The potential and promise of a strengths-based approach to social work practice. In R. Meinert, J. Pardeck, W. Sullivan (Eds.), *Issues in social work: A critical analysis* (pp. 83-104). Westport, CT: Auburn House.

Trutko, J., Pindus, N., and Barnow, B. N. D. (1999). *Early implementation of the Welfare-to-Work Grants Program.* Washington, DC: The Urban Institute.

Weick, A., Rapp, C., Sullivan, W., and Kisthardt, W. (1989). A strengths perspective for social work practice. *Social Work, 34*(4), 350-354.

Chapter 21

Merging a Workforce Investment Board and a Department of Social Services into a County Department of Employment and Human Services

Jonathan Prince
Michael J. Austin

The passage of welfare reform legislation in 1996 signaled a major shift in American domestic policy designed to reduce dependency on public assistance by promoting employment and self-sufficiency. In order to more effectively address the employment issues related to welfare reform, the 1998 federal Workforce Investment Act (WIA) was passed to increase attention on dependency reduction for low-income individuals. Over the past decade, the employment component of social service agencies and the low-income service component of private industry councils (PICs) have shared common objectives and target populations. In some locations the two organizations have actually merged. By partnering, they have provided universal access to integrated services in one-stop employment centers. The purpose of the one-stop center is to increase the continuity of client services, reduce service fragmentation, develop jobs that promote self-sufficiency, and strengthen community capacity to benefit from a growing economy.

Given the shared missions, the two organizations merged in February 1999. They had an existing relationship with PIC job developers in social services agencies, joint responsibility for the planning and delivery of services in one-stop career centers, and the receipt of welfare-to-work funding. To expand understanding of the partnering process, this case study focuses on this unique merger between the PIC and the social services agency in Contra Costa County, California. This case study includes a description of (1) the legislation influencing PICs and social services, (2) the experiences of other counties related to their PIC and social service partnerships, (3) the components of the merger process, (4) the structure of the newly merged organization, and (5) selected issues and lessons learned from the merger process. The merger is viewed by staff as a work in progress, and continues to evolve at a very rapid rate.

LEGISLATION AFFECTING PRIVATE INDUSTRY COUNCILS AND SOCIAL SERVICES

While welfare reform expanded the employment services of social service agencies, the Workforce Investment Act of 1998 created new Department of Labor funding and functions for private industry councils related to creating universal access to employment and other workforce-related services (often in one-stop career centers). Under the WIA, the workforce investment board (WIB) replaced the private industry council (established by the job training partnership act). The WIB is responsible for developing a five-year local workforce investment plan, selecting and overseeing the one-stop career center operators, identifying eligible providers of employment services, coordinating workforce investment and economic development activities, assisting small to midsize employers, and managing youth employment and training services.

WIA requires a multiagency partnership to facilitate the continuity of employment services through one-stop (single location) career centers for businesses, workers, economically disadvantaged persons, veterans, youths, dislocated workers, and the disabled. WIA's increased emphasis on well-planned integrated services for the general population emerged at the same time as welfare reform reinforced the need for social service department collaboration with organizations to enhance employment services for low-income workers. The federal welfare reform legislation called for (1) the promotion of self-sufficiency of welfare recipients by providing a range of employment services, (2) reduction of obstacles to labor-force participation through support services that include child care, transportation, mental health counseling, and substance abuse treatment, and (3) reduction of welfare dependency through the use of time limits and the sanctioning of benefits.

The 1996 welfare reform and 1998 WIA legislation fundamentally changed the delivery of employment services, causing major organizational reassessment in both PICs and social service agencies (named employment and human services (EHS) in Contra Costa County). The next section places the partnership in a larger context by discussing general findings from collaborative efforts in other California locations.

LEARNING FROM OTHERS

To inform the service integration efforts in Contra Costa, members of an ad hoc committee[1] visited and researched counties where PIC and social services were at different stages of partnering (Napa, San Bernardino, Santa Clara, and Sonoma). They also met with representatives of the state departments of social services and employment development. From this research, several general conclusions were drawn from the experiences of other local and state officials in relationship to service delivery, working environment, planning, and oversight as noted in the following list.

1. Service delivery
   - The division of responsibility for workforce development services between PIC and social services can be inefficient and less than optimally effective, and services need to be streamlined through partnership to reduce duplication and overlap.
   - The biggest service delivery challenges are consumer job retention and advancement, promoting employment at a living wage, retraining workers to reflect changing employer needs, biases against welfare recipients, and language and literacy barriers to employment.
2. Work environment
   - The two organizations are not generally accustomed to collaborating with each other and have different cultures and relationships with consumers, with PIC typically being seen as more business oriented and tailored to the private sector and the employer, and social services typically being seen as more government oriented and tailored to the public sector and the employee.
   - Personality clashes and turf battles are usually described as the biggest barriers to service integration.
3. Planning
   - The bifurcation of responsibility for workforce development planning between the PIC and social services is less than optimally efficient, as no county positions coordinate these responsibilities or link workforce and economic development.
   - Consolidation of operations into one location, with extensive cross-agency training, is the most effective strategy for promoting partnership.
   - The oversight of consolidated employment policy under the PIC is beneficial because it increases the consistency and compatibility of welfare and PIC policy.

In addition to analyzing relevant legislation and learning these lessons from locations external to Contra Costa, the ad hoc committee examined the internal resources of the PIC[2] and the social service department in order to structure a unified organization.

Separately, the WIB and the EHS department in Contra Costa County have their own unique strengths. The WIB[3] contains eighteen staff members that administer eleven employment programs, including four programs contracted to EHS before the 1999 merger. In addition to the contractual services for employers and job seekers, WIB staff also specialize in labor-market analysis, strategic economic planning, workforce development, and job creation, and served about 1,250 adults and 1,150 youths in 1997. The much larger EHS department contains over 1,400 staff members that provide assistance to about 12 percent of the county population of over 900,000 residents. It also provides financial resources to support child care, transportation, and treatment for health, mental health, and substance abuse issues in order to assist consumers in removing these common barriers to employment. EHS contains four divisions, including children and family services, adult and senior services, employment services, and the Workforce Investment Board Bureau. At present, WIBs and the social service agencies in Contra Costa and Alameda County jointly operate a new organization called East Bay Works that includes fifteen one-stop career centers which offer a wide range of workforce development services. Welfare-to-work funding for these services is the largest area of overlap between the two organizations. By 2005 the merged WIB and EHS department plans to develop a fully integrated and universally accessible workforce development system that combines comprehensive employment and support services.

Currently the WIB provides labor-market analysis and strategic economic planning, while EHS provides a full range of access to supportive services, such as mental health and substance abuse treatment. Despite these strengths as separate organizations, the considerable service overlap and fragmentation provided the impetus for a more integrated approach.

After taking an inventory of available funding streams, job descriptions, and employment services, the ad hoc committee made several recommendations to the board of supervisors that comprise the merger agenda.

STRUCTURING THE PARTNERSHIP

The nineteen-member PIC staff who had worked previously as employment service planners were given new job titles and responsibilities in a much larger organization with different policies and procedures. Aspects of the merger, as described in the following reflections by two directors who are close to the process, illustrate some of the major issues presented in this case study:

Regarding personnel issues, many PIC staff feel consumed by a much larger bureaucratic structure and, in contrast to social service staff, identify primarily with the private sector and see themselves as more connected with the employer community. In addition, PIC staff are accustomed to doing most things for themselves—from identifying one-stop operators to negotiating contracts, for example—and now these responsibilities lie with other bureaus within EHS. In some ways this should provide a feeling of freedom, but I think it ends up with a feeling of a loss of control and becomes a turf issue. PIC staff are still grappling with their identity in the department, and we are still in the process of deciding what responsibilities will be assigned to the three newly defined bureaus of policy, operations, and administration.

The missions of the PIC and the social service organization were becoming sufficiently similar to justify the merging of the two organizations. In addition, the board of supervisors had specifically designated the PIC to be the policy oversight board for CalWORKs, and leadership in both organizations saw an opportunity to increase efficiency by blending the two organizations. While the logic of the merger was understood by all PIC staff members, several felt that it would dilute adversely the PIC's long and positive history of workforce development and would decrease PIC autonomy. On the other hand, many PIC staff saw the merger as an opportunity to position itself more as a policy and planning group and move away from some of the operational issues that are more appropriately addressed by the one-stop operators. The merger is still a work in progress. The next steps will be to clarify the roles of the merging organizations, to develop multifunctional teams within employment and human services, and to increase everyone's comfort level and the perception that this merger is best for consumers, employers, county staff, and the community.

While the federal government initiated workforce development restructuring and broad partnerships, a wide range of local options were permissible. The committee developed a framework to analyze organizational options ranging from minimal to maximum interdependence of the WIB and EHS. Theoretically, the two organizations could

1. *remain independent,* although recent legislation discourages complete autonomy,
2. *align,* sharing in the planning and delivery of some but not all services,

3. *consolidate* certain services, such as job-search assistance, while maintaining separate functions such as welfare eligibility in EHS and labor-market analysis in the WIB, or
4. *merge,* sharing all functions under one administration.

Many WIB staff, including a retired former director, had expressed preference for the first option. Most EHS staff and the workforce investment board itself,[4] however, supported broader changes, and the Contra Costa County administrator, the director of EHS, and the newly appointed WIB director implemented the fourth option of total merger. In this approach, the WIB generally oversees CalWORKs policy, yet CalWORKs funding flows through the EHS department and the workforce services director oversees program administration. This conforms to provisions in the WIA prohibiting the WIB from assuming responsibility for both policy and program operation. Working as a member of the One-Stop Operator Consortium, the social service department oversees service delivery (operations) and WIB oversees workforce development planning and procedure (policy). Community representatives from adult education, community colleges, EHS, the employment development department, and other local stakeholders are also members of the WIB or assume policy roles.[5]

The final Contra Costa Board of Supervisors action describing the unified organization was approved in February 1999 and included (1) a new workforce services director, responsible for all employment and training operations formerly delivered by the WIB and the social service department, (2) a new workforce investment board executive director, responsible for policy oversight, one-stop career center certification, economic strategic planning, and staffing the new workforce investment board, (3) the renaming of the social service department to the employment and human services department, and (4) an education program for current WIB and CalWORKs consumers and a workforce development transition committee to address transitional issues.

Figure 21.1 highlights the organizational structure of the merged agency, showing the new administrative division between workforce policy, under the WIB executive director, and workforce operations, under the workforce services director. WIB staff were integrated into policy, operations, or administrative bureaus in EHS depending on their particular area of specialization. Some staff reassignments, for example clerical or facility personnel, were relatively straightforward, while others, such as contract negotiation staff, involved considerable time and attention.

Unlike staff, WIB and EHS funding streams have not been integrated and are not as easily categorized. For example, job seekers can receive welfare-to-work funding if they have a low income, veteran's assistance if they

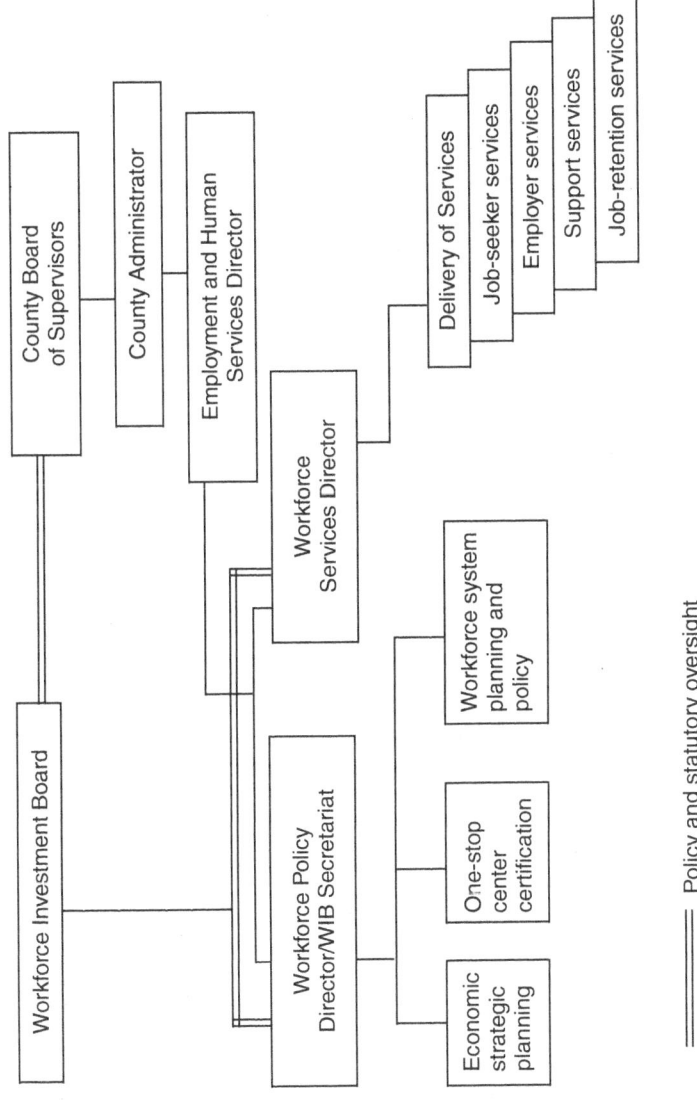

FIGURE 21.1. Organizational Structure of the Workforce Development Organization

served in the armed forces, or supplemental security income if they are disabled. The WIB budget (100 percent federal Department of Labor block grants program funding) was only about 4 percent of total EHS funding ($238,732,293) in 1998-1999 revenues.

The differences between EHS and WIB welfare-to-work service eligibility and funding are described in Table 21.1. For example, unpaid consumer work is an allowable employment activity in the CalWORKs welfare-to-work program in EHS, yet consumer employment in the WIB's Department of Labor welfare-to-work program must be paid in order for it to be considered an allowable work activity. Other EHS funding streams are extremely diverse and do not generally overlap with WIB revenues.

EVOLVING ISSUES

Although EHS has made some structural changes in response to the merger by separating the responsibility for policy and operations within employment services, the WIB staff have had to adapt to many more bureaucratic EHS policies and procedures than were necessary when they operated as PICs. While WIB staff members have felt some real frustrations during the transition process, EHS staff have been less affected by the merger.

Most WIB and EHS staff report ongoing confusion with respect to new policies and procedures that have not yet been fully operationalized, leading one WIB staff member to claim that it was "like moving in before the walls were painted." As a result, a substantial number of meetings were needed to clarify the changing roles in an evolving system. Some of the WIB staff are dissatisfied with the changes in responsibilities created by the merger and others feel that they have lost some of their autonomy and feel less valued in the much larger organization.

In addition, some WIB staff expressed concern that employers would find it difficult to hire the growing numbers of the working poor due to limited job skills. In the past, WIB consumers were referred for job placement only after the successful completion of a literacy examination. Finally, some WIB staff were initially concerned that the larger merged organization would not be able to adapt quickly enough to meet the dynamic needs of the business community and that employers would respond less favorably to the less business-like nature of a social service agency. According to one director, however, these concerns have not materialized. Instead, they reflect primarily the WIB staff identification with the business community rather than actual differences in WIB and EHS employment service delivery.

Although they have been affected less by the merger, some social service staff have felt that the primary identification of the WIB staff with the busi-

TABLE 21.1. Differences Between Social Services and Workforce Investment Board Service Eligibility and Funding

Note: CalWORKs welfare-to-work services is referred to as WTWS. Department of Labor (DOL) welfare to work is referred to as WtW.

In 1996, the federal welfare reform act was passed, eliminating the AFDC and GAIN programs and block-granting funds for these programs in a new funding stream, Temporary Assistance for Needy Families (TANF). In California, the CalWORKs program was created effective January 1, 1998, to replace AFDC and GAIN. CalWORKs is funded by TANF through the federal Department of Health and Human Services.

In 1997, the federal Balanced Budget Act created an additional welfare-to-work program, funded by TANF through the federal Department of Labor and administered in California by the private industry councils. In addition to CalWORKs WTWS participants, the DOL WtW program serves eligible noncustodial parents of CalWORKs participants. The DOL WtW program is specifically targeted to the hard to serve and focuses on placement and postemployment services.

Local social service departments and PICs must develop service models and protocols to serve job seekers who qualify for both programs. Each program has separate eligibility requirements, reporting requirements, funding restrictions, allowable services, and performance outcome mandates.

Note: Pending federal legislation would reduce, but not eliminate, some of the differences outlined in the following table.

Requirement	CalWORKs WTWS	DOL WtW
Eligibility	Income and asset tests; must have a minor child and meet deprivation-of-child standard.	Must be eligible for CalWORKs or an eligible noncustodial parent of a CalWORKs participant when enrolled in WtW. CalWORKs participant must have been on aid thirty months or be within twelve months of the five-year lifetime limit for TANF benefits.
Work activities requirements	Required to participate in work activities if not exempt; may volunteer. Must participate 32 hrs/wk (two-parent families: 35-55 hrs/wk).	In addition to the on-aid-thirty-months requirement, must be hard to serve (meets two of three criteria): no high school diploma/GED and low reading or math skills, substance abuse, and/or poor work history.

TABLE 21.1 (continued)

Allowable activities/ services	Twelve in federal law, eighteen in state law (unpaid is okay) (work, work experience, on-the-job training, community service, education and training, etc.); case management and supportive services.	Placement in employment, work experience, on-the-job training, or community service (must be paid). Postemployment services include case management, education, and training.
Length of participation	Eighteen to twenty-four months.	Funding is for three years and lasts four years; program may be reauthorized. No specific time limit for participation.
Supportive services	Child care, cash aid, transportation, mental health, substance abuse, domestic violence services, other	Child care, transportation, substance abuse services, other
Performance outcomes	Diversion from cash aid exits to increase employment earnings	Placements in employment; length of employment; increased earnings
Funding	WTWS is funded by TANF. Funds come from the Federal Department of Health and Human Services (DHHS) to the California Department of Social Services (CDSS) to local social service departments. States and counties have a maintenance of effort (MOE) requirement.	WtW is also funded by TANF. Base funds come from DOL to local PICs (other WtW funds go to the state or are allocated by DOL in competitive grants). Note: There is a state MOE requirement to this program. In California, the state match funds are allocated to social service departments. Only one-third of the MOE funds have been allocated so far.

Source: Contra Costa County Administrator's Office, 1998.

ness community, rather than with the individual consumer, is elitist in nature. In addition, because WIB employment services have not been as formalized (i.e., less bureaucratic) than social service employment services, some social service staff have expressed dissatisfaction with a service planning and delivery approach that seems on the surface to be less structured.

Despite differences in the formal division of labor, however, both the WIB and the social service department deliver high-quality services, and each benefits from the expertise of the other organization.

A variety of equally important but less tense evolving issues are also present. Regarding service delivery, the merged organization had to first balance the consumer focus of social services with the employer-focused assistance of the former PICs. For example, job-ready consumers should be referred to businesses if services are primarily employer focused, while work-first job placement followed by on-the-job training is the top priority if services are primarily consumer focused. Second, the organization had to decide how to structure multifunctional service delivery teams to deliver a wide range of workforce investment services within the guidelines of welfare-to-work policy. For example, in order for the WIB to receive Department of Labor welfare-to-work funding, employment services must be delivered to hard-to-serve consumers who have a poor work history, low reading or math skills, or a substance abuse problem. Consumers at different levels of functioning are eligible for CalWORKs welfare-to-work funding in EHS.

In relation to policy and planning, the WIB had to adjust to its new role in CalWORKs oversight with very little prior experience. For instance, the WIB has not traditionally reported to the board of supervisors, as social service directors have traditionally been responsible for CalWORKs policy oversight. Second, EHS had to find the best way to collaborate with the Richmond WIB, as it remains autonomous and operates a one-stop employment center in close proximity to a second center operated by the merged Contra Costa WIB. The Richmond WIB, noted for its effectiveness in serving city residents, opted not to merge in order to preserve its current sources of revenue. As the Richmond and Contra Costa WIBs provide identical services to an overlapping consumer population, it is not clear how long the Richmond WIB can retain its autonomy given the service duplication and fragmentation that results from the separation. Third, EHS needed to find the best ways to blend and leverage funding to address unmet consumer needs. For example, CalWORKs consumers with disabilities can benefit from Department of Labor welfare-to-work funding that is targeted specifically for individuals with multiple barriers to employment.

Regarding administration, the unified organization needed to find the best way for the executive directors of EHS and WIB to share leadership under the county administrator and the board of supervisors. The shared goal was to promote the most productive partnership between the two new bureau directors of policy and operations with respect to authorizing contracts and dealing with WIA financial audits.

LESSONS LEARNED

The following lessons have been identified by personnel directly involved in the merger:

1. The social services executive director should select staff for the planning committee that are most committed to promoting significant change and begin by defining the nature of the expected change in order to maximize committee progress.
2. At least one highly placed merger facilitator should begin well in advance to build leadership, consensus, and motivation for partnership with little loss of momentum during the process in order to generate and maintain reform despite staff time constraints and concerns about job change.
3. It is important to anticipate and proactively address merger-related personnel issues with the understanding that they will be eventually resolved, although perhaps not in the immediate future, and that change and risk are inevitable. For example, possible job title, responsibility, and salary adjustments should be discussed with staff so that these changes do not come as a surprise, and they should be reassured that individual concerns will be addressed as they arise in the merger process.
4. Although social service managers have long recognized the importance of involving the business community in public welfare, they have less experience with integrating highly experienced, private-sector employment specialists into public social service organizations without being promoted gradually up the organizational hierarchy.
5. The combined expertise of WIB and EHS personnel has increased the quality of employment service planning and delivery and expanded the potential for pooled funding. Prior to the merger much less communication, cooperation, and resource sharing took place between the two organizations.

Although there was some administrative confusion about the division of responsibility related to policymaking and program operations as well as some staff tension in dealing with new procedures, most staff understand the need for integrated service planning and delivery in order to provide quality employment assistance to the community.

NOTES

1. The ad hoc committee was formed by the county administrator; contained representatives from the PIC, the social service department, the county administrator, and the Contra Costa Economic Partnership; was charged with examining organiza-

tional options that maximize the availability and quality of coordinated employment training and support services; and prepared the Private Industry Council and Social Services Department Ad Hoc Committee Report (Contra Costa County Administrator's Office, 1998).

2. In the remainder of this case study the PIC is referred to by its current (postmerger) name, the workforce investment board.

3. Contra Costa County has two WIBs. The City of Richmond WIB operates independently from the Contra Costa PIC and EHS, and is not a focus of this case study.

4. The workforce investment board oversees employment policy and operations and is differentiated here from WIB staff members who contract and/or deliver employment services.

5. Despite ongoing local restructuring in response to federal guidelines, the merger may take a completely different course if the California legislature initiates new statewide WIB reform. For example, state lawmakers may decide that all WIBs need to conform to a single model, thereby curtailing several unique local restructuring efforts.

REFERENCE

Contra Costa County Administrator's Office (1998). Private Industry Council and Social Services Department ad hoc committee report: Recommendations for effective workforce development in Contra Costa County. Unpublished manuscript.

Chapter 22

Blending Multiple Funding Streams into County Welfare-to-Work Programs

Christine M. Schmidt
Michael J. Austin

In August 1996, the president signed a comprehensive federal welfare reform bill, the Personal Responsibility and Work Opportunity Reconciliation Act, which consolidated the Aid to Families with Dependent Children (AFDC), Emergency Assistance, and Job Opportunities and Basic Skills (JOBS) programs into a single block grant for Temporary Assistance to Needy Families (TANF). The primary focus of the 1996 act was to (1) provide assistance to needy families so that children may be cared for in their own homes or in the homes of relatives; (2) end the dependence of needy parents on government benefits by promoting job preparation, work, and marriage; (3) prevent and reduce the incidence of out-of-wedlock pregnancies and establish annual numeric goals toward this end; and (4) encourage the formation and maintenance of two-parent families.

In response to the federal legislation, states developed their own legislation (CalWORKs) that would adhere to the new federal guidelines while instituting welfare-to-work (WtW) programs within separate counties or statewide. Welfare agencies across the nation relied heavily on their welfare-to-work departments (formerly known as employment and training programs) to propel welfare recipients into economic self-sufficiency (Greenberg and Appenzeller, 1998). By funding welfare in block grants to states, the law provides increased flexibility to states and counties to design their own welfare-to-work programs. This flexibility enables agencies to utilize multiple forms of funding to maximize client eligibility and service outcomes.

Despite the new flexibility, blending funding streams can be complicated to manage due to different service eligibility criteria and methods of accountability. This is a case study of how Sonoma County Human Services Department blended state and federal funding to implement welfare-to-work programs that addressed an array of client needs. The case focuses on

353

the multiple funding streams used to maximize client participation and service outcomes.

LITERATURE REVIEW HIGHLIGHTS

Although literature on utilization of multiple funding for welfare-to-work programs is scarce at best, it is important to focus briefly on the management of multiple funding sources within an environment of resource dependency. While it is well known that nonprofit social service agencies seek multiple resources to accomplish specific goals, it is not always clear which political and economic forces will shape their organizational actions. External forces include the volume and nature of service demand, professional and institutional models of action, structure of available resource streams, and the actions of other similar organizations. Internal forces include agency mission and formal organizational structure (Gronbjerg, 1993). In essence, they are resource dependent.

Using a resource-dependency model for understanding organizational behavior (Gronbjerg, 1993), Gronbjerg argues that funding structures provide the critical context within which nonprofit decision making takes place. Key nonprofit funding sources, such as governmental grants, differ according to their predictability and how easily they can be controlled. Funding sources introduce uncertainty into organizational decision making. They differ in the range and nature of management tasks they require, the effort organizations must devote to these tasks, and the extent to which these tasks can be routinized (Gronbjerg, 1993, p. 32).

A major aspect of obtaining and working with government funding is data collection and cost analysis related to the number of participants, costs per participant, and program costs. The following data items are critical to the cost analysis of ongoing welfare-to-work programs (Greenberg and Appenzeller, 1998) in relationship to the time the participant spends in each program component:

1. Allowances paid to program participants (e.g., day care, clothing)
2. Vendor payments made on behalf of program participants (e.g., day care)
3. Subsidies paid to employers who hire program participants
4. Salary and fringe benefits of each staff member
5. Special purchases (e.g., forms, computers, furniture) for program use
6. Office overhead

Utilizing multiple funding is complex and challenging, as each funding source has different policies and requirements. These include the types of activities that are fundable, the level of funding available, service program requirements, deadlines and grant award dates, reporting requirements, and payment procedures. However, maintaining multiple funding sources can be advantageous to an agency by providing flexibility to meet the demands of a diverse community. The trade-off for blending multiple funding sources involves compliance with continuous monitoring and adjusting, complex client eligibility and/or program guidelines, separate financial accounting, and differing enrollment criteria and monitoring strategies. The organizational structure of Sonoma County Human Services Department made it simpler to blend funding streams because CalWORKs, Job Training Partnership Act (JTPA), and welfare-to-work funds are all monitored within the department, rather than being located in separate agencies. The following sections outline the three main legislative sources and funding streams used by Sonoma County to support programs with broad-based client eligibility and service delivery. The three pieces of federal legislation include the TANF welfare system, JTPA job-training programs, and welfare-to-work labor programs.

CALWORKS/TANF

In 1997, the passage of AB 1542, the California Work Opportunity and Responsibility to Kids Act (CalWORKs), provided a framework for the distribution of TANF funds in California. Statewide CalWORKs rules went into effect on January 1, 1998, requiring counties to phase current recipients into CalWORKs by January 1, 1999. The major changes that came with the new CalWORKs legislation included time limits on benefits, workforce participation requirements, and funding for support services that enhance an individual's ability to participate in welfare-to-work programs. One billion dollars in federal funds are available through the year 2003 as a performance bonus to reward states for moving TANF recipients into jobs.

JOB TRAINING PARTNERSHIP ACT

The federal Job Training Partnership Act authorizes and funds a number of employment and training programs in California. JTPA's primary purpose is to establish programs to provide job-training services for economically disadvantaged adults and youths, dislocated workers, and others who face significant employment barriers. JTPA is divided into four programs designed to serve a specific purpose or group. These programs help prepare individuals in California for participation in the state's workforce, increase their employment and earnings potential, improve their educational and occupational skills, and reduce their dependency on welfare.

In California, the state employment development department (EDD) administers the program and distributes funds among California's fifty-two service delivery areas (SDAs), which are comprised of units of local government and private industry councils (PIC). The PICs consist of representatives from private business, community-based organizations, organized labor, private-sector business, local government, and local educational institutions (California Employment Development Department, 2000).

WELFARE-TO-WORK

The federal welfare-to-work program was authorized in 1998 to complement the major welfare reform provisions set forth in the 1996 Temporary Assistance to Needy Families program. This new funding source complements TANF in that it is designed specifically for work-related activities for those who are least employable and face numerous barriers to employment. Services utilizing WtW funds may also be used to serve noncustodial fathers of children who receive TANF.

Unlike TANF, which is managed by the U.S. Department of Health and Human Services (DHHS), the WtW program is administered by the U.S. Department of Labor (DOL). It is intended to assist states in meeting their welfare reform objectives by providing resources to propel the least employable into sustained, long-term, unsubsidized employment. Some uses of WtW funds include but are not limited to the following (U.S. Department of Labor, 1997):

- Wage subsidies
- On-the-job training
- Job readiness
- Job-placement services
- Postemployment education and services
- Job vouchers for job readiness, placement, or postemployment services, community service, or work experience
- Job-retention services
- Other support services

Seventy-five percent of WtW funds are allocated to states based on a formula that takes into account the number of poor individuals and adult recipients of assistance under TANF in each state. States are required to pass along 85 percent of the money to local private industry councils, which oversee and guide job-training programs in geographical jurisdictions called service delivery areas. A state is allowed to retain 15 percent of the money for welfare-to-work projects of its choice. States must provide $1 of nonfederal funding match for every $2 of federal funding provided under the formula (U.S. Department of Labor, 1999).

BLENDING THREE FUNDING STREAMS

Blending these three funding sources (CalWORKs, JTPA, and WtW) allowed Sonoma County to work within federal guidelines to develop programs that increased the number of participants as well as their success in gaining and maintaining employment. If a willing participant did not meet eligibility criteria for one funding source, then the county would enroll that person using other funding sources. The following are three examples of county-developed programs that blend multiple funding streams to maximize client participation and service outcomes: youth programs, homeless services, and the Sonoma Caregivers Program.

Youth Programs

Sonoma County funded a total of five youth programs in program year 1999, including Circuit Rider Productions (Summer Youth Conservation Corps [SYCC]), Petaluma People Services Center (PPSC), Social Advocates for Youth (SAY), Sonoma County Association for Youth Development (SCAYD), and West County Community Services (WCCS).

Contracts were awarded to nonprofit agencies based on grant proposals selected by the Sonoma County Human Services Department (HSD) in keeping with community needs. Funds were blended for these youth programs in response to cuts in allocations from the previous year. Sonoma County used multiple funds in an effort to maintain their commitment to the community in serving eligible youth participants. Some funds were kept in-house by the county to offset administrative costs, with the balance being distributed through cost-reimbursement contracts for services provided by community-based organizations.

The funding for these programs was blended in the form of 60 percent JTPA and 40 percent CalWORKs. This funding split was based on the goal that 40 percent of the program participants would be members of families receiving TANF. The county prescribed the parameters of participant eligibility, and applicants were referred to the contract agency for selection and enrollment. In keeping with CalWORKs funding restrictions for this county-developed program, 40 percent of youth participants in the programs were required to be TANF eligible. In 1999, all TANF youths were exempt from CalWORKs work requirements.

For these youth programs, JTPA had a funding requirement as well. Thirty percent of total funds received must be spent in addressing the needs of out-of-school youths aged fourteen to twenty-one, who do not meet the criteria of an in-school youth (defined as a youth who has not yet attained a high school diploma and is attending school full-time). Out-of-school youths can therefore be youths that have attained a high school diploma or GED or youths that for any number of reasons are not attending school full-time.

Homeless Services

Homeless Services of Sonoma County is another example of blended funding. It involves contracts with nonprofit agencies related to subsidies. One contract with the California Human Development Corporation (CHDC) provides the homeless with wage subsidies. Another contract with the Sonoma County Community Development Commission (CDC) provides the homeless with housing subsidies. Between the two contracts, Sonoma County annually spends approximately $2 million for homeless services. Under the terms of both contracts, the agencies agree to provide services to any and all county-referred clients, and both are required to coordinate services with the other. Although performance goals are outlined in each of the contracts with the community-based organizations, they are not a requirement of the funding sources.

The following client services are described in the CHDC contract with the county:

- Case management
- Paid work experience
- Temporary unsubsidized employment
- Job-retention work maturity workshops
- Life skills training
- Workshops
- Coordination and facilitation of support services for housing
- Transportation
- Health and human resources
- Individual short-term vocational skills training
- Unsubsidized job placement and retention
- Van transportation service

The county maintains the final word on all services and participant statuses under the contract (California Human Development Corporation, 1999). The CDHC is required to submit a monthly performance report (MPR) as well as a monthly cost report (MCR) for homeless services. Participants of this program are required to develop a community service/work experience training agreement outlining their plan to meet the CalWORKs and WtW work requirements.

Sonoma County's contract with the CDC is similar to CDHC. In the contract, the CDC administers rent subsidies on behalf of county-referred clients, and they are required to submit monthly MPRs and MCRs to the human services department. The responsibilities of the CDC include, but are not limited to, processing applications, providing housing-search support, arranging leases and inspections, and providing program staff supervision. Ongoing training between the CDHC, CDC, and human services staffs occurs as necessary. Human services trains homeless services staff on policies and procedures of the SonomaWORKS/WtW program, and homeless services trains human services staff on services, policies, and procedures of their programs.

Multiple funding of homeless services in Sonoma County makes it possible to reach the most unemployable populations. The welfare-to-work funds target persons with multiple barriers to employment. Its eligibility requirements make it possible to include noncustodial parents of children receiving TANF. The CalWORKs funds provide the cash assistance that welfare-to-work cannot, in addition to support services such as child care and transportation.

Although WtW opens up eligibility for noncustodial parents, it has a rather significant limitation. Eligibility criteria for welfare-to-work funds dictate that 70 percent of funds be utilized for one group of clients, while no more than 30 percent may be used for another. The problem in Sonoma County was that the numbers of clients who fit specifically into the 30 percent eligibility category far outnumbered the limit the county could enroll. As a result, the county used additional unspent CalWORKs money to offset the costs of the additional participants.

Blended funding also has other challenges. Enrollment and monitoring of participants must be done continuously due to separate eligibility requirements and the importance of keeping separate financial accounts. Because the programs rely on state funds, new funding guidelines may require changes in program designs. Monitoring clients, determining eligibility, and adjusting programs to meet funding requirements is an ongoing administrative challenge, involving extensive paperwork and constant change.

Sonoma Caregivers Program

The Sonoma Caregivers Program grew out of the combined efforts in 1997 of staff collaboration inside Sonoma County's human services department, namely the program development manager and county in-home support services (IHSS) staff. There was a need for service providers in IHSS, and this need matched the job-development objectives of SonomaWORKS. It was determined that recruiting welfare recipients as IHSS workers, along with ongoing training and opportunities to advance within the in-home health care system, would create a win-win partnership for both programs. The county would place people in jobs and the IHSS program would have a larger staff and more flexibility. Program participants would learn job skills and have the opportunity to continue their education and receive their license as certified nursing assistants (CNAs) or home health aides (HHAs).

Recruitment was done in two main ways. First, an informational flyer was included in the mailing of the monthly income report forms encouraging interested persons to contact IHSS for job applications. Second, information was shared with potential CalWORKs participants at the mandatory orientation sessions. Those who were interested in the program were asked to fill out a questionnaire that SonomaWORKS and IHSS staff could use to assess a person's suitability for the position. If deemed suitable by SonomaWORKS staff, the application was forwarded to the screening committee. Once they had received an appropriate number of applications, IHSS and SonomaWORKS staff screened applications to select those for formal interviews. The final step came when potential participants met with employers (usually disabled persons or homebound elderly), who had the final say in selecting a person to provide attendant care.

The process continued until there were about twenty suitable participants, enough for a training group. Sonoma Caregivers training included a ten-week program designed to educate participants about the basic skills necessary for IHSS work along with the rights and responsibilities of both worker and client. Participants worked as part-time IHSS workers during the ten-week program and met for four training hours each week to cover topics such as preventive care, effects of aging, communication skills, and nutrition.

With the satisfactory completion of caregivers training, participants were given the option of progressing to the next level—the CNA training. If participants demonstrated satisfactory progress in that area, they were then given the option to participate in the HHA training process. Incentive for the CNA and HHA programs was high; wages and employability increased as participants received higher levels of skill training.

Although generally successful, the Sonoma Caregivers Program encountered several challenges. First, recruitment was difficult due to the relatively low unemployment rate in Sonoma County, and the IHSS minimum wage was lower than other entry-level wages. Second, IHSS is often physically and emotionally taxing, and many people do not want to work that hard for minimum wage.

This training program required multiple funding streams that included CalWORKs (ten-week caregivers training), JTPA (CNA and HHA training), and in-kind services from the existing IHSS program (a nurse for six hours for the ten-week period and a provider coordinator for thirty hours during the ten-week period). Because the funds were blended, the program was free to provide job training, job skills, and support services to men and women, parents and nonparents. In-kind services by IHSS enabled services to be provided that would not normally be covered under typical welfare-to-work regulations.

LESSONS LEARNED

The lessons learned about blended funding are drawn from all three case examples. The following lessons reflect a mixture of issues regarding eligibility, monitoring, training, and continuity of service:

1. It is sometimes necessary to take the risk of using alternate methods of funding client services, especially when the state-allocated funding formula does not always fit the description or needs of clients. For example, although CalWORKs/TANF funds cannot be used to provide services to noncustodial fathers of TANF-eligible children, these persons could meet eligibility requirements for WtW funding, provided that other criteria are met. Counties who see a number of unemployed fathers may do well to utilize this funding.
2. Given the constraints of underspending or overspending allocated program funds, it is necessary to closely monitor client eligibility. For example, CalWORKs has ongoing monthly eligibility monitoring while JTPA continues to fund anyone who was eligible at the onset of services. Therefore, when CalWORKs clients are no longer eligible for benefits, they can be enrolled in JTPA when space is available and eligibility criteria are met.
3. In order to help staff from different programs understand the differences in client eligibility and needs, cross training between welfare-to-work staff and contract agencies is very important. To prevent misunderstandings and potential stereotyping of clients, it is imperative

that both groups fully understand the goals and objectives of each other's programs in order to maximize program and client successes as well as monitor the extent to which personal values may be clouding professional judgments.
4. It is an ongoing challenge for management to convey to staff the importance of administrative tasks for maintaining the continuous flow of funding. Constant documentation, monitoring, and adjusting are crucial to maintaining state and federal funding. Reasons for providing certain information need to be made clear to all involved.
5. Ongoing service integration is needed where staff from programs assisting parents work in cooperation with systems assisting their children. Case managers for both groups need to communicate on a regular basis.

REFERENCES

California Employment Development Department (2000). Job Training Partnership Act. Available at <www.edd.cahwnet.gov/jtpaind.htm>.
California Human Development Corporation (1999). Contract to provide homeless services.
Dess, G.G. and Beard, D.W. (1984). Dimensions of organizational task environments. *Administrative Science Quarterly,* 29:52-53.
Greenberg, D.H. and Appenzeller, U. (1998). *Cost Analysis Step by Step: A How-to Guide for Planners and Providers of Welfare-to-Work and Other Employment and Training Programs.* New York: Manpower Demonstration Research Corporation.
Gronbjerg, K.A. (1993). *Understanding Non-Profit Funding: Managing Revenues in Social Services and Community Development Organizations.* San Francisco: Jossey-Bass Publishers.
Pfeffer, J. and Leong, A. (1977). Resource allocation in united funds: Examination of power and dependency. *Social Forces,* 55:775-790.
Pfeffer, J. and Salancik, G. (1978). *The External Control of Organizations: A Resource Dependence Perspective.* New York: Harper & Row.
Provan, K.G., Beyer, J.M., and Kruytbosch, C. (1980). Environmental linkages and power in resource-dependence relations between organizations. *Administrative Science Quarterly,* 25:200-225.
U.S. Department of Labor (1997). Welfare to Work (WtW) grants: Rules and regulations. *Federal Register,* 62(222):1,6-7.
U.S. Department of Labor, Employment and Training Administration (1999). Welfare to Work: Fact sheet. Washington, DC. Available at <www.dol.gov>.

Chapter 23

Crossover Services Between Child Welfare and Welfare-to-Work Programs

Jonathan Prince
Michael J. Austin

Human service agencies are exploring new ways of assisting individuals with multiple needs by fostering inter- and intra-agency collaboration in this era of welfare reform implementation. Increased staff collaboration is needed to address the needs of *crossover* consumers who receive both employment services in welfare-to-work programs and family maintenance services in child welfare programs. Without intra-agency collaboration, mothers receiving Temporary Assistance to Needy Families (TANF) benefits could lose them at the same time that they could lose their child through foster care placement (Frame, 1999). Carefully planned collaborative case planning and service delivery can address incompatible program requirements.

When jointly coordinated, welfare-to-work services which facilitate economic self-sufficiency and family maintenance services which preserve families can together be viewed as a comprehensive child welfare program. Both services assist children either directly (e.g., cash allocations, child care, foster care) or indirectly (e.g., helping the parent resolve a substance abuse issue and find employment); the term child welfare is frequently used to describe the service system for children who have been abused or neglected by their caretakers. According to Frame (1999),

> family welfare and child protection are viewed from a contemporary standpoint as distinct domains of domestic policy in the United States, protecting children from the vicissitudes of the market on the one hand, and protecting them from their families on the other. (p. 709)

Not all welfare-to-work service participants with children are eligible for crossover assistance. Only parents receiving in-home child welfare services to preserve the family unit (i.e., family maintenance services) qualify for TANF benefits, as parents who have children that are placed outside of the home in foster or group care can no longer receive family-based welfare-to-work services.

This case study examines a pilot project in the Contra Costa County Department of Employment and Human Services (EHS) that addresses the crossover needs of child welfare and welfare-to-work service participants. The case study includes (1) a case vignette of a consumer with service needs related to welfare-to-work and child welfare, (2) a brief review of the relevant literature, (3) the process of crossover service planning, delivery, and funding, and (4) lessons learned in the process. To illustrate crossover assistance from a service delivery perspective, the following case study highlights the experiences of a consumer receiving coordinated care (Frame et al., 1998, p. 12):

In one of her first visits with her child welfare worker, Susan anxiously described her fear of losing her CalWORKs assistance (California's welfare-to-work program) because she could not simultaneously meet the requirements of the child welfare and the welfare-to-work programs, explaining that, in addition to her child welfare obligations, she needed to remain in a job club for six to eight hours every weekday looking for work. Her child welfare worker assured Susan that child welfare and CalWORKs services could be planned and delivered jointly, and later walked down the hall of the human services building to discuss the case with Susan's CalWORKs caseworker. The two staff members agreed that it was a sensitive case—failure to meet child welfare objectives could result in loss of child custody, and failure to meet CalWORKs objectives could result in the loss of primary income.

The two staff members met with Susan to establish a case plan, agreeing that Susan can participate in the job club for four hours every weekday morning and that all child welfare, mental health, and drug treatment services can be scheduled in the afternoons. Furthermore, the CalWORKs division agreed to provide child care assistance while Susan attends to her many out-of-home obligations.

It is apparent from this example that consumers can have multiple, overlapping obligations in human service agencies and that staff members with differing areas of expertise may be unaware of these obligations. Furthermore, intradepartmental staff collaboration can address conflicting consumer obligations through coordinated case planning. Finally, in addition to preventing poor consumer outcomes, communication between intra-agency divisions can prevent inefficient use of resources and duplication or fragmentation of services.

BRIEF LITERATURE REVIEW

Very little has been written on child welfare and welfare-to-work crossover service involvement, yet the literature offers insight in three important areas. They include (1) the potential impact of welfare reform on the child welfare system, (2) the degree to which caseloads overlap, and (3) a strategy for integrating the two service delivery systems into a single system of care. Each area is discussed in turn.

The Impact of Welfare Reform on Children

The welfare reform legislation of 1996 included the responsibility-based Temporary Assistance to Needy Families program (known as CalWORKs in California). This reform of the welfare system is designed to (1) promote the self-sufficiency of welfare recipients by providing a range of employment services; (2) reduce obstacles to labor-force participation through support services which include child care, transportation, mental health counseling, and substance abuse treatment; and (3) reduce welfare dependency through the use of time limits and the sanctioning of benefits.

Because welfare benefits are no longer an entitlement, welfare-to-work sanctions can be detrimental to the child if parents lose their benefits for not complying with program requirements, and many states will discontinue cash allocations to the children if parents are noncompliant (Frame, 1999). Furthermore, many child welfare professionals have expressed general concern that welfare-to-work programs will increase child foster care entry and length-of-stay rates when parents and extended family members begin to reach their time limits for welfare participation and can no longer provide adequate care for children (Berns and Drake, 1999).

Finally, Frame (1999) cautions that the "surveillance" aspects of public assistance have increased with welfare reform, potentially rekindling the "suitable" and "unsuitable" parent distinction of earlier welfare traditions which led to highly subjective and overly intrusive interventions into family life. Frame quotes a TANF policy from the California Department of Services that states:

> You must cooperate with the county, state and federal staff. A county worker can come to your home at any time to check out your facts, including seeing each family member, without calling ahead of time. You may not get benefits or your benefits may be stopped if you do not cooperate.

Because a failure to cooperate could result in benefit loss, there is an increased risk of child welfare involvement if caretaking resources are no longer available (Frame, 1999).

On the other hand, welfare reform can positively affect parents and their children if it promotes employment stability, job advancement, parent sobriety, mental health, and consistent child care and school attendance (Berrick, 1999), and the creative use of TANF funding can help child welfare consumers (Frame, 1999).

Degree of Caseload Overlap

Although a large number of families in the child welfare system receive welfare-to-work services, percentages vary with location and case-tracking methods. Most locations have an average caseload crossover rate[1] of about 40 to 50 percent, yet rates of about 60 percent have been reported in New York and Riverside County, California, and have approached 80 percent in Arkansas (Riverside County, 1998; Zeller, 1999). These rates decrease when only children are studied. In an archival analysis of 63,768 children in ten California counties, Needell and colleagues (1999) found the following:

- Twenty-seven percent of children who began to receive welfare in 1990 experienced a child maltreatment report within five years.
- Twenty-two percent had a child welfare case investigation within five years.
- Eight percent had child welfare cases opened within five years.
- Three percent entered foster care within five years.

The percentage of crossover involvement decreases dramatically, however, when child welfare participation is defined by ongoing service participation (case opening) or foster care entry.

Integrating Child Welfare and Welfare-to-Work Services in a System of Care

Most current conceptualizations of child welfare services and welfare-to-work assistance do not reflect an understanding of the overlap between the two programs. Child welfare services have focused on child protection, family preservation, and permanence, while welfare-to-work programs have been concerned primarily with employment, removal of barriers to labor-force participation, and benefit eligibility. However, the El Paso County Department of Human Services in Colorado has bridged this separation by *conceptualizing welfare-to-work assistance as a child welfare prevention program*. The many service needs that are important in preventing child abuse and neglect are addressed in welfare-to-work programs, including income maintenance, employment, housing, nutrition, medical care, substance abuse, education, training, and child care (Berns and Drake, 1999). The department has integrated the two programs by

- investing $6.5 million in unspent TANF funds, resulting from a decreased caseload, in child welfare prevention services;
- providing child welfare workers with additional resources and supports through TANF funds;
- implementing a TANF-funded program that provides cash and comprehensive support services to grandparents and other kin who are raising extended family members to preserve the biological family and prevent out-of-home placement;
- offering TANF-supported child care assistance to families in the child welfare system; and
- supporting teen parents who are at risk for child abuse and neglect through teen TANF program services that include home visits, crisis intervention, nurse visitation, parenting instruction, continuing education, job training, and mentoring.

In sum, the literature on child welfare and welfare-to-work crossover services discusses (1) the impact of TANF sanctions and time limits on adult benefit loss and the associated risk of child welfare involvement if caretaking resources are no longer available, (2) the implications of overlapping caseloads, as most locations have an average caseload crossover rate of about 40 to 50 percent, and (3) a strategy for integrating the two service delivery systems into a single system of care by conceptualizing welfare-to-work assistance as a child welfare prevention program. The next section describes crossover services in Contra Costa County.

CROSSOVER SERVICE PLANNING

Social services staff recognized the need for crossover service planning soon after the early 1998 implementation of CalWORKs, and to address this need the director formed a crossover team which met several times to define cross-program issues. In an initial training session, the crossover team was oriented by completing a survey to see how much CalWORKs staff knew about child welfare policy and how much child welfare staff knew about CalWORKs policy, as illustrated in Box 23.1.

Administration of these surveys revealed a lack of knowledge on the part of both child welfare and CalWORKs staff. To facilitate greater intradepartmental knowledge and partnership, the crossover team continued to educate each other by distributing a biweekly newsletter discussing cross-program issues and utilized a consultant to identify cross-training needs and recom-

> **Box 23.1. Professional Cross-Program Surveys**
>
> *Examples of Questions for Child Welfare Staff That Relate to CalWORKs Services*
>
> 1. A client who is a domestic violence victim has a three-month exemption before CalWORKs time limits begin. True/False
> 2. A parent about to reunify with his/her child is able to receive that child's CalWORKs grant for two months prior to the child's return. True/False
> 3. Lack of immunizations and poor school attendance will affect a family's CalWORKs eligibility. True/False
>
> *Examples of Questions for CalWORKs Staff That Relate to Child Welfare Services*
>
> 1. CPS has seventy-two hours to investigate a screened-in report of child abuse and/or neglect. True/False
> 2. A typical CPS case plan may include
>   (a) a parenting class requirement
>   (b) visitation guidelines
>   (c) a substance abuse treatment and/or requirement
>   (d) instructions for care of the child
>   (e) a, b, and c
> 3. For children over the age of three, parents have twenty-four months to reunify with their children. True/False

mend strategies for facilitating collaboration. To assist direct service workers, the team then (1) developed examples of collaborative case plans; (2) defined crossover objectives, services, and consumers; (3) defined child welfare assistance, especially court-ordered services, as more pressing than CalWORKs responsibilities, which can be postponed or reduced with less severe consequences; and (4) provided training about assistance offered in both divisions and how to identify and access CalWORKs funds (generally less restrictive than child welfare funding) for serving crossover consumers.

The next step involved the identification of crossover cases. Child welfare and CalWORKs crossover cases are identified by consumer self-report or by the child welfare screening unit clerk who identifies overlapping cases from the management and information system (MIS). The screening unit clerk first identifies all *existing* crossover consumers in the MIS and then identifies *new* cases in child welfare clearances that accompany CalWORKs applications. Once identified, the screening unit clerk alerts staff in both divisions with a "XOVER 1" form. The worker in either division then asks the adult consumer to sign a form authorizing exchange of information among child welfare and CalWORKs staff, in addition to health, mental health, and substance abuse staff if the consumer is in need of assistance in these areas. Different procedures are followed when a CalWORKs staff member refers directly to the child welfare division if (1) the welfare-to-work consumer is a homeless or unsupervised minor, (2) the children of the consumer are not attending school, or (3) when domestic violence or sexual assault issues are involved.

The team then planned the delivery of crossover services. The first step is for staff to contact the co-worker in the other division, discussing the consumer's program needs and developing a coordinated plan of action. The next step involves the staff in making recommendations to the consumer that child welfare and welfare-to-work activities be integrated in the case plan. A discussion of welfare-to-work activity and self-sufficiency is needed in the case plan to justify the utilization of crossover services, and a meeting with a county judge or counsel may be required for these services to be accepted in a court-approved plan. With consumer consent to release information and CalWORKs staff approval, the child welfare consumer is then referred to employment specialists. This staff person is authorized to issue payment for the approved service with knowledge of the service provider's name, address, phone number, federal identification or social security number, description of the service provided, and the case identification number of the consumer. Finally, both staff members monitor the attendance and progress of consumers receiving crossover services.

The crossover team developed outcome measures of success and encouraged child welfare staff to claim welfare-to-work activities, when appropriate, on employee quarterly time studies that are used to secure CalWORKs funding. The service criteria for such claims include the following:

1. communicating with a client, supervisor, co-workers, employment services personnel, or other concerned professionals about CalWORKs;
2. reading about CalWORKs;
3. attending CalWORKs meetings and training;
4. preparing, maintaining, and monitoring an integrated crossover case plan; and
5. evaluating, monitoring, and reviewing case plans from other divisions that directly or indirectly promote employment (including CalWORKs, substance abuse, mental health, and domestic violence).

CROSSOVER SERVICE DELIVERY

In April 1999, the delivery of crossover services began after several months of planning. Previously, direct service staff from both CalWORKs and child welfare divisions within the agency had been surprised to learn that a consumer was a service recipient in the other division. This sometimes led to a revision of the separate case plans and a redetermination of benefit eligibility.[2] It became clear that if these crossover cases could be identified during the intake process, it would facilitate collaborative case planning at the start of service delivery. A child welfare consumer flowchart, redesigned to illustrate where welfare-to-work crossover services are delivered, is shown in Figure 23.1.

In addition to providing services jointly in the areas noted in Figure 23.1, it became evident that cross-program partnership is especially important

1. at the opening, assignment, reassignment, review, closing, or sanctioning of a case;
2. during assessments of financial hardships in areas such as housing, child care, or transportation;
3. during a period of noncompliance with case plans;
4. when the consumer is experiencing difficulty relating to child abuse, domestic violence, substance abuse, or mental health problems or cannot access appropriate child care or housing; and
5. upon the removal, return, or birth of a child, or when a parent or significant other leaves or returns to the home or goes to prison.

It became apparent that effective crossover service delivery can help consumers to retain family members and benefits. Child welfare staff can prevent overpayment or underpayment to the family by notifying CalWORKs staff about changes in household composition, such as when children have been removed or returned to the home. Furthermore, it soon became evident that efficient crossover assistance can reduce service duplication and improve communications between divisions.

CROSSOVER SERVICE FUNDING

Although current Contra Costa County CalWORKs and child welfare funding does not overlap,[3] by claiming welfare-to-work activity on quarterly time studies child welfare staff can collectively demonstrate the need for additional staff to deliver welfare-to-work services that promote employment, such as the following:

- substance abuse treatment, including assessments and evaluations;
- transportation for any consumer attending a welfare-to-work activity;
- child care for any consumer attending a welfare-to-work activity;

- parenting classes and child-parent enrichment programs that address the issues of working parents;
- inpatient or outpatient health or mental health services, including assessments and evaluations;
- anger-management classes that address issues of anger in the workplace; and
- domestic violence services for the batterer.[4]

County TANF funding is granted in capped block payments, yet in order to access these funds counties must first spend their own local share in what is termed "Maintenance of Effort" (MOE). Only after the local MOE is reached can counties receive federal and state government funding. By contrast, child welfare funding is consumer driven in that counties are reimbursed according to the average caseload costs per employee. For example, family maintenance workers in Contra Costa County assist about thirty-five families per month, and federal and state reimbursement is determined by calculating worker salary, supplies, administrative support, and other expenses needed to manage this caseload.

Compared to open-ended reimbursement, counties generally have more difficulty functioning financially within the limits of capped grants, yet as a result of decreased caseloads, TANF funding is currently more available than child welfare funding. For this reason crossover funding is currently unilateral, involving one-way transfers from CalWORKs to child welfare. However this may not always be the case, as TANF funding can easily decrease as a result of an increase in the TANF caseload during the next recession or a legislative decision to reduce underutilized block payments.

NEXT STEPS

Staff have identified several next steps in crossover service planning and delivery, including the following:

- providing for crossover needs in other areas, such as housing and dental work;
- determining permissible CalWORKs funds that are to be used for crossover services by clarifying federal, state, and local laws and budgets;
- dedicating several staff to crossover consumer caseloads and hiring a permanent manager of crossover services;
- helping staff to know with whom to communicate in the other division once crossover cases are identified; and

- considering locating crossover service delivery, planning, and administration at neighborhood-based service integration team sites that offer CalWORKs, substance abuse, mental health, youth, probation, and school services.

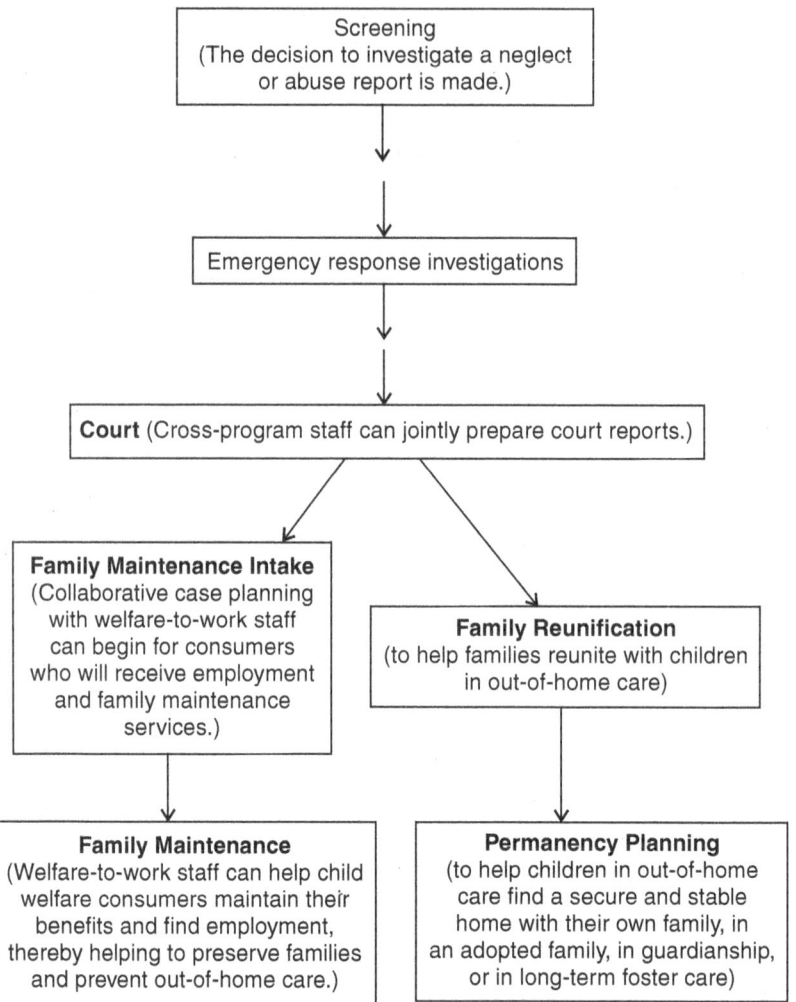

FIGURE 23.1. Welfare-to-Work Crossover Service Delivery in the Child Welfare System

Note: Crossover service delivery areas are typed in bold.

LESSONS LEARNED

Contra Costa County staff members have learned several major lessons from crossover service planning, delivery, and funding. In relation to funding, it will be difficult to maintain CalWORKs crossover funding to child welfare consumers when welfare-to-work funds become less available in the next recession. For instance, when a higher unemployment rate expands welfare caseloads, it will become more difficult to obtain incentive funds for facilitating the self-sufficiency of consumers, and less CalWORKs funding will be available to cross over to the child welfare division. CalWORKs administrators are currently concerned that child welfare staff may rely too heavily on TANF funding that will not be as easily accessible in the future.

In relation to service delivery, it has been difficult to maintain consumer confidentiality, despite having obtained consumer consent to release information, especially relating to highly sensitive child welfare issues. As a result, many surveyed CalWORKs staff reported feeling that Child Protective Services staff did not want to release important client data. The three most important lessons, however, include the following:

1. The early identification of crossover cases is not as straightforward a process as it at first may seem, and staff are still trying to decide why, for example, in March 2000 the child welfare division identified 170 crossover cases while CalWORKs identified 475 cases. These numbers should be the same, as a crossover consumer is by definition receiving services in both divisions.
2. It is a challenge for staff to find additional time to collaborate while maintaining ongoing job responsibilities, and a gradual reduction in staff interest occurs if crossover planning is not steadily reinforced by management. This loss of project momentum reduces coordinated case-planning efforts.
3. It is apparent that consumers can have multiple, overlapping obligations in human service agencies and that staff members with differing areas of expertise may be unaware of these obligations. Intradepartmental staff collaboration can address conflicting consumer obligations through coordinated case planning, and communication between intra-agency divisions can prevent inefficient use of resources and duplication or fragmentation of services.

Effective crossover service delivery can help consumers to retain family members and benefits, and child welfare staff can prevent overpayment or underpayment to the family by notifying CalWORKs staff about changes in household composition, such as when children have been removed or returned to the home. Furthermore, efficient crossover assistance can improve communication between divisions. Finally, child welfare staff can collectively utilize CalWORKs funds for services that promote employment, including health services, substance abuse treatment, mental health services, transportation, child care, and parenting classes.

NOTES

1. Caseload crossover refers to the cross-sectional estimation of the number of individuals on both child welfare and welfare-to-work caseloads.
2. Benefits may have to be discontinued if, for example, the only child of a parent participating in CalWORKs is removed from the home because of abuse or neglect.
3. The federal and state CalWORKs allocations for fiscal year 1999-2000 total $25,117,811. Of this amount, about 23 percent is for eligibility administration, 36 percent is for employment services, 39 percent is for child care, and the remaining 2 percent is for case management. Contra Costa County must first spend $4,126,052 (the Maintenance of Effort) before receiving state and federal funding. Child welfare funding is allocated by categories that include eligibility determination, training, court services, case management, emergency assistance, staff development, and group home visits. Child welfare allocations for fiscal year 1999-2000 total $24,993,568. Of this amount, the federal government contributes about 40 percent, the state government 40 percent, and the county government 20 percent. Each child welfare staff member has a workload standard, or a specified number of consumers that can be assisted each month within service categories. Currently, emergency response staff are funded for 320 consumers, family maintenance staff for thirty-five consumers, family reunification staff for twenty-seven consumers, and permanent placement staff for fifty-four consumers per month. When caseload standards are reduced, the amount of funding remains constant and staff members are given additional time to work with each consumer. Unused funds in one category are shifted as needed, and the county employs additional staff that are not federally or state funded.
4. Victims of domestic violence are exempt from CalWORKs program requirements and related services.

REFERENCES

Berns, D.A. and Drake, B.J. (1999). Combining child welfare and welfare reform at a local level. *Policy and Practice of Public Human Services,* 57(1), 26-35.

Berrick, J.D. (1999). Entitled to what? Welfare and child welfare in a shifting policy environment. *Children and Youth Services Review,* Special Double Issue, 21(9-10), 709-717.

Frame, L. (1999). Suitable homes revisited: An historical look at child protection and welfare reform. *Children and Youth Services Review,* Special Double Issue, 21(9-10), 719-754.

Frame, L., Berrick, J.D., Lee, S., Needell, B., Cuccaro-Alamin, S., Barth, R.P., Brookhart, A., and Pernas, M. (1998). *Child welfare in a CalWORKs environment: An empirically-based curriculum*. University of California: Child Welfare Research Center.
Needell, B., Cuccaro-Alamin, S., Brookhart, A., and Lee, S. (1999). Transitions from AFDC to child welfare in California. *Children and Youth Services Review, Special Double Issue, 21*(9-10), 815-841.
Riverside County (1998). Child welfare services—CalWORKs interface. Unpublished internal document.
Zeller, D.E. (1999). Welfare reform impacts on child welfare caseloads: A research agenda. The Arkansas Department of Human Services, Division of Children and Family Services. Available at <http://www.state.ar.us/dhs/chilnfam/nawrs/wriocwc.html>.

SECTION V:
CONCLUSION
AND FUTURE CONSIDERATIONS

Chapter 24

Managing Out: The Community Practice Dimensions of Effective Agency Management

Michael J. Austin

As seen in all the previous cases, the implementation of welfare reform provides those holding management positions in public social service agencies and nonprofit agencies with new challenges (Austin, 2003). One of these challenges involves the need to expand and refine the community practice skills needed to guide organizational change and reposition public social service agencies in local communities. This analysis builds upon some of the early findings emerging from welfare reform implementation. For example, Chapter 1 describes a study of county social service directors which includes the following challenges facing managers: (1) restructuring the agency's mission to capture the shift from determining eligibility to fostering self-sufficiency, (2) substantial organizational restructuring, (3) engaging in partnerships and collaborations with a wide range of partners, including other county departments, community-based organizations, and for-profit businesses, (4) renewed pressure to integrate services as part of interagency collaborations and interdisciplinary teams, and (5) increased demand for data-based planning and evaluation at all levels of the organization (Carnochan and Austin, 2002). Although strengthening an agency's mission, engaging in organizational restructuring, and data-based planning and evaluation are part of the traditional skill sets of most senior managers, the *building of community partnerships* and fostering *interdisciplinary practice* require community practice skills. This final chapter focuses on community-based interagency partnerships and intra-agency collaboration as a way

---

This chapter originally appeared in *Journal of Community Practice* 10(4): 33-48. Copyright 2002 The Haworth Press, Inc.

of addressing the community practice skills needed for effective networking inside and outside the agency. As cases reflect practice in nonprofit community-based organizations as well as public social service agencies, these managerial skills are relevant for all aspects of managing service delivery, partnership development, and agency restructuring.

MANAGEMENT PRACTICE AS WE KNOW IT

The literature on managerial skills in the human services reflects a primary focus on overseeing the work of others (Austin, 1981; Kettner, 2002; Lewis et al., 2001; Lohman and Lohman, 2002; Netting, Kettner, and McMurty, 1993; Rapp and Poertner, 1991). This focus includes an emphasis on supervising staff, managing financial and information resources, assessing client needs, and evaluating services, service and program planning, and resource acquisition to maintain the agency's viability. This emphasis has its origins in the management sciences, where lessons from the for-profit arena have been adapted and modified for the nonprofit sector (Au, 1994). For the purposes of this analysis, these traditional management functions are defined as *managing down* (Keys and Bell, 1982). In contrast, *managing up* involves middle management and top management influencing the thinking and behaviors of those at higher levels of authority (Austin, 1988). This chapter explores a third domain of managerial practice, namely, *managing out*. Managing out is defined here as the relationship-building process whereby top managers continuously network internally with their senior management group and externally with agency board members or county commissioners as well as with other community leaders and agency executives, and middle managers actively network with other middle managers inside their own agency as well as outside with colleagues in other agencies.

The challenges of reaching out and networking are similar for both agency directors and middle managers. The increased pressure to integrate services, facilitate organizational change, foster interdisciplinary practice, and identify best practices is forcing middle and top managers to refine or add the community practice skills of managing out to their expertise in managing down and managing up. The community practice skills related to managing out include the group work skills of working on an interagency task force, the community work skills of building coalitions *inside and outside* the agency, and the community involvement and development skills needed to address social service issues. When referring to community practice skills, Weil's (1996) definition provides the context for the practice of managing out. She refers to community building as the foundation of community practice that includes the activities, practices, and policies which support and foster positive connections among individuals, groups, organizations, neighborhoods, and geographic and functional communities. Managing out involves all of these connections but uses the service delivery agency as the auspice for reaching out to people inside and outside the agency. From one perspective of managing out, the agency can be viewed as a community unto itself, with its own history, power structure, leadership capacities, communication patterns, and future directions. From another perspective, the agency can be seen as simply one element in a network of agencies and neighborhood/community organizations.

The need for knowledge and skills in the area of managing out emerged dramatically in the early 1980s when social agencies confronted the first major round of budget cuts, resource scarcity, and organizational restructuring (Austin, 1984). The early 1980s were a wake-up call signaling the end of the era of continuous growth in human service expenditures and the beginning of an era of planning for the strategic use of scarce resources. Agency executives began to realize that new leadership capacities were needed to more actively reach out and network with other agencies, funding sources, and governing bodies outside their agencies. Using coalitions to lobby at the local, state, and national levels and expand relationships with board members and community influentials became a top priority for agency directors. Some of the outreach lessons of the 1980s were repeated in the 1990s as public social service agency directors and staff reached out and networked in the rapidly changing environment of welfare reform and managed care.

When it comes to incorporating community practice into management practice, the managing out process can be viewed in terms of Quinn's (1988) leadership domain of boundary spanning. This domain involves the skills of political negotiation and utilizing power relationships to carry out the roles of broker and innovator. *Brokering* includes the resource acquisition skills of developing and maintaining interpersonal relationships, monitoring the community environment, promoting collaborative relations with other organizations in the community, and effectively using power and influence. The *innovator* role involves envisioning and facilitating change by managers seeking out new opportunities, encouraging and utilizing new ideas, and displaying a high level of tolerance for ambiguity and capacity to take risks.

The early signs of the need for middle managers to manage out can be found in the research of Havassy (1990), who noted that successful supervisors are able to accept and deal with differences by (1) dealing with underlying *connectedness* (searching for common ground required of someone in the middle) as a way to tolerate ambiguity, (2) *spanning boundaries* between various systems (departments inside and outside the agency) by maintaining loyalty to multiple groups, and (3) engaging in *cross-system communication* by expressing the needs, expectations, and demands for one system (top management or line staff) in the terms and concepts of another. In a similar way, Floyd and Woodridge (1996) identified the key interpersonal components of middle-management practice: *synthesizing* (gathering new information and understanding the need for change), *facilitating* (preparing for change and nurturing the creative efforts of others), *championing* (stimulating change by matching recognized and unrecognized capabilities with emerging opportunities), and *implementing* (managing the process of changing the way existing capabilities are deployed). Successful efforts to manage out require synthesizing new information, nurturing the creative efforts of others, seizing opportunities to promote change, and bringing people and resources together in new ways.

It is clear that the nature of managerial practice has shifted dramatically over the past two decades, from a primary focus on internal operations to a more external, community focus. As Menefee and Thompson (1994, p. 23) found in one of the few studies of management practice in social service settings,

> No longer are social work managers predominantly concerned with structures, processes, and conditions within the agency; they now give equal if not more attention to the entire context of service delivery by actively monitoring and managing the boundary between the external environment and internal organizational arrangements.

Menefee and Thompson noted that managers actively engage in modeling the values and practices of boundary spanning for their staff as they seek to foster greater staff and community ownership in the service of the agency. They identified the core skills as networking, managing internal and external relationships, lobbying external and internal constituencies, fostering agency-community relations, and effectively using one's own power. They also found that boundary spanning took place at least once a week and was regarded as very important by the managers in their study.

In a follow-up study, Menefee (1998) found that boundary spanning had become the central skill needed for fostering internal and external relationships. The skills for successful boundary spanning include communicating, teaming, facilitating, aligning, and coordinating, which are defined as follows (Menefee, 1998):

- *Communicating:* Exchanging information between the agency and its internal and external stakeholders by keeping staff informed, making presentations in the community, and developing publications and related correspondence.
- *Teaming:* Organizing and enlisting the work of groups to support agency operations and services by developing coalitions to respond to

community needs, organizing and developing staff teams, planning and leading agency/community initiatives, and modeling effective meeting management capabilities.
- *Facilitating:* Enabling others to carry out the work of the agency by helping others (staff and community) to influence agency operations and programs, empowering staff with educational experiences and career guidance, educating the board and community, and serving as a role model.
- *Aligning:* Arranging or rearranging structures, processes, and resources by delegating tasks and responsibilities, organizing tasks into jobs or programs, recruiting and hiring staff, and maintaining staff morale.
- *Coordinating:* Directing and guiding the agency, which includes service delivery and infrastructure development, coordinating units/departments, attending to staff needs and concerns, providing distance supervision in the form of oversight/monitoring, and consulting through the use of advising and supporting staff.

This set of boundary-spanning skills is part of a comprehensive array of managerial skills required to manage in a changing environment. The other skill sets identified by Menefee (1998) include *futuring* (strategic planning), *managing and leveraging resources* (financial, physical, material, and human), *evaluating* (needs, effectiveness, cost-benefit, and capabilities), and *policy practice* (interpreting laws/regulations, translating policies into practices, and representing the agency by lobbying/testifying before policy-making bodies).

FROM THEORY TO INFORMED PRACTICE

Before exploring the major practice components of managing out, it is important to identify some of the critical concepts from interorganizational relations theory to provide a context for understanding the need for managing out. In Reitan's (1998) review of interorganizational relations in the human services, she notes the growing shift in focus from an emphasis on intraorganizational issues to interorganizational relations. Based on an analysis which spans the social sciences, she concluded that interorganizational relations in the human services

1. feature new ways of governing through networks of agencies,
2. represent a continuous changing of intensity and content as agencies actively engage one another in an effort to address such factors as scarce resources and service fragmentation,

3. reflect interorganizational structures (collaboratives, consortia, partnerships) that are designed to ensure goal attainment and efficiency (sharing insufficient resources or providing integrated services),
4. carry significant importance for the recipients of services (accessibility, availability, responsiveness), and
5. seek stability so that they can endure.

The central feature of interorganizational relations theory is the way agency interdependence is managed as the human services increasingly shift back and forth from competition to cooperation (Hasenfeld and Giron, 1993). These issues are viewed differently by social scientists. The sociological literature on interorganizational relations focuses on cooperating relationships (Hall and Taylor, 1996), while the political economy perspective emphasizes the interagency relationship factors of transaction costs, contracting, and accountability (Reitan, 1998). The organizational psychology perspective focuses more on the strategic choices that organizational leaders make as they respond to problems in their environment by maximizing their discretion and producing different kinds of interorganizational relations (Oliver, 1988).

Each of these social science perspectives adds an important dimension to our understanding of interorganizational relations. It is also important to highlight the empirical research on interorganizational relations among human service organizations. In his search for the key ingredients which foster interorganizational collaboration, Bardach (1998, p. 157) found that interagency collaboration was a "joint activity between two or more agencies intended to increase public value by working together" based on "tangible components" (formal agreements) and "intangible components" (expectations of one another). His major contribution to our understanding of interorganizational relations is that successful relationships require a shared capacity to manage joint activity. In so doing, he isolated the following critical ingredients to managing collaboration:

1. an operating system that promotes flexibility around turf issues, cross training to enhance trust and open dialogue, peer accountability, and financial incentives;
2. the sharing of resources (acquiring and allocating fiscal, human, and facility resources);
3. establishing a process of shared leadership to steer a course (strategic directions, customer-centered, shared problem solving, leadership succession planning, and a set of shared values to guide decision making);

4. building a culture of joint problem solving (embracing change, mediating differences, and continuous trust building); and
5. action planning (a structure of specific steps that builds from the bottom up and generates/sustains momentum beginning with early successes).

To foster and maintain the collaborative process, Bardach (1998) calls for "administrative craftsmanship" in the form of seizing opportunities, playing new roles, converting problems into challenges, appreciating the slow pace of developing collaborations, working backward from the goals to be achieved to build action steps, and "muddling through" to address shortcomings and promote continuous process improvement. Many of these elements of interagency collaboration are central to the process of managing out.

In addition to Bardach (1998), it is also important to note the significant empirical work of Alter and Hage (1993) on interorganizational networks and relationships. Their contribution is in the form of an evolutionary theory of collaboration and a set of key questions. The core elements of their theory are as follows:

1. willingness to collaborate (linked to a culture of trust, history and complexity of relationships),
2. need for expertise (linked to innovation, standardization, and task complexity),
3. need for financial resources and shared risk (linked to the political economy of the organizational environment and the specialization of each agency's market niche), and
4. need for adaptive efficiency (linked to the size of collaborating organizations and the pace of change in technology and knowledge).

While they document the complexity of interorganizational relationships, they also provide important guideposts to the continuous search for understanding this complexity. The guideposts are in the form of key questions (p. 261):

- What pushes organizations toward collaboration in spite of the difficulties?
- What are the forms of collaboration and how do they differ?
- What influences the way in which systemic networks (of organizations) are structured and operate?
- What influences the choices of partners and ensures compliance (with shared goals)?

These questions can provide a foundation for evaluating the impact of managing out.

Finally, the search for theory to inform practice needs to include the impact of internal operations on the external agency relationships. In essence, the ability to collaborate successfully with other organizations can be linked to the effectiveness of internal relationships and processes within the agency. This perspective takes us to the important work of Hastings (1993) and Senge (1990). Hastings focuses attention on shifting the organizational culture from a traditional, bureaucratic mode to a new culture of networking. Senge identifies the important organizational roles needed to develop a learning organization.

It has become increasingly clear that leadership at any level in an organization is directly affected by the culture of the organization and the organization's capacity to learn and change (Schein, 1988). Identifying and modifying elements of an organization's culture can be exceedingly difficult. One approach used by Hastings (1993) is to restructure organizations by creating organizational networks and thereby grow a new organizational culture. The first step is to identify the nature of the old, traditional culture in contrast to the new, networking culture. Hastings (1993) identifies four key elements that need to be addressed in order to transform an organization's culture from the old way of doing business to the new networking model of operations, namely, role, relationships, communication, and organizational perspective. Some examples of this transformation include the following:

1. making the *role* transition from one of specialists telling others to one of specialists learning from others,
2. facilitating the *relationship* transition from exclusivity to inclusivity,
3. modifying the *organizational perspective* from top down to inside out and outside in, and
4. transforming the *communication of information* from retaining information to sharing information

Changing the organizational culture is related to transforming human service agencies into learning organizations. Senge (1990) first identified the art and practice of building a learning organization in which staff continually expand their capacities to understand complexity, clarify vision, improve their ability to think creatively, and take responsibility for continued learning. The challenge for the transformational manager is to foster a learning environment by refining one's skills in carrying out the following roles:

1. *designer* or "organizational architect" who constructs learning processes to deal productively with critical issues and develop a sense of mastery whereby all staff can approach their work from the perspective of "What can I learn today?" rather than "What must get done today?",
2. steward who seeks to balance the desire for continuity with the desire for innovation by integrating the big picture into the daily testing of new ideas as well as listening to the ideas of others as a way to demonstrate a willingness to change or modify one's own vision of the future, and
3. teacher who helps staff achieve more accurate, insightful, and empowering views of reality by shifting the focus of attention beyond the daily events and patterns of behavior (reactive) to the organization's purpose for existence and future direction (proactive) to assist others in developing systemic understandings of the role of the agency in the community.

Each of these leadership roles is valuable for building a learning community inside and outside the organization by identifying the forces that contribute to current realities. The gap between current realities and the vision produces the creative tension needed to energize others. For example, the extensive efforts made by some California county social service agencies to involve the community in developing the county's welfare reform plan provided all segments of the community (including the business community) an opportunity to contribute to a new service system as well as share ownership in its processes and outcomes.

This brief literature review provides a foundation of key concepts for exploring the process of managing out. With regard to organizational structures, Bardach's (1998) concepts suggest that new structures inside and outside the organization are needed to create effective operating systems, facilitate the sharing of resources and leadership, and establish mechanisms for linking joint problem solving with action planning. When it comes to redefining organizational processes, Alter and Hage (1993) identify critical concepts that can facilitate collaborative processes, namely, a willingness to collaborate as well as a recognized need for expertise, shared risk, and adaptive efficiency. One way to capture the interrelationships of these structural and process concepts is to frame them as part of the following checklist for those in organizations who are engaged in managing out.

Organizational Structures (Bardach, 1998)

- Do we have the human resource capacities to build operating systems to support interagency collaboration in the community?

- Do we have the mechanisms in place to share resources and leadership in the community?
- Do we have mechanisms for joint problem solving (internal work groups or external advisory groups) that can facilitate action planning and community collaboration?

Organizational Processes (Alter and Hage, 1993)

- Do we have a method for demonstrating our willingness to collaborate and monitor the messages?
- Do we have mechanisms in place to identify our need for expertise, our capacity to share risks, and our commitment to collaboration and change?

In addition to this focus on organizational structures and processes, the literature on organizational collaboration also suggests the need to redefine managerial leadership. As Hastings (1993) noted, traditional organizations need leadership that can foster a networking culture which calls for changes in roles, relationships, communications, and perspectives. In a similar way, Senge (1990) is calling for the new leadership roles of designer, steward, and teacher. Each of these concepts can be reflected in the following questions that address the leadership challenges facing organizations with staff committed to effectively managing out:

Fostering a Networking Culture (Hastings, 1993)

- Is there a capacity to promote *networks of staff* inside and outside the organization where help seeking is seen as a strength by staff who reach out for consultation and advice?
- Are there ways to promote *multidisciplinary teamwork* based on *relationships* that are inclusive, capable of searching for common goals with outsiders, and oriented toward reducing barriers to exchange in the community?
- Can *information* be *shared* on the basis of wanting to know rather than a need to know?
- Can the *organizational perspectives* of staff be altered from a top down to an inside out and outside in viewpoint where boundaries are spanned, ambiguity is tolerated, and responsibilities are shared with others in the community?

Adopting New Leadership Roles (Senge, 1990)

- How do leadership styles need to be modified to become the *designer* of learning processes that deal productively with critical issues?
- How does one's day-to-day work reflect a balance between the need for continuity and the need for innovation that includes actively testing new ideas, listening for new ideas, and demonstrating a capacity to change one's views (*stewardship*)?
- How does one help staff gain new insights about the need to maintain a balance between reactive and proactive behaviors as well as gain a more holistic understanding of the role of the organization in the community (*teacher*)?

These questions, which seek to link theory with practice, provide a context for describing the community practice aspects of managing out in human service organizations.

THE MULTIPLE DIMENSIONS OF MANAGING OUT

Although managing out can be demonstrated at all levels of staff (e.g., secretaries who coordinate effectively with other units in the agency as well as network effectively with agencies and clients in the community), the focus here is on the top and middle levels of management. Irrespective of the level of management, managing out can include the three key functions of leading, managing, and partnering. Using Kotter's (1990) definitions for leading and managing, *leading* relates to coping with change (setting directions, aligning people, and motivating/inspiring) and *managing* refers to coping with complexity (planning and budgeting, organizing and staffing, and evaluating and problem solving). The third concept of *partnering* relates to the governance of human service organizations in a community, such as working with governing boards and interagency advisory boards (public and voluntary) and monitoring changing community needs and building partnerships with a wide variety of institutions and individuals. In order to illustrate the potential array of activities related to managing out, sample activities are highlighted in Table 24.1 for two levels of management (middle and top) and the three domains of management practice (leading, managing, and partnering).

Although the agency director may be able to devote a substantial portion of a typical work week to managing out, the challenge of setting priorities is no different than for anyone else holding a management position in the agency. However, in the case of top management there may be greater freedom and autonomy (often as a result of delegating tasks to others) than can

TABLE 24.1. Sample Activities of Managing Out

Leading: Coping with Change	Managing: Coping with Complexity	Partnering: Building and Maintaining Relationships
Top Management		
• Scanning the local, regional, state, and national environment for issues of potential importance to the organization • Developing a shared vision of the organization's future by involving all key stakeholders • Continuously on the alert for opportunities to promote interagency collaboration	• Continuously seeking client's assessment of the organization • Consistently team building at the top of the organization • Extensive schedule of meetings with key people outside the organization • Conscientiously mentoring those inside the organization	• Consistently fostering improved executive board relations • Coalition building at local, regional, state, and national levels • Seeking public speaking and lobbying opportunities to market the organization • Continuously seizing opportunities to celebrate successes inside and outside the organization
Middle Management		
• Continuously assessing the needs for internal organizational change • Actively participating in setting organizational priorities • Proposing and designing strategies to modify and strengthen operations	• Negotiating and mediating interdepartmental conflicts • Building coalitions inside the organization • Continuously fostering a climate of collegiality and sharing • Repeatedly searching for opportunities for team building • Mentoring others inside the organization	• Building coalitions with colleagues outside the organization • Negotiating and mediating interagency conflicts • Mentoring others outside the organization • Fostering a climate of collegiality and sharing in the community • Continuously seizing opportunities to celebrate successes inside and outside the organization

be found in the middle-management ranks. There is also greater accountability to keep members of the agency's governing board apprised of the director's managing out efforts on behalf of the agency. Although most successful directors understand the importance of networking and relationship building in the community, it has only recently become apparent that proactively seeking and scheduling public speaking engagements with community groups needs to receive higher priority (McDaniel, 1994). These outreach activities address one of the most neglected areas of human service administration, namely community and media relations (Brawley, 1995). By managing out, managers can engage in the continuous process of educating the American public about the nature of human services, sharing the successes emerging daily from excellent staff work, and reminding the community that it is their neighbors who need support from everyone, not just from the public and nonprofit human service agencies (Goldberg, Cullen, and Austin, 2001).

The challenges facing middle managers and supervisors related to managing out can be substantial. Although top management has the authority to manage out, middle managers often need to secure that authority from top management. Even with the delegated authority, middle managers find their managing out activities to be primarily horizontal with peers, relying more on persuasive abilities than any authority to mandate change. Some of the most prevalent challenges facing middle managers engaged in managing out can be (1) getting the right people at the table to foster exchange and collaboration across boundaries, (2) developing common understandings needed to get everyone on the same page in order to sustain momentum, (3) understanding differing agency politics that relate to turf issues in order to reach decisions, (4) dealing with the interests of agencies and communities that may differ, and (5) getting clarity as to who has authority to reach a decision and monitor its implementation. These challenges are organized into the following four areas:

1. Addressing power and leadership issues
   - Letting go of turf issues
   - Building an understanding of who has authority to make decisions
   - Knowing the politics of participating organizations
   - Handling the mutual/competing interests between agency and community
   - Meeting the needs of agencies and clients
2. Forming group structures
   - Getting the right people at that table
   - Identifying an array of stakeholders
   - Finding a time and place to meet
   - Receiving support from above

3. Fostering and maintaining group processes
   - Getting everyone on the same page
   - Getting groups to decide
   - Sustaining momentum
   - Developing common understandings
   - Motivating participants to complete agreed-upon work
   - Maintaining attendance levels
   - Dealing with previous histories that affect involvement (collaboration issues)
   - Handling a variety of issues/interests, especially competing interests
   - Facilitating without dominating
   - Identifying roles to be taken
   - Dealing with a lack of openness
   - Using the expertise of others
   - Saying the right thing (being knowledgeable and not being stereotyped)
4. Engaging in follow-up and implementation
   - Monitoring decision making and implementation
   - Ensuring unified agency position on a given issue (shared understandings)
   - Anticipating program implications
   - Identifying external constraints on implementation
   - Developing creative strategies to make departmental changes
   - Monitoring implementation to see that resources are not spread too thin

CONCLUSION

This discussion of managing out began with the community practice dimensions of spanning organizational boundaries. It was followed by an assessment of interorganizational concepts relevant to the process of managing out. This assessment identified a series of questions for agency managers to use in their ongoing assessment of the external and internal dimensions of their organizational structures and processes as well as the elements of leadership and networking. The questions provided a beginning framework for exploring the organizational dynamics of managing out. Particular attention was given to examples of managing out by those in top management as well as middle-management positions.

For middle managers, managing out to others inside their agency as well as to those in other agencies may require a significant realignment of traditional middle-management job functions (e.g., reducing the amount of time devoted to supervising staff to increasing the amount of time devoted to managing out). For senior managers, managing out may require an expanded commitment to the agency's *external* issues in the larger community as well as the *internal* issues related to promoting the culture of a learning organization (DuBrow, Wocher, and Austin, 2001).

In the cases of both middle managers and top managers, the rebalancing of current job activities to account for more managing out would mean that internal operations might receive less attention while external relations might receive more attention. Ultimately, the role of the middle manager and top manager in human service organizations will need to be redesigned if future managers are going to master the skills of managing out as well as monitor the impact of this increasingly important community practice component of effective agency management. As seen in the lessons learned from implementing welfare reform, top management will be increasingly called upon to build and maintain community partnerships and middle managers will be encouraged to give more attention to interdisciplinary practice inside and outside the agency.

REFERENCES

Alter, C. and Hage, J. (1993). *Organizations working together.* Newbury Park, CA: Sage Publications.

Au, C. (1994). The status of theory and knowledge in social welfare administration. *Administration in Social Work, 18*(3), 27-57.

Austin, M. J. (1981). *Supervisory management for the human services.* Englewood Cliffs, NJ: Prentice Hall.

Austin, M. J. (1984). Managing cutbacks in the 1980s. *Social Work, 29*(5), 428-434.

Austin, M. J. (1988). Managing up: Relationship building between middle management and top management. *Administration in Social Work, 12*(4), 29-46.

Austin, M. J. (2003). The changing relationship between nonprofit organizations and public social service agencies in the era of welfare reform. *Nonprofit and Voluntary Sector Quarterly, 32*(1), 97-114.

Bardach, E. (1998). *Getting agencies to work together: The practice and theory of managerial craftsmanship.* Washington, DC: Brookings Institution Press.

Brawley, E. (1995). *Human services and the media: Developing partnerships for change.* New Brunswick, NJ: Harwood Academic Publishers.

Carnochan, S. and Austin, M. J. (2002). Implementing welfare reform and guiding organizational change. *Administration in Social Work, 26*(1), 61-78.

DuBrow, A., Wocher, D., and Austin, M. J. (2001). Introducing organizational development (OD) practices into a county social service agency. *Administration in Social Work, 25*(4), 63-84.

Floyd, S. W. and Woodridge, B. (1996). *The strategic middle manager: How to create and sustain competitive advantage.* San Francisco, CA: Jossey-Bass.

Goldberg, S., Cullen, J., and Austin, M. J. (2001). Developing a public information and community relations strategy in a county social service agency. *Administration in Social Work, 25*(2), 61-80.
Hall, P. and Taylor, R. (1996). Political science and the three new institutionalisms. *Political Studies, 30,* 936-957.
Hasenfeld, Y. and Gidron, B. (1993). Self-help groups and human service organizations: An interorganization perspective. *Social Science Review, 67*(2), 217-236.
Hastings, C. (1993). *The new organization: Growing the culture of organizational networking.* London: McGraw-Hill.
Havassy, H. M. (1990). Effective second-story bureaucrats: Mastering the paradox of diversity. *Social Work, 35*(2), 103-109.
Kettner, P. M. (2002). *Achieving excellence in the management of human service organizations.* Boston, MA: Allen and Bacon.
Keys, B. and Bell, R. (1982). Four faces of the fully functioning middle manager. *California Management Review, 24*(4), 59-67.
Kotter, J. P. (1990). What leaders really do. *Harvard Business Review, 68*(3), 103-111.
Lewis, J. A., Lewis, M. D., Packard, T., and Souflee, F. (2001). *Management of human service programs,* Third edition. Belmont, CA: Wadsworth/Thomson Learning.
Lohman, R. A. and Lohman, N. (2002). *Social Administration.* New York: Columbia University Press.
McDaniel, R. (1994). *Scared speechless: Public speaking step by step.* Thousand Oaks, CA: Sage.
Menefee, D. (1998). Identifying and comparing competencies for social work management II: A replication study. *Administration in Social Work, 22*(4), 53-63.
Menefee, D. T. and Thompson, J. J. (1994). Identifying and comparing competencies for social work management: A practice driven approach. *Administration in Social Work, 18*(3), 1-25.
Netting, F. E., Kettner, P. M., and McMurty, S. L. (1993). *Social work macro practice.* New York: Longman.
Oliver, C. (1988). The collective strategy of framework: An application to competing preconditions of isomorphism. *Administrative Science Quarterly, 33,* 543-561.
Quinn, R. E. (1988). *Beyond rational management: Mastering the paradoxes and competing demands of high performance.* San Francisco, CA: Jossey-Bass.
Rapp, C. and Poertner, J. (1991). *Social administration: A client-centered approach.* White Plains, NY: Longman.
Reitan, T. C. (1998). Theories of interorganizational relations in the human services. *Social Science Review, 72*(3), 285-309.
Schein, E. (1988). *Organizational culture and leadership.* San Francisco, CA: Jossey-Bass.
Senge, P. M. (1990). *The fifth discipline: The art and practice of the learning organization.* New York: Doubleday.
Weil, M. O. (1996). Community building: Building community practice. *Social Work, 41*(5), 481-499.

Index

AAA (American Automobile Association), 72
Accountability of social service agencies, 43
Ad hoc culture, 28
ADD (American Dream Demonstration), 166-167
Adelante Familia NSSC, 225-226
Administrative craftsmanship, 385
Adopt-A-Family program
  adopted family experiences, 139
  challenges, 140-141
  community partnership, 42
  description of program, 134-136
  development, 132-134
  godparent experience, 137-139
  lessons learned, 139-140
  overview, 131, 141
  purpose, 32
  referring agencies, 136-137
  similar programs, 131-132
AFDC. *See* Aid to Families with Dependent Children
AFIA (Assets for Independence Act of 1998), 167-168
Agency restructuring
  organizational changes, *xx-xxii*, 38-40
  overview, *xxviii*, 17-24
  vision statement, *xxix*
Agnew, Robert, 252
Aid to Families with Dependent Children (AFDC)
  impact of PRWORA, *xvii*, 217, 353
  transportation to work obstacle, 54
  WorkCenter employment, 104, 108

Aid to the Disabled (ATD), WorkCenter employment, 108
Alameda County Neighborhood Jobs Pilot Initiative
  history, 189-191
  literature review, 191-193
  Lower San Antonio/Fruitvale, 190-191, 204-211
  overview, 189
  Prescott, 190-191, 199-204
  South Hayward, 190-191, 194-199
Aligning, defined, 383
Alliance (Assets for All Alliance), 169-172, 173
Alliance for Children and Families, 119
Alter, C., 385, 387, 388
American Automobile Association (AAA) car seat donation, 72
American Dream Demonstration (ADD), 166-167
Aroner, Dion, 169
Assembly Bill 1542, 55, 91
Assembly Bill 2454, 55
Asset building. *See* Individual Development Account
Asset-poor Americans, 165
Assets and the Poor, 166
Assets for All Alliance, 169-172, 173
Assets for Independence Act of 1998 (AFIA), 167-168
ATD (Aid to the Disabled), WorkCenter employment, 108
Austin, Michael J.
  Adopt-A-Family program, 131
  collaboration of human services agencies and community colleges, 285

Austin, Michael J. *(continued)*
  Connections Shuttle transportation, 53
  county department of employment and human services, 339
  crossover services, 363
  family development credential, 317
  Family Loan Program, 117
  Guaranteed Ride Home Program, 65
  hiring TANF participants, 153
  individual development accounts, 165
  introduction, *xvii-xxxi*
  JobKeeper Hotline, 143
  managing out, 379
  multiple funding streams, 353
  neighborhood partnerships, 189
  neighborhood self-sufficiency centers, 217
  nonprofit and county collaboration, 267
  organizational changes, 3
  organizational development in human service agency, 297
  overview of programs and practices, 27
  substance abuse and homelessness, 251
  TRAIN program, 231
  training exempt providers, 77
  welfare-to-work program, 91
  Work centers, 103

Bailey, S., 79
Bailis, L., 192
Banks
  Adopt-A-Family program, 133
  Family Loan Program, 121, 126, 127-128
  impact on Prescott deterioration, 200
  individual development accounts, 169-170
Bardach, E., 384-385, 387-388
Bardales, Judy, 136
Barnow, B., 192
Barriers
  agency-based empowerment, 318-319
  child care licensure, 87-88
Barriers to workforce participation
  child care. *See* Exempt Provider Training Project
  mental health and substance abuse. *See* SonomaWORKS
  removal of, 28-31, 43
  transportation. *See* Connections Shuttle; Guaranteed Ride Home Program
Base Closure Community Redevelopment and Homeless Assistance Act of 1994, 252
BASSC. *See* Bay Area Social Services Consortium
Bay Area Social Services Consortium (BASSC)
  background, *xxvii*, 24-25
  purpose, 3
  vision statement, 17-24
    building community, 17, 19
    career-resilient workforce, 17, 19-21
    changing professional roles, 17, 22-23
    family support, 17, 21
    family-focused, neighborhood-based human service system, 17, 22, 23
    public agency roles, 17-18, 23-24
    public policies, 18, 24
    social development approach, 17, 18
Beall, James T. Jr., 145, 217
Beasley, R. K., 48-49
Bell, C. H., 300
Black Wealth/White Wealth, 166
Blended funding. *See* Funding
Blending Funding Strategies for Youth Project, 213
Bloom, D., *xxiv*
Blue Cross Foundation grant, 273-275
Blumenberg, E., 54, 66

Boundary spanning, 381, 382-383
Bridge Communities, 234
Brokering, 381
Brookhart, A., 366
Bugental, Scott, 62
Burger King, hiring welfare recipients, 154-155
Burke, W., 299

Calhoun, J. F., 144
California Child Care Resource and Referral Network (CCCRR), 78
California Human Development Corporation (CHDC), 358-359
California Work Opportunity and Responsibility to Kids Program. *See* CalWORKs
California Work Pays Demonstration Project, 168-169
CalWORKs (California Work Opportunity and Responsibility to Kids Program)
 Assembly Bill 1542, 55, 91
 base of SonomaWORKS, 91
 child welfare and welfare-to-work crossover services, 364-365, 367-374
 colocation of services for SonomaWORKS, 96
 Connections Shuttle. *See* Connections Shuttle
 coordinating transportation, 67-68
 history, 3, 65, 217
 impact of PRWORA, 143
 JobKeeper Hotline, 146, 149
 legislation background, 355
 pooling funds, 40
 social service agency organizational changes, *xxi*
 SonomaWORKS funding, 95
 transportation problems, 68
 WorkCenters, 104
 youth programs, 357-358

Cameron, K. S., 28
Cañada College, 111, 287, 291
Candleworks, Inc., 155
Career Retention Employment Support Team (CREST), 146, 148, 149
Career-resilient workforce, BASSC vision statement, 17, 19-21
CareerWorks, 60, 61
CARF (Commission on Accreditation of Rehabilitation Facilities), 111
Carnochan, Sarah, 3
Carten, A., 253
Case management
 coordinated service system, 220
 helping welfare recipients keep jobs, 155
 for the homeless, 233-234
 impact of PRWORA, *xviii, xx*
 Transitional Residential Alliance and Integrated Network, 241-242, 244-245
Caseload overlap, 366, 374
Catholic Charities, 234, 240, 243
CBOs (community-based organizations), 190, 194
CCCRR (California Child Care Resource and Referral Network), 78
CDBG (Community Development Block Grant), 119
CDC (Sonoma County Community Development Commission), 358-359
Center for Venture Philanthropy (CVP), 169, 171
CFED (Corporation for Enterprise Development), 166
Challenges
 Adopt-A-Family program, 140-141
 child care provider training, 80
 coalition of nonprofit and county agencies, 281-282
 Connections Shuttle, 62-63

Challenges *(continued)*
  Exempt Provider Training Project, 80, 88-89
  family development credential, 333-335
  Guaranteed Ride Home Program, 73
  human services agency and community college collaboration, 292-293
  JobKeeper Hotline, 150
  Lower San Antonio/Fruitvale (LSAF) Neighborhood Jobs Pilot Initiative, 210-211
  neighborhood self-sufficiency centers, 228
  PeninsulaWorks-Daly City IDA program, 179-180
  Prescott Neighborhood Jobs Pilot Initiative, 203-204
  Pueblo Del Mar, 260-261
  SonomaWORKS, 98-99
  South Hayward Neighborhood Collaborative, 198-199
  of sustaining innovations, 45-46
  Transitional Residential Alliance and Integrated Network, 247-248
  work centers, 106
  WorkCenter, 114-116
Championing, defined, 382
Change. *See also* Organizational change
  nature and pace, 9, 11
  professional roles, 17, 22-23
CHDC (California Human Development Corporation), 358-359
Cherlin, A., *xxiv*
Child care services
  BASSC vision statement, 21
  Exempt Provider Training Project, 84
  obstacle to work, 161
  redefining service delivery, *xxvii*
  training providers. *See* Exempt Provider Training Project
Child welfare services
  caseload overlap, 366, 374
  delivery of services, 369-370, 371-372
  funding, 370-371
  lessons learned, 373-374
  literature review, 365-367
  planning crossover service, 367-369, 371-372
  professional cross-program surveys, 368
  system of care, 366-367
  TANF and, 40, 365-366
  welfare-to-work crossover services, 363-364
CIRCLES (Comprehensive Integrated Resources for CalWORKs Limited English Speakers), 206-207
Civil service tests, 160, 161-162
Civil society, BASSC vision statement, 17, 19
Clan culture, 28
Cleaver, Emanuel, 156
Clinton, Bill, 65, 154, 217
Coaching to address staff resistance to change, 5
Coalition for Workforce Preparation, 55
Coalition of nonprofit agencies
  background, 36-37
  collaboration with county agency background, 267
  challenges, 281-282
  Front Porch program, 278-279
  history, 268-269
  leadership and growth, 271-272
  lessons learned, 282-283
  literature review, 269-271
  mental health committee, 272-275
  new care system, 275-278
  program successes, 279-281
  service delivery, 41
Collaboration
  challenges, 45
  community and organizations, 6-7
  evolutionary theory, 385

Index

Collaboration *(continued)*
  human services agencies and community colleges
    background, 285-286
    certificate program, 288-291
    challenges, 292-293
    curriculum development, 286-290
    lessons learned, 294
    participants, 290-291
    purpose of program, 291-292
  management of, 384-387
  Neighborhood Jobs Pilot Initiative, 194-196, 200-201, 206, 211-212
  neighborhood self-sufficiency centers, 221
  nonprofit and county agencies
    background, 267
    challenges, 281-282
    Front Porch program, 278-279
    history, 268-269
    leadership and growth, 271-272
    lessons learned, 282-283
    literature review, 269-271
    mental health committee, 272-275
    new care system, 275-278
    program successes, 279-281
    Pueblo Del Mar, 256-259
College. *See* Community college collaborations
College of San Mateo, 291
Colocated services
  benefits, 31
  mental health and substance abuse, 96
  redefining service delivery, *xxvii*, 30-31, 41
  scheduling difficulties, 99
  SonomaWORKS, 98
Commission on Accreditation of Rehabilitation Facilities (CARF), 111
Communication
  cross-system, 381-382
  defined, 382

Community
  involvement in organizational change, 6-7, 41-42
  transitional recovery, 36
Community Bridges, 58-59
Community building
  BASSC vision statement, 17, 19
  defined, *xxvi*, 380-381
  lessons learned, 47
  overview, *xxvii-xxviii*, 47
  policy devolution, *xxv-xxvi*
  supporting and aiding families, 17-18, 23-24
Community college collaborations
  challenges, 292-293
  human services agency
    background, 285-294
    certificate program, 288-291
    curriculum development, 286-290
    participants, 290-291
    lessons learned, 294
    overview, 37
    purpose of program, 291-292
Community Development Block Grant (CDBG), 119
Community Reinvestment Act (CRA)
  banking partners, 127
  Family Loan Program, 32
  overview, 167, 168
Community Workforce Partnership, 156
Community-based organizations (CBOs), 190, 194
Community-wide partnerships
  coalition addressing homelessness, 35-36
  coalition of nonprofit agencies, 36-37
  community colleges, 37
  transitional recovery community, 36
Comprehensive Integrated Resources for CalWORKs Limited English Speakers (CIRCLES), 206-207
Concept papers, 220-221, 223

Connectedness, defined, 381
Connections Shuttle
  background of program, 53
  challenges, 62-63
  goals, 58
  history, 55-57
  job training, 58, 60
  lessons learned, 63-64
  literature review, 54
  operations, 58-61
  overview, 29, 41
  program successes, 61-62
  purpose, 53
  training manual, 59
Consolidated Transportation Services Agency (CTSA), 59
Contact Cares, Inc., 146-148
Continuum of Care, 235-238
Contra Costa County social service agency, 339, 341-342, 364
Contracting, community-based organization, xxvi
Coordinating, defined, 383
Cornell University family development credential, 319-320, 323, 327
Corporation for Enterprise Development (CFED), 166
Courtship period, 242
Covent, Edie, 286, 287
CPR/first aid training for child care providers, 83, 88
CRA. See Community Reinvestment Act
Credit reports for Family Loan Program participation, 123
CREST (Career Retention Employment Support Team), 146, 148, 149
Cross-case analysis, 43-45
Crosscutting, 40-43
Crossover rate, 40
Crossover services
  background, 363-364
  caseload overlap, 366, 374
  delivery of services, 369-370, 371-372

Crossover services *(continued)*
  funding, 370-371
  lessons learned, 373-374
  planning, 367-369, 371-372
  surveys, 368
  system of care, 366-367
  welfare reform and children, 365-366
Cross-system communication, 381-382
CTSA (Consolidated Transportation Services Agency), 59
Cuccaro-Alamin, S., 366
Culture
  ad hoc, 28
  clan, 28
  guiding values, 9
  hierarchy, 28
  networking, 388
  organizational, 386-387
  organizational change and, 4-5
Customer service staff training, 5
CVP (Center for Venture Philanthropy), 169, 171

Data-based planning and evaluation, 7-8
Davidson, Deana, 59, 62
Dean Curtis job club model, 195-196
Deichert, Kirsten A., 153, 285
DeLois, K., 318
Department of Defense base closures, 251-252
Department of Labor welfare-to-work (DOL-WtW), 191-192
Department of Social Services, merging with workforce investment board. See Employment and human services
Depression and welfare-to-work programs, 94
Dial-a-Granny program, 132
Director, demands during organizational change, 10-12, 15-16

Disabled rehabilitation, WorkCenter employment, 108, 114. *See also* WorkCenter
DOL-WtW (Department of Labor welfare-to-work), 191-192
Domain of boundary spanning, 381
Downes, Debbie, 53, 251
Doyle, Susan E., 117, 131
DuBrow, Andrea, 297

Early, D., 234-235
Earned income tax credit (EITC), 156
East Bay Asian Local Development Corporation (EBALDC)
  collaborative efforts, 206
  history, 190
  program strengths and challenges, 209-211
  purpose, 207
EBALDC. *See* East Bay Asian Local Development Corporation
Economy
  impact on welfare reform, *xxxi*
  impact on working poor, *xxii*
Edin, K., 31
EHS. *See* Employment and human services
EITC (earned income tax credit), 156
Emergency Assistance, 217, 353
Employers
  employee obstacles to work, 155
  helping welfare recipients keep jobs, 155-156
  human services agency and community college collaboration, 291-292
  neighborhood self-sufficiency centers, 221
Employment
  career advancement opportunities, 156
  hiring clients, 33. *See also* Workforce
  hiring TANF participants, 153-162
  hotlines. *See* JobKeeper Hotline
  postemployment training, 219-220

Employment *(continued)*
  services. *See* Neighborhood Jobs Pilot Initiative
  social service agencies and, 39
  SonomaWORKS. *See* SonomaWORKS
  supported, 106
  work centers. *See* Work centers
Employment and human services (EHS)
  background, 339-340
  evolving issues, 346-349
  impact of legislation, 340
  lessons learned, 350
  organizational structure, 345
  research studies, 341-342
  social services versus WIB, 347-348
  structure, 342-346
Employment Support Initiative (ESI), 148, 217
Environmental scanning, 288
ESI (Employment Support Initiative), 148, 217
Evaluation
  data-based, 7-8
  Guaranteed Ride Home Program, 72-73
  managing out skill, 383
Exempt Provider Training Project
  challenges, 80, 88-89
  financial assistance, 79, 83
  history, 80-82
  incentives, 83
  lessons learned, 88-89
  licensure, 78, 81, 87-88
  literature review, 77-80
  ongoing training, 79
  orientation training, 78-79
  overview, 30, 41, 77-80
  participants, 84-87
  preservice training, 78
  purpose, 82
  quality of training, 79
  services, 82-84
External relations during organizational change, 10, 11

Facilitating, defined, 382, 383
Facilitators' institute, 324
Family child care homes, defined, 78
Family development credential (FDC)
  background, 38-39, 317-318
  challenges, 333-335
  conclusion, 336-337
  facilitators' institute, 324
  field instruction, 324-325
  history, 319-320
  implementation, 323-331
  lessons learned, 335-336
  modules, 328-330
  participation, 327, 330
  program, 325-327
  social service agency restructuring, 38-39
  start-up, 320-323
  strength-based services, 318-319, 334-335
  successes, 332-333
  transformation, 331
Family Fun Night, 226
Family Loan Program
  applicant requirements, 121
  bank support, 121, 126, 127-128
  history, 118-121
  lessons learned, 125-129
  literature review, 117-118
  loan process, 122-124
  overview, 32, 117, 129-130
  participants, 124-125
  reasons for ineligibility, 128
  San Mateo County, 120-121
Family Service America, Inc., 119
Family support, BASSC vision statement, 17, 21
Family-focused human service system, 17, 22, 23
FDC. *See* Family development credential
Federal Transit Authority (FTA)
  Guaranteed Ride Home Program, 70

Financial assistance. *See also* Funding
  American Automobile Association car seat donation, 72
  Blue Cross Foundation, 273-275
  child care training, 79, 83
  David and Lucile Packard, 120, 170, 223
  Hewlett Foundation, 203-204, 211
  McKnight Foundation, 32, 117, 118, 119-120
  Peninsula Community Foundation, 84, 169
  Queen of the Valley Hospital, 274
  Rockefeller Foundation. *See* Rockefeller Foundation grant
Flowchart
  crossover service delivery, 372
  IDA clients, 175
  Oakland neighborhood CIRCLE service, 208
  SonomaWORKS clients, 92
  South Hayward Neighborhood Collaborative, 197
  WorkCenter intake process, 112
Floyd, S. W., 382
Food and Nutrition Services, Incorporated, 58-59
Fort Ord, 251. *See also* Pueblo Del Mar
Frame, L., 363, 365
French, S., 192
French, W. L., 300
Front Porch program, 278-279
FTA (Federal Transit Authority)
  Guaranteed Ride Home Program, 70
Fulfillment on-site work, 111
Funding. *See also* Financial assistance
  agency-based empowerment, 318
  CalWORKs/TANF, 355. *See also* CalWORKs; Temporary Assistance to Needy Families
  crossover services, 370-371
  homeless services, 358-359
  Job Training Partnership Act, 355-356, 358
  lessons learned, 361-362

Funding *(continued)*
  managing and leveraging, 383
  multiple funding streams, 353-355
  neighborhood self-sufficiency
    centers, 211, 221-222
  pooling, 39-40
  Sonoma Caregivers Program,
    360-361
  welfare-to-work, 356-357. *See also*
    Welfare-to-work program
  youth programs, 357-358
Futuring, defined, 383

GAIN program, 157, 162
Gais, T. L., *xvii, xxiv-xxv*
Galinsky, E., 80
Gardner, S., 93
General Assistance (GA) recipients
  Employment Program, 109
  sanctions, 104-105
  work center minimum wages, 111
  WorkCenter employment, 108
Georgia Travis Center, 226-227
Gibson, J. O., *xxvi*
Gift of Love program, 137-138
Glad Tidings Church (GT), 195, 198
Glassman, A., 301
Glavin, Marie, 252
Glazer, S., *xvii-xviii*
GlenMaye, L., 318
Godparents in Adopt-A-Family
    program
  experiences of, 137-139
  matching to families, 134-137
  material support, 133
  overview, 32
  recruiting, 42
  supportive relationships, 131, 136-137
Golembiewski, R. T., 300
Gore, Vice President Al, 154
Goud, N., 144-145
Government
  asset acquisition subsidies, 165
  individual development account
    policies, 167-169
  social development model, 18

Grants. *See* Financial assistance
Grayson, M., 93
GRHP. *See* Guaranteed Ride Home
    Program
Griffin, Mary, 131, 133, 135
Gronbjerg, K. A., 354
Guaranteed Ride Home Program
    (GRHP)
  background, 65, 69-70
  challenges, 73
  enrollment, 70-71
  evaluation, 72-73
  features, 71-72
  lessons learned, 73-74
  literature review, 66-67
  overview, 29, 41
  planning project, 67-69
  successes, 73
Gustavsson, N., 253
Gutierrez, L., 318

Hage, J., 385, 387, 388
Hagen, J. L., *xxv*
Harbaugh, C., 54
Hastings, C., 386, 388
Havassy, H. M., 381
Head Start organization, 275
Health care, BASSC vision statement,
    21
Helplines, 144-145. *See also* JobKeeper
    Hotline
Hewlett Foundation, 203-204, 211
HHAP (Homeless Housing and
    Assistance Program), 234
HHSA (Napa County Health and
    Human Services Agency),
    235
Hierarchy culture, 28
HIP (Human Investment Project), 128
Hiring TANF participants
  history, 153-154
  lessons learned, 161-162
  literature review, 154-156
  Medi-Cal example

Hiring TANF participants, Medi-Cal
example *(continued)*
client obstacles, 159-160
hiring practices, 158-159
impact of program, 160-161
job description, 157-158
overview, 33
program successes, 160
recruiting, 159
training and hiring, 159-160
support for new hires, 157
History
CalWORKs, 3, 65, 217
Connections Shuttle, 55-57
Exempt Provider Training Project, 80-82
family development credential, 319-320
Family Loan Program, 118-121
hiring TANF participants, 153-154
homeless assistance, 251-253
individual development accounts, 166-167
JobKeeper Hotline, 143, 145-146
Napa collaboration of nonprofit and county agencies, 268-269
Neighborhood Jobs Pilot Initiative, 189-191
SUCCESS, 153
Transitional Residential Alliance and Integrated Network, 235
Holcomb, P., 192
Holiday programs, 131-132
Holub, J., 288
Home care providers, defined, 77-78
Home visits
Exempt Provider Training Project, 83
SonomaWORKS, 97
WorkCenter program, 104-105
Homeless
case management, 233-234
community coalition, 35-36
continuum of care, 235-238
factors, 232-233
funding of services, 358-359

Homeless *(continued)*
housing during substance abuse recovery
history, 251-253
lessons learned, 261
literature review, 253-254
participation forms, 262-264
program challenges, 260-261
program operations, 255-259
program successes, 259-260
social model, 254-255
mental illness factor, 233
solutions, 234
substance abuse recovery, 251
TRAIN program. *See* Transitional Residential Alliance and Integrated Network
Homeless Housing and Assistance Program (HHAP), 234
Hotlines, 144. *See also* JobKeeper Hotline
Housing. *See also* Homeless
BASSC vision statement, 21
TRAIN. *See* Transitional Residential Alliance and Integrated Network (TRAIN)
Housing and Urban Development Section 8 vouchers, 245
Howes, C., 80
Human capital, community building, *xxv-xxvi*
Human Investment Project (HIP), 128
Human service agency
family development credential
background, 317-318
challenges, 333-335
conclusion, 336-337
facilitators' institute, 324
field instruction, 324-325
implementation, 323-331
lessons learned, 335-336
modules, 328-330
participation, 327, 330
program, 325-327
start-up, 320-323

Human service agency, family
    development credential
    (continued)
  strength-based services, 318-319,
    334-335
  successes, 332-333
  transformation, 331
  history, 319-320
  management structure, 312
  organizational development
    background, 297-299
    consultant assessment criteria,
      303-305
    lessons learned, 311, 313-315
    literature review, 299-302
    need for specialist, 302-303
    OD consultation, 310-311
    OD entry phase, 305-310
    OD functions, 308-310
    OD job description, 305, 306-308
Human services agency and community
    college collaboration
  background, 285-286
  certificate program, 288-291
  challenges, 292-293
  curriculum development, 286-290
  lessons learned, 294
  participants, 290-291
  purpose of program, 291-292
Hyundai partnership with Los Angeles
    Harbor College, 288

ICPC (Interagency Children's Policy
    Council), 190, 203-204, 213
IDA. *See* Individual Development
    Account
Impact of welfare reform
  AFDC, 217, 353
  CalWORKs, 143
  overview, *xvii-xxii*
  on poor families, *xxii-xxiii*
  PRWORA, 217, *xvii-xxxii*
  SUCCESS, 154
  TANF, 143

Implementing, defined, 382
Implications, research, *xxx*
Incentives
  Exempt Provider Training Project,
    83
  SonomaWORKS compliance, 97
Individual Development Account
    (IDA)
  federal and state policies, 167-169
  flexibility, 182-183
  history, 166-167
  lessons learned, 182-183
  overview, 33-34, 183-184
  participant feedback, 181-182
  PeninsulaWorks-Daly City IDA
    program. *See*
    PeninsulaWorks-Daly City
    IDA program
  personal transformation, 183
  program challenges, 179-180
  program development, 183
  program strategies, 180-181
  program strengths, 178-179
  purpose, 165-166
  resources, 182
  San Mateo County, 169-172
Innovator role, 381
Integration services, 7
Interagency Children's Policy Council
    (ICPC), 190, 203-204, 213
Internal relations during organizational
    change, 10, 11
Internships for former welfare
    recipients, 162
Interorganizational relations theory,
    383-386
Italian Catholic Federation Gift of Love
    program, 137-138

Jacoby, N., 155
Jammin Company, 275
Jenkins, J. C., 271
Job club models, 195-196
Job Opportunities and Basic Skills
    (JOBS), 217, 353

Job training and Connections Shuttle, 58, 60
Job Training Partnership Act (JTPA), 355-356, 358
JobKeeper Hotline
  challenges, 150
  Contact Cares, Inc., 146-148
  history, 143, 145-146
  lessons learned, 150-151
  literature review, 143-145
  overview, 32-33, 148-149
  purpose, 143
  Santa Clara Valley, 145-146
  successes, 149
JOBS (Job Opportunities and Basic Skills), 217, 353
Johnson, J. B., 145
Joint Center for Housing Studies, 232-233
JTPA (Job Training Partnership Act), 355-356, 358

Kaplan, A., 54
Kaplan, T., *xvii, xxiv-xxv*
Karbo, J., 48-49
Keys, P., 301
Kingsley, G. T., *xxvi*
Kontos, S., 80
Kotter, J. P., *xxx*, 389

Landlords and TRAIN housing, 244, 247, 248
Language
  Adopt-A-Family program, 138
  Comprehensive Integrated Resources for CalWORKs Limited English Speakers (CIRCLES), 206-207
  ESL and VESL classes, 195
  Exempt Provider Training Program, 82, 83, 87, 89
  Guaranteed Ride Home Program, 72
  JobKeeper Hotline, 148, 149

Language *(continued)*
  Lower San Antonio/Fruitvale (LSAF) Neighborhood Jobs Pilot Initiative, 205, 210
  skill development classes, 209
  South Hayward diversity, 194
  South Hayward Neighborhood Collaborative, 198
  transportation problems and, 68
LCD (Lenders for Community Development), 169, 171
Leadership demands during organizational change, 10-11.
  See also Managing out
Leading, defined, 389
Lee, S., 366
Legislation
  Assets for Independence Act of 1998, 167-168
  Base Closure Community Redevelopment and Homeless Assistance Act of 1994, 252
  CalWORKs. See CalWORKs
  CRA. *See* Community Reinvestment Act
  Job Training Partnership Act, 355-356
  McKinney Act, 251-252
  private industry councils, 340
  PRWORA. *See* Personal Responsibility and Work Opportunity Reconciliation Act
  Savings for Working Families Act, 167, 168
  WIA. *See* Workforce Investment Act
Lein, L., 31
Lenders for Community Development (LCD), 169, 171
Lenkert, WorkCenter job contract, 108
Les Brown job club model, 196
Lessons learned
  Adopt-A-Family program, 139-140
  blended funding, 361-362

Lessons learned *(continued)*
 changing welfare services, *xxviii,
  xxx-xxxi*
 client services, 46
 collaboration of nonprofit and
  county agencies, 282-283
 community building, 47
 Connections Shuttle, 63-64
 crossover services, 373-374
 employment and human services,
  350
 Exempt Provider Training Project,
  88-89
 family development credential,
  335-336
 Family Loan Program, 125-129
 Guaranteed Ride Home Program,
  73-74
 hiring TANF participants, 161-162
 human service agency
  organizational development,
  311, 313-315
 human services agency and
  community college
  collaboration, 294
 individual development accounts,
  182-183
 JobKeeper Hotline, 150-151
 Neighborhood Jobs Pilot Initiative
  (NJPI), 211-212
 neighborhood self-sufficiency
  centers, 229
 organizational changes, 9-12, 15
 partnerships, 46-47
 Pueblo Del Mar (PDM), 261
 SonomaWORKS, 99-100
 staff, 46
 Transitional Residential Alliance
  and Integrated Network,
  248-250
Libby, Margaret K., 231, 267
Licensing of child care providers, 78,
 81, 87-88. *See also* Exempt
 Provider Training Project
Life counseling, 155

Literature review
 child welfare and welfare-to-work
  crossover services, 365-367
 collaboration of nonprofit and
  county agencies, 269-271
 exempt provider training, 77-80
 Family Loan Program, 117-118
 Guaranteed Ride Home Program,
  66-67
 hiring TANF participants, 154-156
 homelessness, 232-235
 hotlines, 143-145
 housing during substance abuse
  recovery, 253-254
 human service agency
  organizational development,
  299-302
 multiple funding streams, 354-355
 Neighborhood Jobs Pilot Initiative,
  191-193
 neighborhood self-sufficiency
  centers, 218-220
 substance abuse and mental health,
  93-94
 transportation obstacle, 54
 WorkCenter, 105-107
Loans. *See* Family Loan Program
Los Angeles Harbor College, 288
Los Ninos, 275
Lower San Antonio/Fruitvale (LSAF)
 Neighborhood Jobs Pilot
 Initiative
 challenges, 210-211
 clients, 208-209
 collaboration, 206
 history, 190-191, 204-205
 overview, 204-205
 programs, 206-207
 strengths, 209-210
Low-income workers, agency vision
 statement, *xxix*
Lurie, I., *xvii, xxiv-xxv*

Maintenance of Effort (MOE), 371
Management
 adapting to change, 9-11
 WorkCenter challenges, 114-116

Managing, defined, 389
Managing down, 380
Managing out
  boundary spanning, 381, 382-383
  changing focus, 382
  community building, 380-381
  current practice, 380-383
  defined, 380
  fostering networking culture, 388
  interorganizational relations, 383-384
  knowledge and skills, 381
  leadership domain of boundary spanning, 381
  leadership roles, 389
  managing collaboration, 384-387
  middle managers, 381-382, 389-392
  organizational processes, 388
  organizational structures, 387-388
  overview, 379-380, 392-393
  sample activities, 390
  skills required, 382-383
  top managers, 389
Managing up, 380
Martin, Madelyn, 286
Martinko, M., 301
"Master Your Money" IDA class, 176-178
Material assistance. *See* Adopt-A-Family program; Financial assistance
McCoy, S., 301
McKinney Act, 251-252
McKnight Foundation's Family Loan Program, 32, 117, 118, 19-120. *See also* Family Loan Program
McLean, G., 298
McNeely, J. B., *xxvi*
Medi-Cal
  hiring TANF participants, 153, 157-161
  Prenatal to Three Initiative, 80-82, 83, 88
Menefee, D., 382, 383

Mental health
  assessment and treatment for SonomaWORKS participation, 96-97
  coalition for care, 270-271
  coalition mental health committee, 272-275
  employment and. *See* SonomaWORKS
  literature review, 93-94
  Napa new care system, 275-278
  WorkCenter participation, 113-114
Mental illness and homelessness, 233
Mental models, 13-14, 16
Mentors
  Exempt Provider Training Project, 84
  helping welfare recipients keep jobs, 155-156, 162
Mergers, organizational restructuring, 42-43
Metropolitan Transportation Commission (MTC), 65, 67
Midgley, J., 43, 44
Mission statement, guiding values, 8-9
MOE (Maintenance of Effort), 371
Monsanto, hiring TANF participants, 154
Moore Iacofano Goltsman (MIG), Inc., 67
MTC (Metropolitan Transportation Commission), 65, 67
Multiyear contracting, *xxvi*

Nakashima, Jim, 252
Napa County coalition. *See* Coalition of nonprofit agencies
Napa County Council for Economic Opportunity (NCCEO), 235, 239
Napa County Health and Human Services Agency (HHSA), 235

Napa County Transitional Residential
  Alliance, 41. *See also*
  Transitional Residential
  Alliance and Integrated
  Network
Napa Emergency Women's Shelter
  (NEWS), 235, 239
Nathan, R. P., *xvii, xxiv-xxv*
National Association of Homes and
  Services for Children, 119
NCCEO (Napa County Council for
  Economic Opportunity), 235,
  239
Needell, B., 366
Neighborhood Jobs Pilot Initiative
  (NJPI)
  history, 189-191
  innovative service delivery, 41
  lessons learned, 211-212
  literature review, 191-193
  Lower San Antonio/Fruitvale
    challenges, 210-211
    clients, 208-209
    collaboration, 206
    history, 190-191, 204-205
    overview, 204-205
    programs, 206-207
    strengths, 209-210
  overview, 34-35
  Prescott
    challenges, 203-204
    clients, 202
    collaboration, 200-201
    history, 190-191, 199-200
    programs, 201-202
    strengths, 203
  South Hayward
    challenges, 198-199
    clients, 196-198
    collaboration (SoHNC), 194-196
    description, 194
    history, 190-191
    programs, 195-196
    strengths, 198

Neighborhood self-sufficiency centers
  (NSSCs)
  background, 217-218
  challenges, 228
  future directions, 228
  lessons learned, 229
  literature review, 218-220
  North County Consortium, 224-225
  program requirements, 222-224
  proposal requirements, 221-222
  request for concept papers, 220-221
  Resource Net, 226-227
  South County (Adelante Familia),
    225-226
Neighborhood-based human service
  system, 17, 22, 23
Nelson, G., 271
Network Center, 112-113
Networking culture, 388
New York family development
  credential, 319-320
NEWS (Napa Emergency Women's
  Shelter), 235, 239
Nightingale, D., 192
NJPI. *See* Neighborhood Jobs Pilot
  Initiative
Nonprofit, community-based
  organizations
  coalition. *See* Coalition of nonprofit
    agencies
  impact of PRWORA, *xx*
Norman, A., 301
North County Consortium, 224-225
NOVA Private Industry Council
  (NOVA PIC), 217
NSSC. *See* Neighborhood self-
  sufficiency centers
Nuestra Esperanza, 275

Obstacles to employment
  child care, 161
  civil service test, 160, 161-162
  employer identification of, 155
  solutions, 155-156

Obstacles to employment *(continued)*
 transportation, 54
 workplace issues, 161
Ong, P., 54, 66
Ongoing training, child care providers, 79
Organizational change
 agency restructuring, *xx-xxii*, 38-40
 BASSC vision, supporting low-income workers, 17-24
 challenges, 45-46
 community involvement, 6-7, 41-42
 conclusion, 15-17
 cultural change, 4-5
 data-based planning and evaluation, 7-8
 family development credential, 321
 guidance, 3-4
 guiding values, 8-9
 implication of change, *xxx*
 integration and teamwork, 7
 lessons learned, 9-12, 15
 mental models, 13-14, 16
 personal mastery, 13, 14-15, 16
 restructuring, 5-6, 28, 42-43
 Senge's five learning principles, 13-15
 shared vision, 13, 14, 16
 systems thinking, 13, 16
 team learning, 13, 16
Organizational culture, 386-387
Organizational development (OD)
 consultant assessment criteria, 303-305
 defined, 297, 302
 function of specialists, 38, 308-310
 goals, 298-299
 hiring process, 303-305
 lessons learned, hiring OD specialist, 311, 313-315
 literature review, 299-302
 need for specialists, 302-303
 OD consultation, 310-311
 OD entry phase, 305-310
 OD functions, 305-310

Organizational development (OD) *(continued)*
 specialist job description, 305, 306-308
 steps in intervention, 298
Organizational processes, 388
Organizational structures, 387-388
Orientation training, child care providers, 78-79
Osborne, S., 79
Ouchi, W. G., 145
Our Family organization, 275
OUTREACH, 71-73

Packard, David and Lucile, Foundation
 Family Loan Program, 120
 Individual Development Account, 170
 NOVA PIC, 223
 Resource Net funding, 227
Participants
 CalWORKs, 56-57
 Exempt Provider Training Project, 84-87
 Family Loan Program, 124-125
 work center, 106-107, 112-116
Partnering
 with the community, 34-35, 46-47
 defined, 389
NJPI. *See also* Neighborhood Jobs Pilot Initiative
Pavetti, L., *xxiv*
PCF (Peninsula Community Foundation), 84, 169
PCPC (Prescott Community Parent Collaborative), 201
PDM. *See* Pueblo Del Mar
Peninsula Community Foundation (PCF), 84, 169
PeninsulaWorks-Daly City IDA program
 challenges, 179-180
 client flowchart, 175
 course topics, 176-177

PeninsulaWorks-Daly City IDA
    program *(continued)*
  IDA pilot, 170-172
  overview, 183-184
  participant feedback, 181-182
  program, 174, 176-178
  resources, 182
  start-up, 172, 174
  strategies, 180-181
  strengths, 178-179
Personal mastery, 13, 14-15, 16
Personal Responsibility and Work
    Opportunity Reconciliation
    Act (PRWORA)
  addressing barriers to work, 65
  benefit limitations, 154
  creation of TANF grants, 353
  impact, *xvii-xxii*, 217
  implementation, 317
  individual development accounts,
    167
  key provisions, *xix-xx*
  shift in focus of welfare system, 143
Planning
  crossover services, 367-369
  data-based, 7-8
Policy devolution, *xxv-xxvi*
Policy practice managerial skills, 383
Political environment, organizational
    changes, 10
Pooling funding streams, 39-40
Population, TANF recipients, *xxii-xxiii*
PPI (Progressive Policy Institute), 166
PRC (Prescott Resource Center),
    201-202, 203-204
Preassessment phase, SonomaWORKS,
    92
Prenatal to Three Initiative, 80-82, 83,
    88
Prescott Community Parent
    Collaborative (PCPC), 201
Prescott Neighborhood Jobs Pilot
    Initiative
  challenges, 203-204
  clients, 202
  collaboration, 200-201
  history, 190-191, 199-200

Prescott Neighborhood Jobs Pilot
    Initiative *(continued)*
  programs, 201-202
  strengths, 203
Prescott Resource Center (PRC),
    201-202, 203-204
Preservice training, child care
    providers, 78
Prince, Jonathan
  crossover services, 363
  innovative programs and practices,
    27
  merging services, 339
  training exempt providers, 77
  WorkCenters, 103
Private industry council (PIC). *See also*
    Workforce investment boards
  employment and social service
    agencies, 39
  partnership structuring, 342-343
  purpose, 339
Progress Foundation, 239
Progressive Policy Institute (PPI), 166
PRWORA. *See* Personal Responsibility
    and Work Opportunity
    Reconciliation Act
Public policy
  impact of reforms, *xxxi*
  low-income family support, 18, 24
  research on welfare reform, *xxiii-xxiv*
Pueblo Del Mar (PDM)
  background, 251-252
  homeless status preferences, 263-264
  lessons learned, 261
  literature review, 253-254
  overview, 36
  program challenges, 260-261
  program operations, 255-259
  program successes, 259-260
  residency covenant, 262-263
  social model, 254-255

Queen of the Valley Hospital grant, 274
Quinn, R. E., 28, 381

Referrals, Exempt Provider Training Project, 84
Rehabilitation
  disabled and low-income. See WorkCenter
  vocational, 106-107
  WorkCenter success, 115
Reitan, T. C., 383-384
Rental subsidies, TRAIN, 245
Request for concept papers (RFCP), 220-221
Research on welfare reform
  future, *xxx*
  overview, *xxii*
  population, *xxii-xxiii*
  public policy, *xxiii-xxiv*
  service programs, *xxiv-xxv*
Resistance to change
  agency staff, 5, 11-12
  coaching by senior managers, 5
  director's response, 11-12
  role modeling, 5
  staff training on customer service, 5
Resource Net, 226-227
Resources, managing and leveraging, 383. *See also* Funding
Restructuring
  agency. *See* Agency restructuring
  goals, 5
  organizational, 5-6, 42-43
RFCP (request for concept papers), 220-221
RIDES for Bay Area Commuters, 67
Rockefeller Foundation grant
  community support for workforce development, 193
  Jobs Initiatives models, 212
  Neighborhood Jobs Pilot Initiative, 34, 190, 191, 206
  Prescott Neighborhood Jobs Pilot Initiative, 200, 203
  South Hayward Neighborhood Collaborative (SoHNC), 195
Role modeling, addressing staff resistance to change, 5

Rosenbaum, A., 144
Rothwell, W., 298
Rycraft, J., 253

Safety Net As Ladder, The, 166
Samaritan House, 169
San Mateo County
  family development credential, 318, 320-323
  Family Loan Program, 120-121
  hiring TANF participants, 157-161
  human services agency and community college collaborations, 285-294
  human services agency organizational development, 297-315
  individual development accounts, 169-172
  WorkCenter, 107-109
Sanctions
  General Assistance (GA) recipients, 104-105
  impact of PRWORA, *xxiii-xxiv*
  TANF, 104
Santa Clara County
  employment support initiative, 145-146
  GRHP. *See* Guaranteed Ride Home Program
  Savings for Working Families Act (SWFA), 167, 168
Schmidt, Christine M.
  Guaranteed Ride Home Program, 65
  JobKeeper Hotline, 143
  multiple funding streams, 353
  neighborhood self-sufficiency centers, 217
  welfare-to-work program, 91
School bus license requirements, 62
Seefeldt, K., 192
Self-sufficiency
  neighborhood centers, 35, 217-229
  substance abuse recovery, 254
  support services

Self-sufficiency, support services *(continued)*
  Adopt-A-Family program, 32, 42, 131-141
  agency-based empowerment, 318-319
  Family Loan Program, 32, 117-130
  hiring TANF participants, 153-162
  hotline services, 143-151
  IDA. *See* Individual Development Account
  Individual Development Account (IDA), 165-184
  overview, 31-34
  work centers, 103-116
  Transitional Residential Alliance and Integrated Network, 242
  values, 9
  WorkCenters, 103-116
Senge, P., 12-13, 14, 15, 386, 388, 389
Service delivery
  challenges, 45
  child care. *See* Exempt Provider Training Program
  innovations, 41
  redefining of, *xxvii*. *See also* Barriers to workforce participation
  self-sufficiency. *See* Self-sufficiency
  transportation. *See* Connections Shuttle; Guaranteed Ride Home Program
  welfare-to-work. *See* Welfare-to-work program
Service integration and teamwork, 7
Service programs, research on welfare reform, *xxiv-xxv*
Shared Undertaking to Change the Community to Enable Self-Sufficiency. *See* SUCCESS
Shared vision, 13, 14, 16
Sheltered workshop, 31
Sheltering of work center participants, 106-107
Sherraden, Michael, 166

Silicon Valley Private Industry Council (SVPIC), 217
Single Parent Loan Program, 119
Skyline College, 291
Smith, T., 54
Social Advocates for Youth, 39, 357
Social capital, community building, *xxv-xxvi*
Social development
  BASSC vision statement, 17, 18
  cross-case analysis model, 43-45
  defined, 43
  types of programs, 44
Social isolation
  adopt-a-family programs, 132
  hotlines, 145
Social model approach to substance abuse recovery, 254-255
Social service agency
  employment and, 39
  lessons learned, 46
  merging with workforce investment board. *See* Employment and human services
  organizational changes, *xx-xxii*
  Workforce Investment Board versus, 347-348
Social service workers, changing roles, 17, 22-23
Social Services Agency (SSA)
  Neighborhood Jobs Pilot Initiative, 190, 211
  welfare reform, 217
Soft skills
  hiring TANF participants, 155, 162
  South Hayward Neighborhood Jobs Pilot Initiative, 195
SoHNC (South Hayward Neighborhood Collaborative), 194-199
Sonoma Caregivers Program, 360-361
Sonoma County Community Development Commission (CDC), 358-359
Sonoma County multiple funding streams, 353-362

SonomaWORKS
　client assessment and treatment, 96-97
　client flowchart, 92
　incentives, 97
　lessons learned, 99-100
　literature review, 93-94
　overview, 91-93, 94-95
　program challenges, 98-99
　program successes, 97-98
　screening and referral, 95-96
　Sonoma Caregivers Program, 360-361
　substance abuse and mental health treatment, 96-97
South County (Adelante Familia), 225-226
South Hayward Neighborhood Jobs Pilot Initiative
　challenges, 198-199
　clients, 196-198
　collaboration, 194-195
　description, 194
　history, 190-191
　programs, 195-196
　SoHNC, 194-199
　strengths, 198
Spanning boundaries, 381, 382-383
Sprint, hiring welfare recipients, 154-155
SSA. *See* Social Services Agency
SSI (Supplemental Security Income), 108
Stacey, R., 298
Staff
　agency-based empowerment, 319
　lessons learned, 46
Stewart B. McKinney Homeless Assistance Act, 251-252
Strength-based interdisciplinary services, 318-319, 334-335
Stress management training for child care providers, 79
Stringari, Tim, 285, 286

Substance abuse
　assessment and treatment for SonomaWORKS participation, 96-97
　employment and. *See* SonomaWORKS
　homeless services
　history, 251-253
　lessons learned, 261
　literature review, 253-254
　participation forms, 262-264
　program challenges, 260-261
　program operations, 255-259
　program successes, 259-260
　social model, 254-255
　literature review, 93-94
　transitional recovery community, 36
SUCCESS (Shared Undertaking to Change the Community to Enable Self-Sufficiency), 133
　development of Adopt-A-Family program, 133
　family development credential, 321-323
　history, 153
　impact of PRWORA, 154
　Medi-Cal client employment success, 160
　Medi-Cal job advertising, 159
Successes
　collaboration of nonprofit and county agencies, 279-281
　Connections Shuttle, 61-62
　family development credential, 332-333
　Family Loan Program, 125
　Guaranteed Ride Home Program, 73
　hiring TANF participants, 160
　housing during substance abuse recovery, 259-260
　JobKeeper Hotline, 149
　SonomaWORKS, 97-98
　Transitional Residential Alliance and Integrated Network, 246-247
　WorkCenter, 115

Sullivan, R., 298
Summer Youth Conservation Corps, 39, 357
Sun Street Centers, 251, 255. *See also* Pueblo Del Mar
Supplemental Security Income (SSI), 108
Support groups, Exempt Provider Training Project, 83
Support services
  Adopt-A-Family program, 32, 42, 131-141
  agency-based empowerment, 319
  Family Loan Program, 32, 117-130
  hiring TANF participants, 153-162
  hotline services, 143-151
  IDA. *See* Individual Development Account
  Individual Development Account (IDA), 165-184
  overview, 31-34
  work centers, 103-116
Supporting Low-Income Workers in the Twenty-First Century, 17-24
Svihula, Judie, 165, 189, 317
SVPIC (Silicon Valley Private Industry Council), 217
SWFA (Savings for Working Families Act), 167, 168
Synthesizing, defined, 382
System of care
  child welfare and welfare-to-work crossover services, 366-367
  Napa coalition, 279-280
Systems thinking, 13, 16

TANF. *See* Temporary Assistance to Needy Families
Taylor, B. D., 66
Team learning, 13, 16
Teaming, defined, 382-383
Teamwork and service integration, 7
Teglia, Al
  dependency of Adopt-A-Family program, 141

Teglia, Al *(continued)*
  founder of Adopt-A-Family program, 131, 133, 140
  Gift of Love program, 137-138
  matching families and godparents, 134-136
Telephones. *See* Hotlines
Temporary Assistance to Needy Families (TANF)
  CalWORKs framework for distribution, 355
  child welfare services and, 40, 365-366
  employment sanctions, 104
  impact of PRWORA, *xvii*, 143
  PRWORA block grants, 65
  purpose of policy, 27-28
  youth programs, 357-358
Thoits, P. A., 145
Thompson, J. J., 382
Time limits, impact of PRWORA, *xxiii-xxiv*
Tolchinsky, P., 301
TRAIN program. *See* Transitional Residential Alliance and Integrated Network
Transformation, organizational, 86-387
Transitional Child Care, 156
Transitional Medicaid, 156
Transitional recovery community, 36
Transitional Residential Alliance and Integrated Network (TRAIN)
  background, 41, 231-232, 240-241
  case plans, 244-245
  challenges, 247-248
  client follow-up, 246
  client limitations, 245
  continuum of care, 235-238
  finding housing, 243-244
  function, 241-242
  history, 235
  implementation, 239-240
  lessons learned, 248-250
  literature review, 232-235

Transitional Residential Alliance
and Integrated Network
(continued)
program proposal approved by
HUD, 238-239
referrals, 242
rental subsidies, 245
successes, 246-247
Transportation
AFDC recipients, 54
BASSC vision statement, 21
Connections Shuttle. See
Connections Shuttle
employment and, 118
Exempt Provider Training Project, 83
Guaranteed Ride Home Program.
See Guaranteed Ride Home
Program
needs of CalWORKs participants, 56-57
options for low-skilled workers, 66-67
redefining service delivery, xxvii
Transportation Planning Project, 67-69
Transportation Task Force, 55
Trustlined, 83
Trutko, J., 192

Union transit drivers conflict with shuttle drivers, 63
United Airlines, hiring welfare recipients, 111, 154-155
Unity Council, 206-207, 209-211, 213
Unlicensed child care providers. See Exempt Provider Training Project
UPS, hiring welfare recipients, 154-155

Valley Transportation Authority (VTA), 65, 67
Values, organizational changes, 8-9
Visier, L., 105-106
Vision statement, xxix, 17-24

Vista Imaging, 111
Vocational Rehabilitation Services (VRS), 112
VTA (Valley Transportation Authority), 65, 67

Ways to Work, 120. See also Family Loan Program
WEAP (Women's Economic Agenda Project), 200, 201, 203-204
Weil, M., xxvi, 380-381
Welfare reform
impact. See Impact of welfare reform
implementation, 317
organizational change. See Organizational change
research, xxii-xxv
Welfare to Work Partnership, 154-155
Welfare-to-work program
background, 356-357
CalWORKs. See CalWORKs
cost analysis, 354
crossover services
caseload overlap, 366, 374
child welfare, 363-364
delivery of services, 369-370, 371-372
funding, 370-371
lessons learned, 373-374
literature review, 365-367
planning, 367-369, 371-372
system of care, 366-367
literature review, 93-94
multiple funding streams, 353, 356-361
neighborhood self-sufficiency centers, 218-219
SonomaWORKS. See SonomaWORKS
TANF. See Temporary Assistance to Needy Families
WIA. See Workforce Investment Act
WIBs. See Workforce investment boards

Wilson, Pete, 193
Wocher, Donna, 297
Women's Economic Agenda Project
  (WEAP), 200, 201, 203-204
Woodridge, B., 382
Work centers
  challenges, 106
  literature review, 105-107
  on-site versus supported
    employment, 106, 111
  overview, 103-105
  purpose, 104
  types, 106
  vocational rehabilitation. See
    WorkCenter
WorkCenter
  administrative challenges, 114-116
  background, 31, 107-109
  challenges, 114-116
  client experience, 109-110
  innovative service delivery, 41
  intake process flowchart, 112
  operations, 110-111
  participant assessment, 112-113
  participant challenges, 114
  participants, 113-114
  purpose, 107
  services, 112-113
  successes, 115
Worker Trainee Program, 154
WorkFirst, 191, 195, 317
Work-first policy, impact of
  PRWORA, *xviii, xxiv*
Workforce
  barriers
    child care. See Exempt Provider
      Training Project
    mental health and substance
      abuse. See SonomaWORKS
    removal, 28-31, 43

Workforce, barriers *(continued)*
  transportation. See Connections
    Shuttle; Guaranteed Ride
    Home Program
  career-resilient, 17, 19-21
  development system, 189, 212
  hiring clients, 33. See also Hiring
    TANF participants
  JobKeeper Hotline, 32-33. See also
    JobKeeper Hotline
Workforce Investment Act (WIA)
  background, 37, 39
  human services agencies and
    colleges, 285-286
  neighborhood self-sufficiency
    centers, 228
  purpose, 339
  requirements, 340
Workforce investment boards (WIBs)
  merging employment and social
    service agencies, 39
  merging with department of social
    services. See Employment
    and human services
  pooling funds, 40
  purpose, 340
  social services versus, 347-348
Working poor, impact of economic
  slowdown, *xxii*
Workshop, sheltered, 31
Wraparound services for the homeless.
  See Pueblo Del Mar

Yin, R. K., 48
Young, N., 93
Youth program funding, 357-358

Zawacki, R. A., 300